THE **GENDER BEYOND** SEX

Two Distinct Ways
of Living in Time

Robert Pos, MD
DPsych, FRCPC, PhD, FAPA

Cover concept & design: Ion Design Inc. www.iondesign.ca
Photography: David Coates FGDC

Note for Librarians: A cataloguing record for this book is available from Library and Archives Canada at www.collectionscanada.ca/amicus/index-e.html
ISBN 1-4120-8843-7

Printed in Victoria, BC, Canada. Printed on paper with minimum 30% recycled fibre. Trafford's print shop runs on "green energy" from solar, wind and other environmentally-friendly power sources.

TRAFFORD
PUBLISHING™
Offices in Canada, USA, Ireland and UK

Book sales for North America and international:
Trafford Publishing, 6E–2333 Government St.,
Victoria, BC V8T 4P4 CANADA
phone 250 383 6864 (toll-free 1 888 232 4444)
fax 250 383 6804; email to orders@trafford.com
Book sales in Europe:
Trafford Publishing (UK) Limited, 9 Park End Street, 2nd Floor
Oxford, UK OX1 1HH UNITED KINGDOM
phone 44 (0)1865 722 113 (local rate 0845 230 9601)
facsimile 44 (0)1865 722 868; info.uk@trafford.com
Order online at:
trafford.com/06-0599

10 9 8 7 6 5 4 3

FOREWORD

In 1958, I became involved in psychiatric research and administration, and maintained a private practice in long-term psychotherapy. This counseling experience led me to discover a pervasive duality in people's personality based on how they relate to time (their time gender). I call these two mutually exclusive classes of people alphas and betas,[1] (or sometimes Jungians and Freudians since their personality structure fits the basic one described and owned respectively by Jung and Freud). The alpha personality is situation-bound, completely immersed in the present (the past is "no longer present;" the future "not yet present"), while betas relate to a coherent, personal past and future reality which is continuous with the present ("their timescape").

Over the years I integrated the alpha-beta duality in my counseling practice with men and women from many different walks of life. Most found the time gender model easy to grasp and often they could readily recognize their own time gender and the time gender of others who figured in their lives. This was not simply a matter of intellectual insight, but became a guideline in dealing with problems in alpha-beta interfacing. It also facilitated adjusting to more realistic expectations of themselves and others. Someone made the observation that "Although the world is divided into men and women, it is perhaps equally, if not more important to divide the world into alphas and betas." Many have pressed me to put this new model before the public. However, my scientific inclination made this more time consuming than originally thought. I found myself moving back and forth between an academic and a shorter version. In the end I have two versions: an academic e-book version (which may be obtained through my Internet's website <www.robertpos.info>). It serves as the resource back-up for the shorter version in book form, which you have here.

Creating this version took more than a year. It differs from the e-book in three aspects:

1. Appendix 3 *(About personality inversion and bifocal identity)* which may be of interest to some psychiatrists and psychologists is omitted. Readers who are interested in this may consult the e-book version. As a result, Appendix 4 in the e-book (CD-book) version *(Summary of time gender features)* has become Appendix 3 in this amended version.

2. This version differs from the e-book version in the specifics of genetic transmission of one's time gender. In the CD-book (e-book), I tentatively suggested that marriages between two alphas produce only alpha children, and between two betas only beta children; and that half of the children from marriages between an alpha

and beta are alphas, the other half betas. Recently published research on the DNA sequence of the human X-chromosome[2] made me arrive at the explanation that a dominant gene on the X-chromosome is responsible for the alpha time gender and a recessive gene for the beta time gender. Details are discussed in Chapter 11 of this book.

NOTES

1   I borrowed the alpha-beta terminology from my old high school, the Barlaeus Gymnasium in Amsterdam, the Netherlands, where those majoring in Latin and Greek and arts were called *alphas* and those who minored in Latin and Greek and majored in sciences *betas*. My use of the alpha/beta terminology has, however, nothing to do with the division between arts or sciences or, for that matter, with the classic A and B personality dichotomy, or with recognizing dominant alpha males among animals, or with any use of the alpha-beta terminology introduced by others.

2   Ross et al (2005); Carrel & Willard (2005).

ACKNOWLEDGEMENTS

From a theoretical point of view I would not have been able to create this work without the writings of Sigmund Freud and Carl Gustav Jung, both of whom created "a psychology of emotions without intelligence," and of Jean Piaget, who introduced "a psychology of intelligence without emotions."[1] I must also acknowledge the influences of men like Julius Thomas Fraser,[2] Gerald M. Edelman,[3] Julian Jaynes,[4] Howard Gardner,[5] and John Rowan.[6]

The practical development of the time gender model greatly benefited from the significant input from three friends. David Aris, a Dutch engineer and good friend, reviewed and critiqued The Gender Beyond Sex while I returned the favor concerning his book-in-the-making Brainwaves: Building Blocks for Psychology. His contribution to my thinking is considerable. Dr. E. Michael Coles, Associate Professor of Psychology, Simon Fraser University, Vancouver BC, Canada, presently retired, and a reliable friend since 1982, not only edited each chapter of the book meticulously while suggesting significant changes, but also was a source of encouragement over the years. My friend Donald Lidstone, a prominent constitutional and municipal lawyer, not only functioned as co-editor, but deserves credit for the idea of first placing this work in electronic form on the Internet for interested parties.

I am very grateful to Dr. Janette Pelletier, Associate Professor, Department of Human Development and Applied Psychology, the Ontario Institute for Studies in Education, University of Toronto, who amidst her busy work schedule took the time to read the entire manuscript and file a thorough review. It is a pleasure working with her.

I am much indebted to Mark Aultman, Attorney-at-Law, Legal Ethics, Columbia OH, who is a well-established member of the International Society for the Study of Time (unlike myself who joined only recently). Mark, who scrutinized the e-book, influenced this version a great deal through his extensive constructive criticisms.

Susan Curtis, M.Ed. Counseling Psychology, CEAP (Certified Employee Assistance Professional), a consultant to the Continuing Studies Women's Resources Centre, University of British Columbia, and to Career Connections, has a private practice in Vancouver. In supervising her work over a number of years she convinced me that other clinicians could be taught to put the time gender model to efficient use in their counseling practices.

I am grateful to Dr. J. M. Friedman MD, PhD, Professor of Medical Genetics, University of British Columbia, Vancouver BC, who reviewed the genetic data of my clinical cohort and wisely advised me to significant caution in interpreting them. Concerning my statistical data analysis an internationally recognized authority in statistical genetics, David F. Andrews, PhD, Emeritus Professor of Statistics, University of Toronto, wrote that the chapter on Time Gender and Sexuality, Partnering and Parenting which summarizes the associations found between type (alpha/beta) and a number of sexual behaviors showed a consistent pattern to support the major theses of the book.

I promised our three children, Steven, Gabriella, and Max Becker-Pos that I would not publish this theory in book form unless the three of them had understood it. Steven, a computer technologist with a BA, courageously cut out parts of the e-book version which he considered too academic; Gabriella, an artist, with a BA, a Diploma of Fine Arts and a degree of the Ontario College of Arts and Designs, molded the result to her taste through further editing; and Max, an English teacher and editor with a MA in International Studies, ended up putting the dots on the i's and crossing the t's. For their efforts I thank all three from the bottom of my heart.

My foremost gratitude goes, however, to Marie Becker-Pos, the only person who for seventeen years believed in what I was doing and sustained me throughout with her counsel and love.

Vancouver BC, winter 2005-2006.

Robert Pos, MD

NOTES

1   Anthony (1956).
2   See, for example, Fraser (1966) and Fraser, Lawrence and Haber (1986). Dr. J. T. Fraser, who founded the International Society for the Study of Time in 1966, wrote some 40 years ago: "Tell me what you think of time and I will know what to think of you" [Fraser (2004)].
3   Edelman (1989).
4   Jaynes (1976, 1982).
5   Gardner (1985).
6   Rowan (1990).

CONTENTS

CHAPTER I

The Hidden Gender: Are You An Alpha Or A Beta?

My aim in this work is to show that beyond our obvious sexual gender another "gender" lies hidden. This gender influences as much of the way we think, feel and behave as being female or male does. While our sexual gender reflects an *obvious* biologic duality, our time gender which mirrors two distinct ways of relating to time, is a *hidden* biologic duality.[1]

I have written this work not for some privileged professional group. Rather, I have intended it for the general public in the expectation that readers will gain confidence in identifying their own time gender and that of others, and put the time gender model to some practical use in their lives.

About time perspective

Modern humans take it for granted that their lives divide into three time zones: past, present and future. But some people live predominantly in their private past. Greta Garbo, for example, did not appear able to leave her glorious past. She lived in solitude, hiding from her present reality and a future which seemed empty. Others live most of their lives in their future time zone, persistently fighting or fearing futurethreats or focusing on future rewards. Then there are those who, as the Latin saying " carpe dies" goes, seize the day.

Whether we relate more to our past, present or future may seem like a trivial thing. But our preferred orientation toward any one of these time zones has a powerful influence on what motivates us, how we deal with problems, how we relate to others and how we see ourselves. For example, if today affects me more than tomorrow, I may attend to an important personal matter that has just come up, rather than devoting myself to working on a critical business meeting scheduled for tomorrow. On the other hand, I may be someone who takes care of tomorrow at the expense of present priorities. And some people with a rather troubled past can enjoy living their present life to the fullest, while others are simply unable to walk away from past failures and mistakes and hurts.

Clearly, we do not all share the same time zone orientation, even though the past, present, and future are equally important to everybody. The internationally acknowledged scientist in the domain of time, J. T. Fraser, observed already in 1966 "that a person's view of time is a method of discerning his personality." "Tell me what you think of time," he wrote, "and I shall know what to think of you."[2]

Is our relation to the three time zones learned or inborn?

It is often tempting to associate people's time perspective with their stage of life. When we are young and have most of our life ahead of us, it is reasonable to assume that we will have a future orientation. Conversely, when we are old and the finality of death is looming, it will be more pleasant to orient ourselves to our past.

The conventional view among psychiatrists, psychologists and sociologists is that how a person relates to the three time zones is learned. Most experts say that a person's time perspective is the product of many influences, including the particular orientation toward past, present and future in that person's family of origin, social class and culture. Our time orientation is—they say—our unique way of adjusting to our particular social and ecological niche. If the future in that niche is rather attractive, of course some will be future-oriented. For others the past may be more meaningful. According to this view, there is no such thing as people who are either purely past-oriented, present-oriented or future-oriented; we are not stuck with a particular time orientation.[3]

The conventional view suggests that, although we each acquire our own unique set of relationships with the past, present and future, we all share the same basic potential to experience and relate to time. It concludes that we all have the ability to balance an appreciation of the past with a sense of the future, blended with an involvement in the present.

This book will present a radically different point of view. I will show that we can reduce this diversity in time perspectives to two contrasting ways of experiencing time and, therefore, personal reality. This is responsible for a hidden yet fundamental duality in personality that divides people into what I call alphas and betas. Because this classification into alphas and betas is mutually exclusive (like classifying people into men and women) and derives from the way we experience time, I have come to refer to it as our "time gender."

About alphas and betas

Alphas live one day at a time. The main theater in which the alpha scenario is played out is the collective, public reality in the here-and-now, the reality we all own and share. It is not that alphas have chosen to live a day at a time, they can live only for today. For them, the past is "no longer the present" and the future "not yet the present." On closer examination, they often appear functionally disconnected from their personal past and future.

Betas, on the other hand, are like people who have sprung two invisible time cones from their head, one pointing forward into their personal future, the other extending backward into their personal past. They do much of their living in this hidden, individual temporal world, a timescape well beyond the horizon of today. As a result, betas often seem inattentive to the world of the here-and-now.

Alphas and betas each have both impressive strengths and crippling weaknesses. Alphas are dependent for their mood and self-esteem on what is happening now. They are therefore naturally motivated by opportunities in the present and, for this reason, become true tacticians in dealing with the immediacy of social reality and its opportunities and challenges. However, their emotional dependence on the here-and-now makes them vulnerable to ongoing adversities. The ongoing alpha strategy is to strive relentlessly for optimal control over their social environment, but they are deep down never sure of their success. This makes an alpha like a bullfighter who constantly scans the ring for opportunities, and remains ever vigilant and wary of unexpected threats and challenges.

By contrast, the mood and self-esteem of betas depend largely on what has happened before and especially on what the future holds. Therefore, what generally preoccupies and motivates betas are past successes or failures and future promises or threats. Long-term planning is a natural beta strength. In their personal lives, betas are thus strategists rather than tacticians.

Alphas are more vulnerable to current problems and difficulties, because they cannot see the light at the end of the tunnel. Betas, however, are more resilient to present challenges because they can see the light. Betas, by contrast, are far more susceptible to past hurts and failures than alphas. A loss of a loved one, for example, may continue to be a source of sadness for quite some time, even if the present is full of positive experiences. Under similar circumstances an alpha may just walk away from such anguish. Betas are also more likely to be affected by a serious future threat, such as not having the money to pay income tax a few months down the road. Thoughts of this will constantly block their enjoyment of the present. Alphas will only be upset on the day the tax message arrives and then get on with life. A beta without a promising future is a deeply distressed beta. Alphas put past and future displeasures out of their mind. There are fundamental differences in how alphas and betas regulate their mood and self-esteem and how they relate to past traumas and achievements and future threats and promises.

The way alphas and betas see themselves is reflected in their internal dialogue. In an alpha, this silent self-talk is often like an unruly group session; in a beta, more like a one-sided conversation between two people.

Since alphas give priority to their current reality, they are in their personal life generally motivated by short-term goals, and also more focused on public outer reality. Betas, by contrast, tend to give priority to their future and past, are mainly motivated by long-term goals, and more focused on their hidden private inner world. As a result, alphas and betas behave and relate to other people in contrasting ways.

While alphas live in the world and betas live in their head these two groups also think differently. Alphas are more tolerant of apparent contradictions between contexts which permits them to be multifocal in their thinking. Betas are quite intolerant of intellectual contradictions between contexts. They always search for some overall coherent system. Hence, they are monofocal in their thinking and values (see Chapter 8).

It is clearly useful to become aware of who is an alpha and who is a beta because with a reasonable understanding of the alpha-beta duality, many aspects of one's own and other people's behavior become more understandable and predictable. Without time gender awareness, human behavior can sometimes appear age-bound or sex-bound, whereas in fact it is wholly tied to time gender.

Time gender interfacing: alphas and betas interacting

The strengths of the alpha time gender correspond to the weaknesses of the beta, and the other way around. This holds great creative promise not only for the individual but also for society. For if one person is a specialist in operating in the present, and the other a specialist operating in the past and future, then their combined product would likely be superior to that of a pure alpha-alpha or beta-beta combination.

Time gender interfacing between alphas and betas, however, is more often than not full of misinterpretation and conflict. This is so because we do not recognize time gender differences for what they are. Time gender differences, then, often become misunderstood and personalized. We all know what it is like when we become acutely aware of a polarity in the relationship with an important other; that the other person is surprisingly different from what we had originally assumed.

Human history is replete with the drama of alphas and betas interfacing and the creative and destructive impact brought about by this. The plots of novels, movies, and soap operas play on the excitement generated by time gender differences between main characters.

Empirical support for the time gender duality

Empirical support for the time gender theorycomes from research data of people from the Greater Vancouver area in British Columbia, Canada. Those interested in the exact numbers can find them in table 1.1.

Period	alph M	alph F	alph T	beta M	beta F	beta T	all M	all F	TOTAL
1987-1989	58	103	161	67	45	112	125	148	273
1989-1991	33	49	82	32	18	50	65	67	132
1987-1991	91	152	243	99	63	162	190	215	405

alpha = alpha   M = male   F = female   T = Total

Table 1.1: The Vancouver Research Sample

Fortunately, my sample of 405 consecutive clients, collected between 1987-1991 showed by chance the same sex distribution as the 1986 Canadian Census of Greater Vancouver: slightly more than 50% women and slightly less than 50% men. Of these 405 subjects, I classified 60% as alphas and 40% as betas.[4] In addition, statistical analyses of the first 273 subjects showed other corresponding demographics between the sample and the general population age 20 and over,[5] suggesting that the sample approximately represented the general population of Greater Vancouver, the realization of a researcher's dream. The results of these data analyses presented in this book amassed into a consistent, coherent body of facts in support of the proposition that time gender, notwithstanding its masked nature, is as real as sexual gender.[6]

Some of this research results may impress as "ah hah" knowledge, if not pop-psychology weighed down by statistics. It is, however, precisely because of this potentially pop psychology aspect that I felt that scientific proof was needed.

The alpha-beta ratio among men and women is different

Originally I assumed that sexual gender and time gender are completely independent of each other. I thus predicted that I would find about the same proportions of men and women among alphas and betas. This turned out to be invalid, for I found a strong and stable statistical connection between sexual gender and time gender.[7]

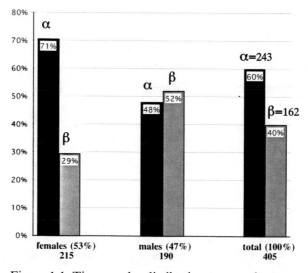

Figure 1.1: Time gender distibution among the sexes

Figure 1.1 shows that, although 60% of my overall research population are alphas and 40% betas, among women the time gender distribution was 70%-30% and, among men virtually 50%-50%. In other words, being female made it 10% more likely to be alpha and 10% less to be beta than expected; and being male made it 10% more likely to be beta and 10% less likely to be alpha than one might expect.

In the CD-book version of this work,[8] I stated that I could not explain this connection between time gender and sexual gender and, more particularly, why the ratio of alphas to betas in my 405 subjects was about 50% 50% among men, but around 70%–30% among women. Even so, concerning the genetic transmission of time gender, I tentatively offered the suggestion that alpha-alpha marriages produce only alpha children; beta-beta marriages only beta children; and that half of the children from marriages between an alpha and beta are alphas, the other half betas. But I was not in a position to indicate the exact genetic mechanics of such time gender transmission. Although I remain totally committed to the genetic basis of the time gender duality, it turned out that the method of obtaining preliminary data in support of the suggestion of the pattern of its transmission is unreliable.

Recently published research on the DNA sequence of the human X-chromosome[9] led me to accept an alternative version of time gender transmission which not only accounts for the difference in alpha-beta ratios among the men and women of my research cohort but, in addition, offers exact details as to how the time gender transmission from parents to children is achieved. This explanation is based on recent evidence supporting the importance of the X-chromosome for various, uniquely human brain functions, and on the fact that women have two X-chromosomes (one inherited from their father and one from their mother), and that men have only one X-chromosome (which they inherit from their mother). According to this explanation a *dominant* gene on the X-chromosome is responsible for the alpha time gender and a *recessive* gene on the X-chromosome for the beta time gender. The time gender of women with their two X-chromosomes is therefore determined by both parents. Since men receive their single X from their mothers, it is the mothers who determine the time gender of their sons. As a result, female alphas may either have the dominant alpha gene on both X-chromosomes (AA), or have one X-chromosome with the dominant alpha gene and the other with the recessive beta gene (Ab), while female betas must carry the recessive beta gene on both their X-chromosomes (bb). Male alphas have an alpha mother (AA or Ab), while male betas may have an alpha mother (Ab) or beta mother (bb). Details are discussed in Chapter 11.

About alpha brains and beta brains

During the course of my practice as a clinical psychiatrist, I found out about time gender by observing that some people have difficulties putting their life story in chronological order (alphas), while others do so with relative ease (betas). In due course, I concluded that this apparent difference in mapping autobiographic long-term memories in the brain mantle accounts for all time gender-specific differences in the behavior and experience of alphas and betas. Thus, it is the biologic underpinning of time gender.

If our time gender is genetically determined, and thus anchored in the biologic make-up of the brain, research in brain structure should eventually verify this. We have known for some time there are subtle but significant differences between male and female brains.[10] Why not subtle and significant differences between alpha and beta brains?

The following chapters will make clear that each time gender is characterized by great strengths and great weaknesses. Even so, some will accuse me of considering one kind of memory or brain superior to the other or that my thesis is racist. To respond to these inevitable accusations I searched for an alpha and a beta of equal standing and unquestionable greatness and fame, admired the world over. Each example would serve as a true-to-life model, if not an advocate, of the two time genders. I found these two types right on my professional doorstep, in two of the greatest twentieth century psychiatrists. They are Carl Jung of the alpha gender,[11] and Sigmund Freud of the beta gender.[12] Both went exhaustively into introspective self-study and analysis, using the structure and dynamics of their own personalities as the basis of their theories of how the mind works. Both made fundamental contributions to modern psychiatry, founding their own schools of thought and creating their own characteristic method of psychotherapy. Jung's life and his theory on personality structure are a superior declaration on the meaning and nature of being an alpha, just as Freud's life and general theory on personality structure are a symphony on beta functioning. I will document these views in due course. The insights into the time genders of those great masters of my profession brought me immense relief. And I decided that as epitaphs to their memory, I would henceforth also refer to alphas as "Jungians"; and to betas as "Freudians."

Why time gender remained hidden behind a mask of uniformity

If the alpha-beta duality determines so much of how we function and experience reality, how is it possible that it has until now remained hidden behind a mask of innocent uniformity? The answer is obvious. Our physical characteristics show our sexual gender but tell us nothing about our time gender. Furthermore, experiences and behaviors that stem from time gender do not stand out rigidly against the background of our overall behavior. They disappear in the rich variety of behaviors and experiences that have little or nothing to do with our time gender and so remain hidden to the untrained eye. The likelihood of a spontaneous discovery of the masked time gender duality was therefore very small.

Remaining unaware of the hidden alpha and beta time gender, layperson and scientist alike continue to assume naturally that we all share the same universal potential of relating to time. This completely unrealistic yet popular myth of temporal sameness haunts us. Everyone carries the weight of one's time gender handicaps. No matter how hard we try, or how many self-help books we read, or how many hours of counseling we have, we cannot change our time gender. If you desperately dislike your sexual gender, you can at least have a sex change operation. Time gender-bending is not an option. Mental health professionals often try—without knowing they are doing so—to help alphas change a particular alpha weakness into a beta strength, or some beta weakness into an alpha strength. Such efforts end by necessity in frustrating failure and a sense of increased inadequacy. To become familiar with the time gender duality and in particular with one's own time gender helps unload the baggage. Once we answer the question of whether we are an alpha or a beta, we become aware of our natural strengths, and we are more free to use them. Once aware of our time gender, we may stop berating ourselves for what are essentially the natural limitations of our genetics. We then may be more inclined to deal with them by looking for compensatory strategies.

Beyond time gender

The notion of time gender is as black and white as that of sexual gender: you are either female or male, and you are either an alpha or a beta. The differences between alphas and betas are exhaustive and mutually exclusive. Time gender, like sexual gender, is one important dimension in the explanation of human behavior. On the other hand, just as we do not expect being male or female to explain all there is to being humans, time gender will not account for all human behavior either. Alphas and betas come in an unlimited assortment, just like men and women.

NOTES

1   While current popular usage tends to equate *gender* with sex, its dictionary meaning is more general, defining it as class or category: "Gender basically means category, and sexual ones provide only a few of them." [Orasanu, Slater & Adler (1979): vii-x].

2   Fraser, J. T. (1966), p. xix.

3   Gonzalez & Zimbardo (1985).

4   I refer people who question my methodology of classifying people as alpha or beta to the discussion of my criteria for arriving at a person's time gender in Chapter 2 and Chapter 11 of this book, and to Appendix 2 *(The chronologic biographic interview)*.

5   See Appendix 1 *(The research sample)*.

6   For example, an internationally recognized authority in statistical genetics, David F. Andrews, Ph.D., Emeritus Professor of Statistics, University of Toronto, wrote that Chapter 7 *(Time gender and Sexuality, Partnering and Parenting)* which summarizes the associations found between type (alpha/beta) and a number of sexual behaviors showed a consistent pattern to support the major theses of the book.

7   A standard logistic analysis by David F. Andrews, Ph.D., Emeritus Professor of Statistics, University of Toronto, showed that there is considerable evidence that women have a greater chance of being classified as alpha ($p=0.0001$) and that there is no evidence that this tendency changes over time ($p=0.997$) [deviance residuals: [1] 0 0 0 0; null deviance: 2.2609e+01 on 3 degrees of freedom; residual deviance: 4.4394e-1 on 0 degrees of freedom; AIC: 27.624; number of Fisher Scoring iterations: 2].

8   Pos (2004).

9   Ross et al (2005); Carrel & Willard (2005)

10   For example: Flor-Henry (1978) and, in terms of imaging of the brain, Del Parigi et al. (2002), Van Laere and Dierckx (2001), Bengtsson et al. (2001), Sadato et al. (2000), Ragland et al. (2000), Kimbrell et al. (1999), Nishizawa et al. (1997), Azari et al. (1995), Gur et al. (1995), Shaywitz et al (1995), Leutwyler (1995), Andreason et al. (1994), Wong et al. (1988), for example.

11   Carl Gustav Jung (1875-1961), Swiss psychiatrist and founder of analytical psychology.

12   Sigmund Freud (1856-1939), Austrian psychiatrist and founder of psychoanalysis.

CHAPTER 2

The Alpha-beta Difference: When, How, And Why

When time gender enters the picture

Sexual gender differences between men and women emerge very early in our development.[1] Time gender differences, however, do not emerge until around six or seven, when young boys and girls who are genetically beta begin branching off from the developmental pathway they previously had shared with alphas-to-be.

When a kindergarten teacher promises the children a reward tomorrow if they will behave themselves today, chances are that no child will earn next day's reward. A 5-year old cannot relate to something one day in the future. And yesterday no longer belongs to their reality. In kindergarten, all children live one day at a time.

The first indication of an awareness of yesterday and tomorrow and, with it, a time gender difference, usually happens around age seven. By grade two, a number of the children will—without further need for reminding or encouragement—get to their next day's reward. These children are becoming betas. But the alpha children do not respond to notions of tomorrow and continue to live one day at a time. If the class is reminded in a gentle, quiet manner of their misbehavior the day before, the faces of some beta children will now twitch here and quiver there. These beta children are clearly extending today's reality into yesterday. But young alphas continue their immersion in today, and listen with a facial expression as pleasant as that of the teacher who is gently chiding them about yesterday.

For young betas, a new reality is opening up. What will happen tomorrow and has happened yesterday become as real as what is happening in the present. It is as if they are sprouting two invisible time cones from their head: an *anterior* time cone pointing from their forehead into the future and a *posterior* cone, pointing from the back of their head into the past. As the beta children get older, these budding time cones will slowly extend their uniquely personal time frame even further backward into their past and even forward into the future.

Around age twelve, toward the end of elementary school, the time cones of these beta children have grown season-deep, spanning three months backward and three months forward. By the time adolescents reach September in the last year of high school, betas will be worrying about their upcoming graduation. Now, their time cones span around nine months. But alpha teenagers will continue taking life a day at a time.

Without any conscious effort, a temporal reality of past and future has spontaneously unfolded before the inner eye of young betas. This process, which I call *betacization,* results in an inner timescape of personal imagery as real and constant as any physical landscape. As a result, betas' personal future and past begin to play an important role in their motivation. This would, ideally, lead to a flexible balance between the various motivating forces (the present, past and future). In reality, from the start, young betas heavily favor their time cones over the present and usually continue living much of their lives in these time cones.

Because alphas are free of time cones, and betas restrained by theirs, each time gender experiences time in distinctly different ways. As a result, this induces dissimilar time gender under similar circumstances, making each person's experiences time gender specific.

How alphas experience time

Other than broadly experiencing memories a part of their past, alphas experience these past episodes as islets in a sea of timelessness. They sample past events as moments or scenes that took place at indistinct points in time, as myths take place "..once upon a time.." For alphas, the past is not yet the present; it is not a coherent inner reality. As a result, alphas cannot stroll back into a timescape of their past, although they can undoubtedly consciously reconstruct their own life story by using external information and logical thinking. But *learning* that the house of one's early years had a red roof is different from *remembering* that the roof of the old familiar house was definitely red and not green or black. Reciting a learned, reconstructed past is not the same as reviewing a spontaneously evolved inner timescape of the past. When alphas recite such a deliberately reconstructed autobiography they, and sensitive listeners too, often feel as if they are telling someone else's story.

What applies to alphas experiencing their past also applies to their experiencing the future. For alphas, the future is "not yet the present"; they do not inwardly perceive a future timescape. Instead of experiencing future events in a personal timeframe, they envision these will happen in the future "one day."

A highly intelligent alpha who is very conversant with the time gender model once told me:

> *"My boyfriend has asked me to marry him!"*

> "When is that going to be?"

> *"In six months."*

Then she was silent for a few moments and, turning both hands inside out while shrugging her shoulders, she added:

> *"Six months...six years...six weeks... it is all the same to me... It will be real when I get there!"*

Alphas do not pre-live their future nor experience it as a pre-recorded reality. This is not to say that alphas may not have spontaneous visions of their future, or fantasize about it, or that they cannot plan their future. They can through deliberate thinking construct a coherent timeframe of their personal future, just as they can reconstruct their past. This is not the same as spontaneously evolving an inner future reality. Their plans only reflect the future as it is perceived today. Tomorrow, a change of circumstances may trigger a review or change of those plans.

Given the ever-changing present t without an enduring past and without a stable view of the future, nothing is unchangeable for alphas. Everything is transient and dynamic. Historic time is only an idea. The only real time is the raw here-it-comes-and-there-it-goes flow of time.

Since alphas do not place the present t moment in the context of a timescape stretching from their personal past through the present into their personal future, their motivation is first and foremost based on their present t situation. In comparison with those who cannot forget about the past or insist that future considerations must prevail, alphas may appear more flexible, open-minded, inventive and mature. Exclusively concentrating on the present t, however, may win the battle but lose the war. In this case, alphas may be judged as having been too shortsighted, opportunistic and impulsive.

How betas experience time

Betas also experience the here-it-comes-there-it-goes flow of outer events. But as their time cones evolve they gain a sense that, once real time passes through Point Zero of the present, it then flows into their past and future time cones and settles there as historic time in a continuous, static, linear timescape. Unlike alphas, betas live perpetually weighted down by their past and future.

Because betas experience both historic time and real time as a continuum, their past and future are psychologically as concrete as their present. This enables them to walk into, and relive their past as far back as their posterior cone reaches. They can also enter the reality ahead and feel their way forward into the future, responding to foreseeable events as real ones rather than as some "what if" vision. They therefore respond much earlier and more concretely to anticipated events than alphas. The time distance perception of betas is far more acute than in alphas. Metaphorically speaking, when betas see a distant car coming their way they get out of its path well in advance, while alphas may jump out of the way just in the nick of time.

Since betas invariably experience current situations as enmeshed in their inner timescape, their primary motivation is not situational, but time-oriented. Unlike alphas, betas cannot say with conviction "It is all water under the bridge!" or "Don't worry, we will cross this bridge when we come to it." In contrast with the tactical approach to life of alphas, the usual beta outlook is strategic. Filtering the present through their time cones, however, may either clarify or muddle their vision. Depending on circumstances, and on who is judging, critics may either view betas as admirably determined, steadfast, solid, stable, consistent, mature or highly principled, or, conversely, as inflexible, rigid, narrow-minded, stubborn, unyielding, or neurotic.

Alphas and betas both capture time as it flows through the present. But then alphas let go of it and attend to their next catch, while betas go on to domesticate time in their cones.[2]

Discovering the difference in the autobiographic memory of alphas and betas

n taking a person's life history, one taps into that part of a person's long-term knowledge memory which contains emotionally colored recollections that make up one's life story. This *autobiographic* knowledge memory is not the same as one's *general* knowledge memory with the impersonal, information about one's reality. For example, retaining important personal events usually requires only a single exposure, while retaining impersonal knowledge involves as a rule repetitive exposures to the relevant data. Furthermore, one's general knowledge memory starts functioning at birth, if not sooner, while one's autobiographic memory (which is responsible for one's life history) begins functioning only around age 5 or 6. Thus autobiographic and general knowledge memory are two separate functional divisions of one's long-term memory.

I discovered time gender by *not* following the traditional subject-oriented method of taking a life history. This method focuses on relevant subject areas—early family setting, education, occupational background, sexual history, and so on—and leads to a compartmentalized, fragmented life story, consisting of a multitude of parallel sub-histories. The traditional method portrays a person as a youngster, a student, a working person, a sexual being, and so on, without integrating these subject areas into a single biography. Instead, one teacher taught me to approach a person's past as a sequence of personal milestones stretching from birth to the presenting problem, with in-between-events also embedded in sequential fashion. It structures someone's unique past as a highly personalized calendar of significant memories and produces a single, integrated life story,[3] rather than a collage of multiple sub-biographies.

Taking such a timeframe-oriented life history involves a 60-minute structured interview divided into three parts. The first is an introduction of about 5 minutes for an initial talk about the client's reason for seeing me. The second is constructing a personal calendar or chronology of personal milestones that becomes the backbone of my chronologic, biographic history. It subdivides a client's life into a series of circumscribed life episodes. This usually takes 25-30 minutes. The third part is the stress and strain history, which takes up the final 25-30 minutes. It consists of taking the client through each of the life episodes in the personal calendar, from birth until the history of the present problem. This is done by first soliciting spontaneous memories, and then following through with a subject-oriented grid of questions, which is appropriate to each life episode. Personal data which emerge are inserted into the personal calendar. This completes the client's integrated life history.[4]

While constructing several thousand personal calendars over some thirty years of professional practice, and fleshing them out with a stress and strain history, I took for granted that everyone relates to time the same way I do. In the late 1980s, however, I began to wonder upon meeting a new client: "Will this hour of constructing a personal calendar and fleshing it out with a stress and strain history be easy or difficult? Will the client be able to place unrelated memories in a stable, personal time frame? Or will I have to work like a detective trying to solve a puzzle of time sequences?" In the latter case, clients often would apologetically say: "I am sorry, Doctor, I never seem to know what comes first and what later...I am not very good at keeping track of time." It turned out that some people recall unrelated personal events in a loosely organized, changeable timeframe (alphas), while others recall unrelated autobiographic memories in a rather fixed and linear sequence (betas). This must have its roots in the fact that the autobiographic memories of alphas and betas are different.

Alphas' autobiographic memory is apparently free of before-after connections between unrelated life events; while the one of betasevidently contains some system of spontaneously arising before-after connections between unrelated life episodes. Since the autobiographic memories of alphas and betas and, thus, the beginning of their life stories, emerge early in middle childhood, the time gender-specific behavioral styles of alphas and betas — time gender differentiation — must also begin evolving during this developmental period.

Introducing the autobiographies of Carl Jung and Sigmund Freud

This human duality in storing, retaining, and remembering unrelated past memories appeared more and more a black or white proposition. I could not find any transitional states, such as people with both alpha and beta traits, or people who had changed time gender over the years. This definitely favored a genetic rather than learned underpinning. Genetic theories of behavior, however, can prove controversial. In order to defend myself against possible charges that I thought one type to be superior to the other, I decided to choose an equally famous and respected alpha and beta as models for my theory.

In order to assess the time gender of potential candidates, I looked in my library for autobiographies. Among these were the ones of Sigmund Freud (1856-1939) and Carl Jung (1875-1961). This was no surprise for both were pioneers in exploring and modeling human personality and played major roles in my professional development. During my training and as a young psychiatrist, Freud had greatly influenced me. As I grew older, Jung's teachings began adding their weight, perhaps because Jung preferred, unlike Freud, treating people over age forty. He felt that younger people were still too busy making their mark with career-building and creating a family to devote sufficient time to the process of self-realization.

When I had previously read Freud's and Jung's autobiographies, I had, in retrospect, considered everyone, including Freud and Jung, a beta like myself; I had been *betacizing* everyone. At this point, however, my focus was on the way Freud and Jung appeared to recall their lives in writing their autobiographies. Had they been able to do so in the context of an orderly time frame? For the one who would have had a problem in this regard, writing his autobiographies would have been far more difficult than writing an innovative but impersonal knowledge paper. With this in mind, I took a fresh look at Jung's autobiography, *Memories, Dreams and Reflections,*[5] which he began when he was 82 years of age.

Jung experienced enormous difficulties in putting his autobiography together. Indeed, one of his pupils, the Jungian psychoanalyst, Aniella Jaffé, had to come to his rescue, and began meeting with him about one afternoon per week, with her asking questions and noting down his replies. She also became his editor, and, where needed, his ghost-writer.[6]

By the end of the first year, Jung had told Jaffé, among other things, many of his earliest memories. But there remained great gaps in his story.[7] Jung was aware of this and it preoccupied him. He wrote to a friend that when asked to answer some questions about his personal life he had found that with but a few exceptions he barely could recollect the very things that make up a sensible biography, such as "people one has met, travels, adventures, entanglements, blows of destiny, and so on." Instead, all his vivid memories had to do with emotional experiences that arouse uneasiness and passion and were hardly fit to render an objective account of his life.[8] Jung clearly made the point that he had profound problems in framing his past and demonstrated that he (unlike a beta with a posterior time cone) had no conscious orderly access to his past. He furthermore indicated in his autobiography that, rather than experiencing time as an orderly timescape, stretching from early memory through the time cone of the past into the present and then extending into the time cone of the future, his time experience reflected instead the here-it-comes-and-there-it-goes flow of real time in Point Zero. He described his conscious personal reality as a fleeting, transient conscious personal here-and-now which makes it a miracle that anything can exist and develop at all, saying:

> "In the end the only events in my life worth telling are those when the imperishable world [of the unconscious] irrupted into this transitory one [of the conscious]. That is why I speak chiefly of inner experiences, among which I include my dreams and visions...All other memories of travels, people and my surroundings have paled beside these interior happenings... Recollection of the outward events of my life has largely faded or disappeared ...I cannot tell much about them... I can understand myself only in the light of inner happenings...[which] make up the singularity of my life, and with these my autobiography deals."[9]

There can be no doubt that Jung is of the alpha time gender. As a result, his personal time frame was so loosely organized that, despite his profound thinking and prolific writings in the impersonal knowledge arena, constructing an account of his own life became an agonizing challenge. It took him four months to deliberately reconstruct his childhood, school days, and years at university.[10] It took him and Jaffé almost five years to complete an autobiography that remains without the backbone of an orderly personal time frame. In the end Jaffé wrote somewhat apologetically (remarks in brackets mine):

> "The chapters are rapidly moving beams of light that only fleetingly illuminate the outward events [personal milestones] of Jung's life and work. In recompense, they transmit the atmosphere of his intellectual world and the experience of a man to whom the psyche was a profound reality. I often asked Jung for specific data on outward happenings (personal milestones), but I asked in vain. Only the spiritual essence of his life's experience remained in his memory."[11]

There is no doubt about it: taking a personal history of Jung would have been a very challenging procedure. Discovering during my early prospecting for a famous alpha-beta pair that Jung was an alpha was like striking gold. After this extraordinary discovery, I took a second look at Freud's autobiography, hoping that my luck would last and that I would find him to be a beta.

When he was 69, Freud published *An Autobiographical Study*.[12] This was part of a collection of short studies by various members of the medical profession designed to give a picture of the present state of medicine as revealed in the autobiographies of its leaders.[13] His autobiography stresses Freud as a professional person. It is not devoid of private personal milestones. But I really pricked up my ears when I noted that Freud said in the opening chapter:

> "...I must endeavor to construct a narrative in which subjective and objective attitudes, biographical and historic interests, are combined in a new proportion."[14]

He is talking about wanting to unfold important aspects of his timescape. He wrote a coherent autobiographical narrative that clearly suggests a facility in recalling autobiographic vignettes in a time-ordered manner. He furthermore tended to be preoccupied with keeping track of his past—his posterior time cone—since he had already published a little known autobiography of himself when he was 45 years old.[15] He continued from there on in various autobiographic reviews of his development.[16] Apparently, writing an autobiography was for Freud no more difficult than his innovative writing in the impersonal arena.

Constructing a personalized calendar of personal milestones, dressed up with a stress and strain history, would in Freud's case certainly have been much easier than with

Jung. No doubt, Freud was of the beta time gender. I was elated! I had reached my goal of finding an alpha and a beta who were equally famous and respected because of comparable achievements which should offset the potentially nasty political implications of the genetic nature of my time gender model.

Relating Freud's and Jung's theories to their time gender

Finding that Jung was an alpha and Freud a beta had unexpected spin-offs. While both Freud and Jung were working on their respective *magna opera* during their late thirties, early forties—Freud on *The Interpretation of Dreams*[17] during the late 1890s, Jung on *Psychological Types*[18] during the 1913-1918 period—each went through some kind of creative mid-life crisis. Both handled their period of emotional upheaval through self-analysis. Freud's self-analysis became the foundation of his psychoanalytic theory and the Freudian model for psychoanalyzing others. Jung's self-analysis became the basis of the Jungian personality model and the exemplary model of exploring other people's minds.

Both theories and methods are generalizations of how Freud and Jung came to view their own personality and psyche, and how they investigated them. As a result, each model and method would carry the stamp of its maker's time gender. This is why these two personality models become relevant to our discussion.

Indeed, Freud's beta-centric psychoanalysis ended up aiming for harmony between the past and the present. His psychoanalysis sought to identify causal connections between present problems and past experiences through free association; and then to clarify and interpret these causal connections to the client. Acquiring these fresh insights plus emotionally re-experiencing the past reality would then enable the client to transcend the past by developing more healthy adaptive patterns in the present.

Instead of giving the present a backward-looking meaning through exploring its connections with the past, the aim of Jungian alpha-centric analysis became to give a new, forward looking, goal directed meaning to the present.[19] To achieve this, he used dream analysis (identifying directed associations that surround dream themes with the analyst actively participating) and active imagination (one's myth-making fantasy or day dreaming). He felt that in this way an all embracing, psychic complex of associative connections that is self-realizing (goal-directed) and thus forward-oriented looking would be identified as the underpinning of the present. He named this all embracing, self-realizing complex "the Self." Once identified, the Self would give a fresh, forward-looking meaning to the present, and a new, lasting harmony between the present and the unconscious, self-realizing Self would result.

Freud and Jung each lived well into their 80s and were very prolific in publishing their explorations of the human psyche. This makes the alpha-centric *Collected Works* of Jung and the beta-centric *Collected Works* of Freud [20] a gem-packed mine for comparative time gender research.

More about Freud

Freud suffered from a mid-life crisis that began around age forty and lasted about five years. It was intimately connected with anxious concerns about how his budding theory about the role of sexuality in early development applied to himself. His mid-life upheaval drove him in July 1897 to begin an intense period of self-analysis.[21]

In self-analysis Freud used free association, especially on his own dreams in order to have these dreams lead him into his own past to end up in his childhood. He reported many details of the analysis of his dreams in *The Interpretation of Dreams,* which was published in 1900, and became a pioneering, standard-setting work for dream analysis.

However, Freud had introduced the main features of his innovative psychoanalytic technique of free association well before starting his self-analysis. First, he had started using hypnosis in patients to trace the history of a neurotic symptom such as a phobia or hysterical paralysis, back to its starting point in the patient's past, in the posterior cone. He obviously took implicitly for granted that everyone has a coherent past embedded in a linear personal time frame. He soon concluded that his hypnotized subjects would not stop their recollections at the point of origin of their symptom but would carry on further back into their past, and end up in their childhood.[22] His early theoretical position, based on hypnosis, was that while the origin of a symptom was triggered somewhere in the past, the potential for this triggering was rooted in what actually happened in early childhood.

Some patients were hypnosis-resistant. In these cases Freud began developing an alternative technique to get at the past origin of neurotic symptoms. Instead of trying to induce a trance while having them in a reclining position with their eyes closed, he would press them on their forehead while convincingly suggesting they could remember where the symptom had started. After some success he began gradually to drop suggestion, pressing on their head, and questioning, and eventually ended up with only encouraging spontaneous, uncensored free association while reclining on the couch with their eyes closed. To his surprise he found that this, too, led his patients beyond the origin of their symptoms deeper into their past. In due course he found this free association so superior that, by 1896, he abandoned exploratory hypnosis altogether.[23]

When eventually Freud began his self-analysis, he applied this technique of free association on himself, to lead him into his own past, specifically his early childhood. This is how he became convinced that sexuality played a major role in his own, and, therefore, in everyone's early childhood. Conversely, his self-analysis also made him realize that the conflicts and irrationalities he observed in his patients were present in himself. He therefore became reluctant to accept the validity of any hypothesis unless he had tested it out on himself. As a result, he continued his self-analysis throughout his life and amended his personality theory accordingly.[24] In the 1920s, when he developed his final personality model of id, ego and superego this clearly showed his beta time gender, as I will demonstrate in due course.

More about Jung

In April 1906, Jung was 31 and lived in Zurich, Switzerland. At that time he began a correspondence with the then 50-year old Sigmund Freud in Vienna.[25] They developed a mutual admiration society that soon led to intimate friendship. They analyzed each other's dreams, for example, when in 1909 they traveled together to the United States to give lectures at Clark University in Worcester, Massachusetts.[26]

Alphas like Jung and betas like Freud not only experience themselves in distinctly different ways, but they also think differently. Accordingly, as Jung began maturing as an explorer of the psyche in his own right, he naturally began feeling uncomfortable with the beta-centric personality model Freud was offering. It did not fit him, and he therefore had to free himself from Freud's powerful grip and create his own alpha-centric model.

In 1912, there was a parting of the ways with Freud. The following years (1913-18) turned into a protracted episode of emotional upheaval, a highly imaginative, yet deeply disturbing mid-life crisis a creative illness,[27] comparable with Freud's troublesome, yet inventive midlife crisis during the late 1890s.

As Jung began his self-analysis, he first fell back on dream analysis through free association as Freud had done, expecting this would lead him into his past toward some retrospective meaning of the problem he was facing. He soon discovered that, no matter what he began free-associating on, he always ended up in the same complexes of memories. The free association failed to lead incrementally into his past. "Free association will get me nowhere, any more than it would help me to decipher a Hittite inscription," he said later, "It will of course help me to uncover all my own complexes, but for this purpose I have no need of a dream—I could just as well take a public notice or a sentence in a newspaper [and free-associate on those instead of free-associating on a dream]."[28]

Despite his failure to get into his past through unfocused free association, Jung initially persisted in his adherence to Freud's beta-centric view that the answer to his problems must lie in his past. Thus, he deliberately went over his past, especially his childhood memories, to see whether he might have overlooked the cause of his problems. However, these efforts only led to a renewed acknowledgment of his ignorance in this regard, whereupon he decided he simply would willingly submit himself to any impulses coming from his unconscious.[29]

Therefore, he began giving free reign to what seemed an inexhaustible chaos of timeless fantasies and daydreams in which he personified the creations of his imagination, experiencing them as real people, giving them a voice and an identity in their own right. He continued to pursue this technique of active imagination throughout the years 1913-1918. During these years, he found himself facing an alien reality which seemed difficult to grasp, often feeling as if "gigantic blocks of stone were tumbling down" upon him. While doing his best not to "lose his head" and trying to find some way to understand these strange experiences, he felt himself in a constant state of tension.[30] To stay sane, he had to draw heavily on the real life in his family and profession.[31]

Jung remained convinced that he would eventually bring order to this chaos and that understanding the meaning of it all would then not only change his own mental state for the better, but also open the human psyche to him.[32] Hence his unswerving pursuit of the stream of mental imagery that his unlimited day dreaming produced. To help him to grasp the meaning of this image stream, he consistently kept track of it by translating it as best he could into words, and, occasionally, in graphic, colorful pictures.

It was not until 1917 that his surge of fantasies from within began to ebb away. Only then was he able to take reflect on what had happened to him. Jung came to view his self-observations during the critical 1913-1918 years as the core of the theories that emerged in his published work. He considered these years of pursuing his inner images the most important of his life, for during these years all essential material came into focus. As a result, he began to infer the presence in our psyche of an organizing, all-embracing, self-realizing, goal directed unconscious Self, quite distinct from the conscious executive ego that Freud had introduced and Jung would continue to make use of.[33]

Jung's emphasis on day dreaming and active imagination does not mean he had completely lost faith in the analysis of night dreams. In his case, however, free-associating on any dream component would (because of the absence of a posterior time cone) repetitively lead to the same set of memory complexes. He understandably generalized this to everyone's psyche—alphacizing everybody—concluding that in dream analysis free association was never all that helpful. He found it far more useful to take each single point of the dream as a central theme and explore all its possible directed associations.

This approach results in a radial configuration of associations around each dream theme, like the spokes of a wheel around their axle, a Jungian memory islet, so to speak,[34] as demonstrated by Figure 2.1. Jung eventually came to refer to this approach as directed association,[35] implying that, in order to make sense of their unconscious associative connections, alphas need some direction.

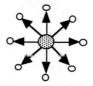

Figure 2.1: A Jungian memory islet of directed associations

By way of further illustration, the Jungian analysis of a dream with, let us say, five themes may be represented by figure 2.2. Each theme is represented by a cluster of associations—Jungian islets—which analysts will then interpret, leaning heavily on mythological themes.

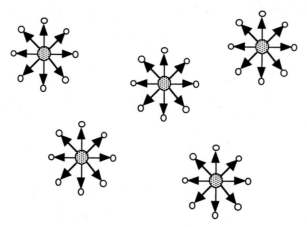

Figure 2.2: The representation of Jungian analysis of a dream with five themes

Jung's directed association contrasts with Freud's free association. As an alpha, free association did not get him anywhere. In betas, however, free association follows a rambling pathway of consecutive free associations that may move them incrementally farther and farther away in time from the reference point. Figure 2.3 represents such a Freudian memory chain, metaphorically, and Figure 2.4 the result of Freudian analysis of a dream with five themes.

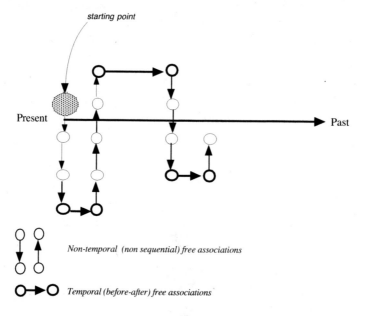

Figure 2.3: Freudian memory chain of free associations

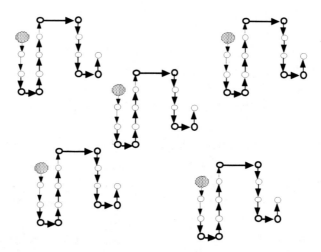

Figure 2.4: The representation of Freudian analysis of a dream with five themes

Martha, the non-believer

I will illustrate these points through the example of Martha, a sophisticated alpha lawyer who had become very conversant with the time gender model. However, the idea that her autobiographic memory was different from mine (a beta's) troubled her. One day she challenged me:

> "When I, an alpha, think about my first year in law school, I clearly remember where I went, the sequence of the subjects I took that year, my various professors, many of my fellow students, my boyfriends, and what not."

To underline this she then spontaneously produced some personal stories from that time in her life. Martha clearly began by deliberately focusing on the first year in her professional school, producing a Jungian memory islet, a radial arrangement of personal vignettes that were associatively connected with her "First Year in Law school." This is metaphorically depicted in figure 2.5, a typical instance of what Jung deliberately went after with his method of directed association in dream analysis.

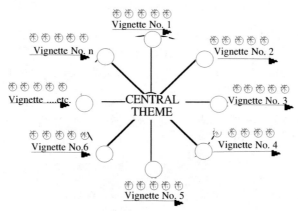

Figure 2.5: A Jungian memory islet of personal vignettes clustering around a central theme

This is not to say that Martha's attention did not soon wander away from her chosen central theme "The First Year in Law school." Of course it did. After all, the Jungian memory islet of the "First Year in Law school" was not a freestanding memory complex but part of a mega-network of interlocking Jungian islets. When discussing a classmate in Law school who was also her boyfriend that year she spontaneously shifted away from her law school complex and began talking about other boyfriends—an associative shift in this case from one central theme (First Year in Law school) to another (Boyfriends). Then she spontaneously free associated to something else. Her shift from her initial directed associations toward spontaneous, unfocused, passive autobiographicassociations mirrored her mega-network of parallel and telescoping Jungian memory. Figure 2.6 is a metaphorical interpretation of this timeless associative mega-network of Jungian memory islets in alphas, and also demonstrates the pathway that unfocussed free association will follow in Jungians.

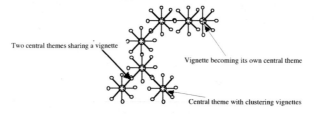

Two central themes sharing a vignette

Vignette becoming its own central theme

Central theme with clustering vignettes

The mega-network of interlocking Jungian memory islets in the the autobiographic memory bank of alphas

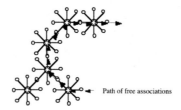

Path of free associations

Pursuing free-association in the alpha network of Jungian memory islets

Note: *All associative bonds are perceptual - conceptual - emotional in nature*

Figure 2.6

As mentioned, Jung experienced early in his self-analysis that such free associations repeatedly led him into the same set of dominant memory islets, no matter from which point he entered the network. However, we did not get that far with Martha. She stopped at some point and asked:

> *"So how is my alpha memory different from your beta memory starting at your First Year in Medical School?"*

I closed my eyes to let these memories come freely and said:

> "I remember my first year in medical school, all right,"

and I began verbalizing some relevant vignettes that came to mind while initially stuck at "My First Year in Medical School" as central theme and thus developing, so to say, my own Jungian Islet. But soon I found myself saying:

"But that was also the time when [such and such] happened to my father."

After talking about this a bit, I then found myself spontaneously shifting to a rather important event that, I recalled, happened shortly after and involved a certain experience with a friend. In other words, before realizing it, I first shifted to a vignette about my father, and then to one about a friend—vignettes that were neither conceptually, perceptually nor emotionally related to "My First Year in Medical School" nor to each other. Instead, they were structured as personal milestones that progressed in a long, quasi-linear time frame.

When betas are free-associating, they are not only dancing around from one interlocking Jungian islet to another; they are also intermittently moving backward, or forward, through the timescape of their posterior time cone. Figure 2.7 represents this associative pathway of betas diagrammatically.

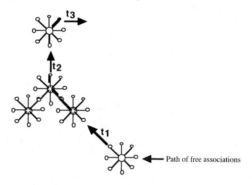

Note: All associative bonds are perceptual , conceptual , or emotional in nature , except the thick-lined arrows which represent temporal bonds   that lead incrementally into the past (posterior time cone)

Figure 2.7: Pursuing free association in the beta version of
the autobiographic network of Jungian memory islets

In summary, this exercise reaffirmed that a Jungian alpha like Martha did not produce any temporal associations between unrelated life events. Later, when we examined her Jungian islet of her first year as law student, we also found that she could not spontaneously come up with the time sequence within this particular Jungian memory islet unless an obvious calendar connection, say the opening ceremony (in September), or the Christmas holiday, provided time coordinates.

The exercise further evidenced that betas supplement their "timeless" autobiographic network of Jungian memory islets with a network of time bonds, which is the underpinning of their past and future time cones.

Free association has limits, even in betas

Originally Freud used hypnosis to track the origin of his patients' neurotic symptoms to some point in the past. He then found his patients would move beyond this point into their early childhood. Of course, the first five to six years of life is a period of which we all have, at best, only a spotty memory, something Freud called infantile amnesia.

When Freud replaced hypnosis with free association, he ran into the same phenomenon of patients moving in their early childhood. He remained for some time convinced that his patients' revelations about their early childhood — frequently involving incestuous child abuse — were a genuine part of their early childhood history, and that such traumatic experiences were, indeed, the actual cause of their neurosis (the traumatic origin of neurosis).

Using in all patients, alphas and betas alike, completely uncensored free association to trace present mental activities into early childhood, Freud assumed that everyone has a sequential autobiographic memory, or in my terms, a posterior time cone through which free association will progressively lead back into one's past. However, Jung the Master Alpha had realized that free association did not lead him into the past, but got him going around in circles of memory complexes. So, the first question becomes: what happened with the alpha patients with whom Freud supposedly applied his technique of free association?

Freud furthermore assumed that, in my terms, the tip of the posterior time cone of his beta patients reaches into to the point of birth, well prior to the age of six when time binding begins between unrelated life vignettes (betacization). Early childhood is not included in a beta's timescape, so free association cannot possibly lead betas into their early childhood. The second question therefore becomes: what happened to Freud's beta patients for whom he thought that free association would lead into memories of early childhood?

In answering these two questions, it is of interest to note that, whatever the time gender of Freud's patients, they all seemed to end up with stories about incestuous sexual abuse in early childhood which, for some years, he assumed to have really happened. However, in due course Freud came to realize that his patients' revelations did not reflect actual childhood events, but childhood-like fantasies. As a result, he replaced the theory of the traumatic origin of neurosis with the theory of psychic reality origin of neurosis. When all of Freud's patients, alphas and betas alike, were supposedly going back to early childhood, they were not purely free-associating but shifting into what Jung later substituted for free association, namely active imagination, or what I call personal myth making. Jung described this active imagination as: "The art of letting things happen, action through non-action, letting go of oneself, as taught by Meister Eckhart..."[36] He saw creative fantasy as expressing the mythopoeic imagination of the mythmakers, our early ancestors.[37] Freud's transition from hypnosis to free association unwittingly left the door open to a mixture of pure free association and active imagination.

In Freud's case active imagination led to idiosyncratic interpretations of a single myth, namely that of Oedipus, while in Jung's case it led to equally idiosyncratic interpretations involving the entire human mythology. This difference in interpretation may now be seen in the light of their time gender in which their thinking was rooted, as will be discussed in Chapter 8.

Alphas and betas often display no clear differences in their pasts

There are many complex reasons why Carl Jung and Sigmund Freud did not recognize the alpha-beta duality in our autobiographic memory. Let me conclude this chapter by mentioning two.

Betas' ability to walk back into and relive their past provides for an opportunity to act and respond concretely to specific past events. But, while remembering the good things of life is a delight, there also will be past pains that make for a living hell. The same holds when betas pre-live their future. Past guilt or anxiety about the future is why betas may wish they could get rid of their cones. Sometimes alcohol will do the trick for them, for, with alcohol in their blood, their cones fall off. To betas alcohol is like "alpha juice." It temporarily turns betas into chemical alphas and that easily gets them into hot water. Of course, next morning the cones are back on again.

The more usual routine for betas, dealing with hurtful sectors in their time cones, is to develop mental tricks — defense mechanisms — to avoid access to painful time cone sectors. Some become masters in denying or repressing both past and future hurts. As a rule, betas cannot freely navigate through their cones. More often than not, there are unconscious signals all over the place that read "Do not enter!" " Danger zone!" "Detour!" "Look somewhere else!"

Thus, we have betas who have access to an orderly past but often avoid that access, while for alphas, having empty spots in their history is normal. Sometimes they may fill in some of these empty spots with their creative imagination. As a result, in alphas and betas, the picture of their past appears frequently not all that different: empty spots and filled in spots. No wonder that humankind generally overlooked the possibility of some fundamental difference in the way people view and recollect their past, or, for that matter, envision their future. Even Sigmund Freud and Carl Jung, who analyzed their own psyche and the minds of others, overlooked the time gender duality.

We need a basic model to work with

Now the reader knows that time gender emerges early in middle childhood as a difference in experiencing and relating to time, and that this mirrors a difference in the time structure of the brain's autobiographicmemory.

My next task is to begin translating this difference in time gender into the private experiences and publicly observable behaviors that are unique to alphas and betas. But before I can present a coherent discussion of the many practical implications of time gender, I must offer a mind-body (psyche-soma) model in which to fit the two time genders.[38] I will introduce such a model in the next chapter, which will require some patience from the reader. Once introduced, however, the reader will be able to confidently tackle the rest of the book and turn the perplexing mysteries of time gender into "Aha...now I see!" knowledge.

NOTES

1   Flor-Henry (1978).
2   Kastenbaum (1975).
3   Pos (1978.) The principle of the method was introduced by Adolph Meyer (1866-1950) [Lief (1948): 418-422.
4   See for further details *Appendix 2: The chronologic biographic interview* .
5   Jung (1965)
6   Jaffé (1965), p. v.
7   Jaffé (1965), p. vi.
8   Jung, quoted by Jaffé (1965), p. viii-ix.
9   Jung (1965), p. 4-5.
10   Jaffé (1965), p. v-ix.
11   Jaffé (1965), p. vi-vii.
12   Freud (1950).
13   Freud (1950), p. 9
14   Freud (1950), p. 12.
15   Jones (1955), vol. 2, p. 11.
16   Freud (1950), p. 11.
17   Published in 1900; Jones (1953), p. 321.
18   Published in 1921; Jung (1977), Vol 6.
19   Jacobi (1951).
20   Freud (1959); Jung (1953-78).
21   Jones (1953).
22   Jones (1953), p. 240, 247.
23   Jones (1953), p. 244.
24   Jones (1953), p. 244. 320, 327.
25   Jones (1955), p. 459.
26   Jung (1965), p. 158.
27   Stevens (1990), p. 7; Ellenberger (1970), p. 447
28   Jung (1977), vol. 16, p. 149.
29   Jung (1965), p. 173.
30   Jung (1965), p. 176-177, 184-187.
31   Jung and Jaffé (1965), p. 214; quoted by Jacoby (1990), p. 48.
32   Jung (1965), p. 170-199.
33   Jung (1965), p. 196, 199, 206-20;.Jacoby (1990), p. 49.
34   Jung, (1977), vol. 16, p. 42, 58, 148-149.
35   Jacobi (1951).
36   Jung (1962), p. 93, quoted by Stevens (1990) p.201
37   Jung (1965), p. 188.
38   To give the interested reader a flavor of this general model, here are the last few lines of my Ph.D. thesis *The Psyche-Soma Complex: Its Psychology and Logic* (1963*)*: '...one day the physician will look upon "psychosomatics" as the physicist looks upon "wavicles"; then the relation between the mental system (psyche) and the physical system (soma) will no longer be a mystery but history. And, on the question whether the human being should be considered matter or mind, he finally and confidently may answer: "never mind, it does not matter."'

CHAPTER 3

The Time Gender Model

This chapter is devoted to creating a theoretical model that allows for discussion of both subjective mental experience and objective physical behavior in general, and of time gender-specific expressions thereof in particular.[1]

Our mind and brain reflect a complex of many subsystems. The global map of relations between and within these subsystems changes about twenty times per second.[2] In this process attention plays a major role. It reflects not only a snapshot of the brain's global map of ever-changing relations between and within its subsystems, but also the focused state of our conscious mind.[3] Accordingly, changing the focus of our attention means, on one hand, that we are re-allocating and re-distributing the functional priorities between and within the brain's subsystems, and, on the other hand, shifting our particular private conscious focus of the moment. Attention rooted in a combination of instinct and memory mediates the highest level of our immensely complex brain operation, as well as the coherent unfolding of our conscious stream of experience.

Our attention fluctuates between the conscious flow of outer events in the surrounding world of real time, and the conscious flow of inner events in our mind. These outer and inner flows of consciousness portray two basic, contrasting attention modes. They are the two constituent units of my model of which, as I will demonstrate, time gender becomes a natural extension.

The conscious flow of outer events: the world in 4–D

When you are sitting in a chair paying attention to your physical environment, you are in real time, in the objective reality of the here-and-now. This physical world you are in is not a three-dimensional but a four-dimensional theater. Why four dimensions? First, there are the three dimensions of conventional space, as illustrated in figure 3.1.

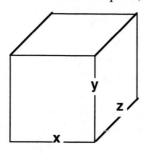

Figure 3.1: Three-dimensional space

However, we do not experience our reality as a three-dimensional still picture. We see it, instead, as a three-dimensional movie. If we want to pinpoint a past event, we must not only state where it happened by assigning it a particular location in the three dimensions of space; we also must say when it took place by locating it in the fourth dimension of time, with a clock and a calendar (Figure 3.2).

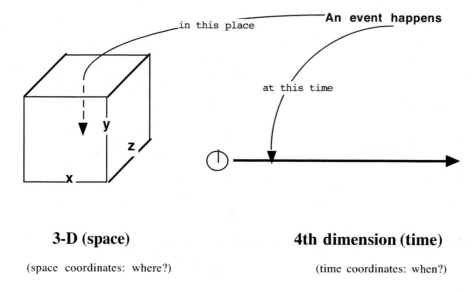

3-D (space)   **4th dimension (time)**

(space coordinates: where?)   (time coordinates: when?)

Figure 3.2: Four-dimensional time-space

Therefore, we experience the world in which time ticks away not just as a three-dimensional reality in space (3-D), but rather as a four-dimensional time-space world (4–D). I use a simple square, as seen in figure 3.3, to symbolize the transient, momentary experience of this reality in 4–D. It represents a snapshot of our reality movie in 4–D; a still picture of the present.

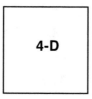

Figure 3.3: The reality of 4-D

While focusing on the conscious flow of outer events — when your attention is in the 4–D mode — your dominant mind-brain activity is perception. A perception is a conscious, real-time display of the 4–D reality. Figure 3.3 simultaneously represents the present (the here-and-now) and the current perception. The duration of this 4–D snapshot depends on the simplicity or complexity of the current perception. A simple perception such as the hue and color of a single light flash, or the loudness and pitch of a single beep, requires only one attentionswitch so that its present (4–D) lasts only 50 milliseconds. More complicated perceptions that need multiple attention shifts create a present duration of multiples of 50 milliseconds. The duration of the present in 4–D has, however, an upper limit of about 500 msecs (half a second),[4] the time span of the brain's display memory (the memory function that keeps the various individual features of a conscious perception in focus until the display is completed).[5]

Our body is part of the 4–D world

No matter what you are concentrating on in 4–D, your body is always somewhere in the picture. For example, when you are studying a painting, you may find you are stretching your neck and fixing your eyes on the picture. While concentrating on a sound you may be holding your hand behind your ear, turning your head toward it. Your body is clearly part of the 4–D reality.

How does your body in 4–D differ from its physical-social surroundings in 4–D? The 4–D world is largely a public reality. We all can see, hear, touch, smell and taste it. However, your own body belongs to 4–D's public domain only in as far as anyone can see, hear, smell, taste, or touch it. But, a pain in your chest, some peculiar feelings in your right foot, or a hunger sensation, belong to the purely private, hidden domain of your 4–D rather than to its public sector. Only you can experience these bodily perceptions. Figure 3.4 represents this differentiation in 4–D between your body and its physical-social surroundings.

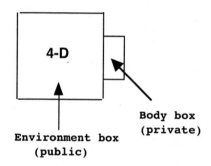

Figure 3.4: Body and environment in 4-D

In this figure the environment box stands for the public sector of 4–D, and this includes the borderline separating it from the body box. This borderline between body and environment represents the public body surface which you and others may see, hear, smell, taste and touch as opposed to the rest of your body box which represents 4–D's private sector, the 4–D only you can experience.

The conscious flow of inner events: the world in 5–D

Our conscious experience goes far beyond perceiving our body and environment. When we try to fall asleep or prepare for meditation, we close our eyes, stop listening to sounds, and keep perfectly still. We try to lock out 4–D reality. As we withdraw from this external flow of conscious images in 4–D, we find ourselves entering the internal flow of conscious images in another, purely private dimension of experience.

This internal stream of consciousness may vary from focusing on some isolated detail like an apple to an unfolding scene such as driving one's dream car. Displays in this internal flow of events are analogs of 4–D displays. They may have colors, shapes, a voice, a taste, or a smell and have feelings. That is why I call the dominant brain activity in this attention mode concrete mentation. Yet, as our dreams dramatically show, this imagery is only quasi-4–D-like, quasi-perceptual without any actual location in real space or real time. Rather than being plugged into the time-space grid of 4–D, our internal stream of consciousness flows outside the four dimensions of 4–D, in a spaceless and timeless fifth dimension of our existence: 5–D.

5–D is the internal mind-space in which we introspect and experience a private reality that exists in parallel with the objective reality in 4–D. Figure 3.5 includes this introspective fifth dimension, 5–D, in my unfolding model.

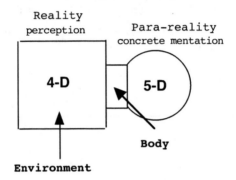

Figure 3.5: The reality of 4-D and parallel reality of 5-D

If I now were to say to someone who seems lost in day dreaming or seems otherwise preoccupied: "Are you in 5–D?---Hey, get out of 5–D. Come back to 4–D!" then my meaning would be clear. After all, while day dreaming or fantasizing, we are predominantly in 5–D, yet we can easily get back to the 4–D attention mode.

Generally, when awake, we shift our attention back and forth constantly between the flow of external events in 4–D and the flow of internal events in 5–D. But when we fall asleep, both worlds in 4–D and 5–D fade out, except in our night dreams. Then the private internal stream in 5–D may re-emerge. In that case our concrete mentation is on automatic; we cannot will our attention back to 4–D. Dreaming means to be locked into 5–D.

5–D: medium of creativity

Because 5–D imitates the real 4–D world so well, we can use its images as building blocks for a whole new world of our own making. In addition, what happens in 5–D remains hidden from the public eye, so we are also free of the social restraints in the 4–D world. We have an almost unlimited, magical power over an extremely flexible medium. We can use 5–D as a heavenly playground for day dreaming or as a private hell in which to fantasize our worst fears.

The reality in 5–D reflects a universe that is subjective, fleeting, lasting only as long as its conscious displays. It must be created repeatedly in contrast to the reality in 4–D which is objective, lasting and stable. This often leads modern humans to treat the subjective psychic reality of 5–D as somehow less real, less important, than the objective physical reality of 4–D. But the people in primitive cultures often call being in 5–D "dream time" (as opposed to real time in 4–D). They treat 5–D with much more deference, if not awe. And rightly so, for 5–D often turns out to be a powerful medium for our most profound religious, meditative, artistic and scientific creativity.

The only way to perpetuate the transient 5–D reality is by writing our thoughts down on paper, transforming its imagery into paintings, sculptures or architecture, or translating its sounds into a music score, thereby translating 5–D's private displays in some suitable public 4–D medium.

5–D: about working memory and knowledge memory

4–D displays derive from the brain's current analysis of environmental and bodily input. All current 5–D displays are present in our working memory into which they are imported from either 4–D, or from our long-term general or autobiographic knowledge memory.[6] The working memory keeps displays in 4–D and 5–D temporarily available for re-display in 5–D, to bring them "back to mind." This makes the working memory the functional backbone of our 5–D world—the blackboard of our mind.[7] It keeps our stream of consciousness coherent.

The storage capacity of our working memory is limited. In adults it has a time span of about 30 seconds. In order to take on new meaningful items it must, therefore, either discard items that are no longer worthy of attention or, in case of possible future significance, initiate their transfer into our knowledge memory.

We are not born with 5–D

Freud and Jung both concluded that, from the moment we are born, we all fantasize silently in 5–D, although admittedly at a primitive level. However, our present knowledge indicates that at birth the working memory is still dormant and therefore there is no 5–D as yet, nor even the slightest sense of past or future. The newborn's conscious state reflects as yet a completely unstructured 4–D world,[8] an undifferentiated scene of sensory impressions and biologic tension states.[9] William James described these as "blooming, buzzing confusion."[10] During the first eight months or so the baby is passively at the mercy of the flux of signals from its body and immediate surroundings and does not even recognize the fundamental distinction between sensory input from its body self and its surroundings. Therefore, this developmental period is often referred to as the "adualistic phase" during which a structure in the body box of 4–D and its environmental near-space develops.[11] This early perceptual structuring is based on associating two 4–D displays that regularly occur *simultaneously* at a time, and leads to a rudimentary, entirely 4–D triggered, general knowledge memory.

Not until around 8 months does a kind of momentary snapshot memory kick in which allows two displays that regularly occur *consecutively* to become connected. This widens the baby's time window on the 4–D reality from a single perceptual display to two consecutive ones.[12] Because the momentary snapshot memory retains a 4–D display for a moment in an incipient, snapshot-type 5–D, the infant can begin to grasp repetitive before-and-after events, first between immediate past (A) and present (B), and next between present (A) and immediately anticipated future (B). This has, among others, two major consequences:

Instead of just recognizing and relating to a mother's breast or a father's voice or the nipple of the baby bottle, a glimpse of a person or object now allows the baby to respond to the sounds and parts of the parents and others as cues of their physical presence in 4–D. When presented with the bottom of the baby bottle, it immediately anticipates the top to be there, for it rotates the bottle straight away to get at the nipple.[13] The new momentary snapshot memory provides objects and persons with a familiar display constancy. This development is often called "the birth of the object."

The momentary snapshot memory also allows the baby for the first time a measure of active participation in its surrounding world. Because the baby can now experience rewards like mother's cuddling that regularly follow certain behaviors, next the baby will anticipate and then invite these rewards. For example, stretching out its arms, followed by mother lifting it up turns into stretching out its arms to get mother to lift it out of its crib. The same applies to learning to avoid such anticipated punishments as mother's warnings and reprimands. Soon we witness a baby that actively experiments in unfamiliar situations with all kinds of tricks toward immediate needs, just like our pet cat or dog learns to do.

However, the momentary snapshot memory also has as result that "out of sight" (out of 4–D) means "out of mind" (out of 5–D). Although the mother, for example, is now apprehended as a physical entity, when her image disappears out of 4–D, it also disappears after a moment or two out of 5–D, because the recall of long-term knowledge memories into consciousness (independently from 4–D) has not yet evolved. Mother is just a situational, albeit recognizable mother with as many reincarnations as she makes reappearances in 4–D.[14] Recognizing when significant others disappear from 4–D not only makes the baby increasingly aware of the fundamental separateness of its own from the parental bodily states, it also begins invoking repeated states of frustration and separation anxiety which results in a process of mutual bonding (the earliest evidence of a baby's interpersonal intelligence). Hence the name "bonding phase" for this period of 8-18 months when the baby's momentary snapshot memory is all the conscious memory it has to rely on.

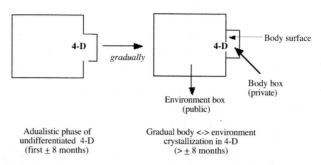

Figure 3.6: From an adualistic undifferentiated 4-D (at birth)
to a 4-D with a gradual body-environment recognition (bonding phase)

That the baby now knows that, in certain situations A leads to B, indicates an extending, but still entirely 4–D-triggered knowledge memory. At around 12 months, this knowledge memory also becomes word-triggered. For, amidst its babbling, the baby begins to exhort its first words—picked up from a parent—verbal labels of things like "Teddy" and close persons like "mama" or "dada." First it will use the name when presented with the object or person. Next, the word "Teddy," for example, spoken by the mother, triggers its 5–D display in the baby, so that the baby will look around for the Teddy bear and, upon seeing it, grab it. By the age of fifteen months, a child (who until now has been crawling) is trying to climb stairs and walk alone, carrying and hugging dolls, and helping when getting dressed. It will have a vocabulary of between three and twenty words and respond to "show me your eyes."[15]

Between 15-18 months there are early indications that 5–D displays no longer reflect solely 4–D events just gone by or immediately anticipated. They begin to spontaneously come from knowledge memory (independent of what is happening in 4–D). This increases incrementally until by 18 months the baby's conscious display of long-term general knowledge memory (independent of what is happening in 4–D) has become operational; and, as well, a knowledge-mediating working memory. In addition to the child's outer stream of consciousness in 4–D, a totally new psychic dimension—an inner stream of consciousness in 5–D—is thus emerging. With this new representational medium the child enters a new era in which symbolic activity will increasingly play an important role in her or his cognition.[16] No wonder this early appearance of representational or symbolic activity in 5–D goes hand in hand with the introduction of language.

Instead of living with a 5–D that is reactive to 4–D—externally directed—the baby henceforth experiences an internally directed 5–Dwith which to proactively manipulate 4–D. It intuits that what is in 5–D can sometimes be had in 4–D. Soon the baby's internally supported 5–D includes its conscious wishes, what it wants in 4–D. Around 19 months it commands "Pajamas on!" for example.

The period between 18-24 months consolidates this internally directed 5–D.[17] The conscious recall of long-term memories in 5–D goes hand in hand with a fundamental transformation in the mother-child relationship. Now when she is out of sight, out of 4–D, the baby can continue her presence by calling her back into 5–D, bringing her back to mind. This reassuring experience obviates the need for her continuous availability in 4–D. The "situational" mother becomes a "permanent" mother. As a result, the baby's confinement to the emotional bonding with her begins to slacken, and it becomes receptive and motivated to exploring the wider social reality of its surroundings. Thus, the bonding phase dissolves. This new level of continuing existence, independent from 4–D and derived from the display of long-term memories in 5–D, applies not only to people the child is familiar with, but to whatever else has become familiar to the child (e.g., toys). This is called object permanence.[18]

By age two the baby may utter "Jesse wants bottle!" using its first grammatically correct sentences and referring to itself by name.[19] Clearly the baby's will is born. Its ego, primitive as it may be, has entered 5–D. The peaceful bonding phase is over. The Terrible Two's have begun.

5–D: the preschool years

It is important to understand, however, that between two and six years of age — the preschool period — the child's *display memory* can only accommodate two features of a perception. When experiencing a ball in 4–D, for example, a preschooler's display memory cannot contain its shape, and color and design and size and position, all at once, but only two features, like its shape and color, or its shape and design.[20] The display memory can only span two attention points.

The *working memory* of children also continues to remain very short-spanned, perhaps only two displays wide. Since children are unable to keep a sizable series of displays available for redisplay in 5–D, 4–D and 5–D clearly remain intertwined rather than being distinct. What happens in 4–D and 5–D is, therefore, equally valid or real.[21] Preschoolers do not yet experience 4–D as reality and 5–D as in the mind. They cannot yet compare what happens in 4–D with what happens in 5–D or discriminate facts from fancy.[22]

Since they cannot yet keep track of silent thoughts or fantasies in 5–D, action in 4–D continues to play a leading role in a preschooler's cognition. Until age six or seven, children think aloud in 4–D, rather than silently in 5–D. A spoken monologue accompanies their actions like a running commentary on what they are doing. Some adults misinterpret this by saying, "This child never stops talking!" Yet the child is not talking in the sense of communicating but is thinking aloud. In other words, when talking aloud, the child sometimes is thinking aloud, at other times it is attempting to communicate.[23] Similarly, preschoolers cannot yet fantasize silently in 5–D. Rather, they use 4–D to playfully act out their fantasies, for they can only superimpose 5–D images onto 4–D displays, pretending, for example, that a cloth with fringed edges is a pillow although it hardly looks like one.[24]

Finally, a preschooler cannot separate "foreground" and "background" in 5–D. Because 4–D and 5–D are still interwoven, a preschooler cannot in 5–D lift an object or person out of their perceptual background in 4–D and consider them independently as a single, fused display in 5–D. There does not exist for the preschooler one doll independent of the child's involvement in 4–D, but only images such as "doll under the armchair" or "doll in the hammock," and images such as "dog in the kitchen" or "dog in the garden." The child has as many memories of the doll or dog as there are perceptual environments in which he or she saw them. Standing in the garden and having seen the dog in the kitchen, the child who is asked whether the dog is in the house may say "doggie (contaminated with the garden perception) is not here." Objects reappearing in different practical positions are recognized and endowed with permanence, yet remain contaminated with the perceptual matrix in which they appear in 4–D, which gives objects a nature between unity and plurality.[25] What holds true for a simple object like a doll, also goes for people, so that their personifications in 5–D are also contaminated by various perceptual backgrounds in 4–D.

5–D: the elementary school years and internalization

Early in elementary school, the child's working memory increases its span considerably. This increase in the span of the working memory's enables the child to keep a sizable series of displays available for redisplay in 5–D, so that 4–D and 5–D are no longer intertwined but become distinct from each other; 5–D matures into a truly autonomous para-reality, side by side with 4–D and becomes an alternative attention mode to 4–D. As a result, counting and thinking aloud and the child's visible and audible fantasy life gradually move from the public, outer conscious stream of events in 4–D into the silent inner conscious stream of 5–D that is only accessible through introspection.[26] This is called "internalization." Because 4–D and 5–D are no longer intertwined, what takes place in 4–D and 5–D is no longer equally valid or real. What is happens in 4–D becomes "the reality" and what happens in 5–D occurs "in the mind." The elementary schooler becomes capable of discriminating facts from fancy.

Internalization involves far more than shifting thinking, counting and fantasizing from 4–D into 5–D. Because 4–D and 5–D become separate, the child can begin to distinguish "foreground in 5–D" from "background in 4–D." Hence objects and persons in 5–D can be considered without background contamination. No longer does the child relate to " the ball under the table" or "the ball in the hammock" but only to "the ball." The child's awareness of objects and persons is further refined by the fact that, in addition to an increase it the child's working memory span, the span of its display memory also increases noticeably. As a result, multiple (rather than only two) aspects of an object or person can be grasped at once. The child becomes able to deal with multiple features of, and relations between people and objects. This enables relating parts to a whole, ordering events in a series, and classifying and sub-classifying objects.[27] Thus internalization enhances the child's general knowledge memory that is based on repetitive exposure to data, and transforms the child's awareness of the

familiar physical and social world in 4–D into recallable, detailed mental versions in 5–D.

So far, iconic imagery has prevailed in 5–D but, with the internalization of language, verbal imagery gradually gains ascendancy and allows thought processes to occur at a much faster rate. Henceforth, the child will no longer do much of its mental labor in 4–D but rather in the silent, timeless, spaceless, much faster world of 5–D, in its head. Indeed, 5–D becomes the child's instrument of natural reasoning, although this thinking remains of the concrete, trial and error variety. It cannot yet move beyond the immediacy of 4–D. For problem solving that is completely free from 4–D to occur has to wait until the arrival of abstract, hypothetical thinking in adolescence.

No wonder that elementary school starts as the internalizing leap in mental development begins. Preschoolers do not yet possess the requisite cognitive processes. Any failure at this age in the maturation of display and working memory functions will result in lowered performance on standardized tests of intelligence.

5–D: self-talk and relating to oneself

A preschooler's monologue in 4–D may not only be an example of thinking aloud, it may also portray publicly acting out a scene of imaginary social interaction, such as an imaginary conversation with mother. With her out of the room, the child may go to the cookie jar and then, suddenly imitating mother's voice, exclaim: "No, don't!" It may even slap its own hand.

How does internalizing 4–D into 5–D affect this? It transforms the many habitual, real and imaginary interpersonal scenarios in 4–D—particularly judgmental ones—into intrapersonal, soundless dialogues and pantomimes in 5–D, which is our judgmental self-talk. This self-talk is, therefore, derived from interactions between the nurturing, socializing adult—usually and predominantly the mother—and the child itself. In other words, self-talk is a repetitive judgmental dialogue between Internalized Parent (Freud called it superego) and Internalized Child (the Freudian ego). Consequently, internalized self-talk is never deliberate, voluntary, or intentional, but always automatic, repetitive, and quasi-rational.

Indeed, the relationship between Internalized Parent and Internalized Child in self-talk is like the one between ventriloquist and puppet based on a set script. The act presents a picture as if the ventriloquist and puppet each take turns in talking and then seriously listening to the other. But it is the ventriloquist who does all the talking and who is in reality not doing any listening at all! The same holds when I get into self-talk in which I criticize myself. I cannot at the same time both talk and listen to myself in 5–D. I can only alternate roles between one "I," the Internalized Parent, and the other "I," the Internalized Child. Both parts follow the same script. No matter how seemingly genuine and open-minded my self-talk, it basically remains repetitive like the internalized habitual interaction scenarios it mirrors. Thus, self-talk is by

definition without any credible emotional detachment. But, as I will discuss later in this book, we are able eventually to amend it with what I will call the Voice of Reasonor paraego.

Since we all have to listen to it for the rest of our lives, this inner show is usually all too familiar. In the final analysis, 5–D as the dimension for self-talk between Internalized Parent and Internalized Child really becomes the dimension in which we praise and criticize, encourage and dissuade, love and hate ourselves—the dimension in which we emotionally relate to ourselves. (The way in which self-talk is different in alphas and betas will be discussed in Chapter 5.)

Internalization: the ego gets into the driver's seat

I previously noted that at around 18 months the child's 5–D, now sustained by knowledge and working memories, begins containing images of what the child wants in 4–D, its conscious wishes, its conscious intentions. This does not mean that henceforth the child can act voluntarily and deliberately. On the contrary, it only knows what it wants, and this conscious display is but an impulse on which to act immediately without giving it any further thought. This remains so until the elementary school years, when true internalization begins.

While the child gradually internalizes its thinking aloud in 4–D, the role of the Internalized Child (ego) goes far beyond its participation in judgmental self-talk. For this internalized ego, "I," is now often thinking silently in 5–D about means and ends before it acts, instead of thinking aloud in 4–D while intuitively acting. As a result, voluntary action begins to gain ascendancy over impulsive acting. We are getting into ego-scenarios of forming intent, and consciously goal-directed behavior.

Such anticipatory 5–D scenarios of ego-thinking may well include feared consequences that will block the execution in 4–D of the relevant action scenario in 5–D. Furthermore, the child's ego may, of course, respond to self-talk in which the superego comments in strong negative terms on what the egois doing or intends to do. Whatever the case, the Internalized Child introduces a new level of impulse control that is no longer situation-reactive (as during the preschool years) but internally proactive and under ego-direction. This naturally enhances the child's socialization.

Elementary school children no longer think only intuitively, but for the first time begin to behave voluntarily and deliberately, based on conscious motives, intentions, reasons and means for guiding their actions in 4–D. An executive ego is emerging in 5–D that will increasingly gain dominance in controlling the child's behavior.

Internalizing the clock and calendar (social time)

All children internalize the time of clock and calendar—4–D's social time—in similar fashion. They gradually learn to handle a rich variety of time concepts pragmatically. A bright five-year-old, asked about the meaning of the words past and future, may say "the future has not happened, the past has happened." Yet, the child remains somewhat confused by the distinction between her or his own future and past activities. And the child certainly does not view past, present and future as zones in a time continuum.[28] Between age three and seven, children begin making correct and consistent use of time words as "yesterday," "today," and "tomorrow."

Children also learn to work, hands-on, with time pieces like the clock with its hours, minutes and seconds; and the calendar with its days, weeks and months. By age eight they can use both clock and calendar competently. "Mummy, it is 8.30, time to go to school!" " Next week is my birthday!" By age nine, most children use the main time words correctly. The past, present and future now assume sequential cohesion: "The past comes before and the future follows the present."[29] They also realize that each clock does not carry its own time but that time on one clock is the same as on another. By age eleven they can use a stopwatch to measure time. Even so, they cannot yet put the rich variety of time concepts they use into a single unified system of time, for this requires abstract logical thinking that only emerges in adolescence. Only around age 12 may the adolescent highschooler begin to acknowledge the abstract features of the past and future and say: "We have knowledge of the past but are ignorant or uncertain of the future."[30] In both time genders, comprehension of time reaches an abstract, conceptually unified level around age 15.

Awareness (in 5-D) of social time in the public domain of 4-D (clocks and calendars) is learned pragmatically and equally by alphas and betas. Social "time" is, however, not the same as personalized "time" as in the sequential, personalized "timescape" of betas, or the personalized fragmented time frame in the 6-D of alphas.

In this regard, the question may arise whether there is any difference between betas and alphas in the way they organize memories according to socially significant events. Wars, catastrophes, or when leaders led countries, may not have had much personal significance for a person but can be, especially with mass media, common social reference points for memories. When someone says: "I graduated from college when Truman was President," then this does not make clear whether the speaker is alpha or beta. Most people can tell where they were and what they were doing when they learned that President Kennedy was shot. But alphas are not good at saying whether a relatively important event in their life occurred before or after that moment. Certain significant social events, or even important personal events ("We moved from a small house to a large house after my father came home from the war") may serve as a calendar-type of social clock and may be associated with personal events, but when one goes into the detailed sequence of personal events the difference between alphas and betas becomes rapidly clear.[31]

6–D: internalizing personal milestones into one's life story

The working memory of preschoolers is still so narrow that it can only deal with two items at a time. The preschooler has as yet no conception of sequential order (backward or forward).[32] As a result, the child cannot keep a story straight but gets distracted by perceptual associations—referred to as centering—rather than following logical connections between one segment and the next to its logical ending.[33] Without a consistent story, there can be no stable memory of it. Naturally, this also applies to personal vignettes. The child cannot yet review and record the sequential contents of autobiographic bits and pieces.

As elementary school begins, the dramatic widening of display and working memories changes all this. The child's working memory can henceforth handle multiple items at a time (rather than only two) and seriate them in a flexible two-way fashion. He or she can get the overall concept of the itemized series. This naturally overcomes the perceptual distractions in telling stories. For the first time the child can keep the internal sequence within a story straight. They are able to grasp the story's coherence (the story line) and move freely back and forth between its parts.

This applies also to their personal experiences. Keeping their personal life vignettes coherent and consistent makes it possible to spontaneously memorize them. Thus begins the internalization of *once-only,* uniquely personal life experiences in 4–D in a newly emerging *autobiographic* knowledge memory. As a result, future alphas and betas occasionally become aware of a retrospective memory and sometimes of a prospective memory (a persistent anticipation) as early expressions of a budding past and future, displayed in a new, sixth dimension of their existence, "6–D," a dimension which soon is to become the medium of their life stories and the implicit foundation of their identities. In other words, internalization not only involves shifting significant aspects of the physical and social reality in 4–D into 5–D (which expresses an increase in the child's *general* knowledge memory of the environment through repetitive interactions with 4–D). Internalization also provides the internalized ego and superego with the appearance of the autobiographic memory which enables youngsters to begin filling the void in personal memories that, until this point, existed universally with a few spotty exceptions.

6–D and time gender

Since we already discussed that alphas and betas store their autobiographic memories in different ways, the differences between alphas and betas begin to appear as internalization develops. I will discuss more details of this process in Chapter 5 on identity. Suffice to say here that what is important for remembering a story is being able to grasp its overall concept (the orderly before-after progression of events). This does not mean, however, that the overall collection of unrelated past memories in every person shows a time-wise coherent before-after sequence. Here is, indeed, where time gender enters the picture.

The autobiographic memory of alphas is like a library of situational short stories by a single author. To this author, it is unimportant to keep these short stories in their original publishing order. Instead, the author follows perceptual, cognitive and/

or emotional associations between individual vignettes. As a result, alphas do not spontaneously order their life vignettes in time. Without such before-after sequencing we may therefore depict their past and future as time spheres with a network of perceptually, cognitively and/or emotionally interconnected autobiographic vignettes, which are like Jungian memory islets floating in a seascape of mythological time. Figure 3.7 depicts this alphacization of autobiographic memory leading to the 6–D of alphas.

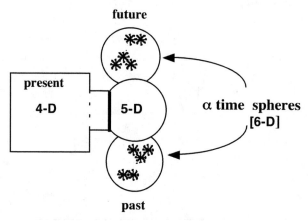

Figure 3.7: The alphacization process

process. By using logic to figure out their puzzle of relevant time sequences, alphas or others studying their biography can deliberately (rather than spontaneously) develop a timescape, but. this cannot occur prior to adolescence since it requires using 7–D. Only a few alphas are motivated to do so. When these alphas recite their life story in a time-ordered fashion (often reading from notes), they do so without much emotion, as if reciting someone else's story.

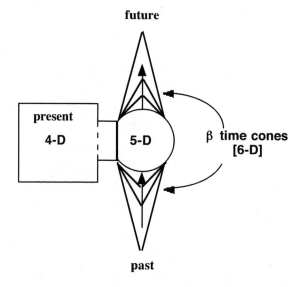

Figure 3.8: The betacization process

The autobiographic memory of betas is, by contrast, more like chapters in a novel that shows a sequential development over time. Young betas spontaneously begin weaving into the associative autobiographic memory network they share with alphas a complimentary linkage system of time bonds, thus introducing a linear sequence (rather than an exact chronology) of personal milestones in their past and future. Thus, betas are inclined to see their life's story in a linear fashion (which is not necessarily chronologic). This replaces the time spheres of Jungian memory islets, floating in a seascape of mythological time, with time cones in a timescape of historic time. Figure 3.8 portrays the betacization of autobiographic memory leading to the 6–D of betas.

The nature of 6–D imagery

When internalizing the world of 4–D into 5–D, and the highlights of one's personal 4–D experiences into 6–D, the verbal mode of memorizing gains ascendancy over the quasi-perceptual image or iconic mode. As a result, not only our general knowledge, but also most of our autobiographic knowledge eventually ends up in the verbal rather than image mode.

This is not to say that remembering a personal story is necessarily a purely intellectual affair without a feeling component. After all, personal experiences have a feeling component as well as a cognitive one. But each is mediated by a different brain division. The upstairs brain specializes in processing and retaining perceptual-cognitive information;[34] the downstairs brain in the affective-feeling information of emotions and appetites.[35] This upstairs-downstairs interaction reflects the interaction between intellectual and affective information. When deeply involved in purely intellectual, impersonal endeavors, the upstairs brain directs our behavior and dominates the interaction with but little participation of the downstairs. Indeed, to study for a test or exam we need to be emotionally unruffled, calm. Being anxious or excited makes it hard to concentrate. Furthermore, we need to rehearse the data well to entrench them in our upstairs knowledge memory. However, when experiencing an intensely emotional event, for example a highly dangerous or wildly passionate one, the downstairs brain determines our behavior with the upstairs playing only a triggering role. This type of experience takes only a single rehearsal to access our autobiographic memory, yet is quite resilient to extinction.

Most life experiences are not that polarized, however. Instead, our upstairs and downstairs brain divisions appear to be teeter-tottering around a center position. These unpolarized experiences fall somewhere between being intensely emotional and unforgettable, on the one hand, and full of information worth adding to our general knowledge, on the other. Yet, notwithstanding the single passage through awareness of these unpolarized experiences, we remember some of them for some time, if not for a lifetime. I say we retain only some, for we do not retain the vast majority of what passes through our awareness.

6–D: alpha amnesia and beta hypermnesia

Scientists already know certain things about the brain's long-term memory selection unit. Whatever personal experiences this selection unit chooses and commits to autobiographic memory in alphas, it treats life vignettes as part of a library of situational short stories. It is far more important to let perceptual, cognitive and/or emotional connections play a role than to keep them in their original publishing order. However, the absence of an overall time line in their life story between unrelated vignettes renders alphas vulnerable to overlook, if not altogether forget some of them because of the lack of reinforcing recall.

Let me quote Carl Jung in this context:

> "...I have spoken with many famous men of my time, the great ones in science and politics, with explorers, artists and writers, princes and financial magnates; but if I am to be honest I must say that only a few such encounters have been significant experiences for me. Our meetings were like those of ships on the high seas, when they dip their flags to one another... I have retained no memories of them, however important these persons may be in the eyes of the world. Our meetings were without portent; they soon faded away and bore no deeper consequences..."[36]

While Jung could vividly recall the intensely emotional experiences in his past and the substance of his own well-rehearsed intellectual world,[37] his words clearly demonstrate that, as time progresses, alphas tend to lose many situational vignettes. In hindsight, I had already, early in my history taking career, often encountered people who had periods in their life virtually void of information. I used to comment to my students: "You know, some people's life history has large barren spots like a desert." Only much later did I realize that such extinction of personal vignettes is not at all uncommon in alphas. This I now call alpha amnesia.

By contrast, the long-term memory selection unit of betas picks particular vignettes for autobiographic storage as chapters in a single chronologically written novel. When betas reflect on their life history they are inclined to follow a time-bound sequencing of unrelated events which reinforces their encoding. The implicit time line in their life story certainly appears to be one reason why their retrospective vignettes are more resilient to extinction than those of alphas. Betas have fewer holes in the chain of their personal memories. This is beta hypermnesia—a more detailed recall of their past history.

Explaining alpha amnesia and beta hypermnesia with the absence or presence of time binding relates to my original observation that taking life histories in alphas is like playing a detective trying to fit their personal memories into some orderly sequence, while in betas the task is much easier. There is, however, another important observation to further explain alpha amnesia and beta hypermnesia. When alphas recount a certain experience it is not uncommon to notice its affective component is rather flat, if not missing altogether. It is not unusual for them to say, upon reflection: "I know what happened, but I cannot feel myself back into it!" They often do not re-live such past events emotionally. It is as if their personal memory lost its feeling component and what is left is descriptive-cognitive. Occasionally, some cover this up by role-playing with exaggerated emotions. But far more common is that after finishing their life story and being asked: "How do you feel having taken a bird's eye view of your own life?" they say: "Hmn...you know...it is almost like listening to someone else's story..."

I already noted that the more intense an emotional experience, the more likely its commitment to autobiographic memory, and the more resilient to extinction. We all know, however, that the affective component of memorized events, even of the most intense ones, tends to fade with time. So, in turn, the dimmer the emotional component of a memory, the more cognitive the memory becomes, and given its original single (rather than multiple) passage through awareness, the greater the likelihood of it fading out. Since in alphas the emotional component of personal vignettes goes flat sooner than in betas, the selection unit of alphas appears to filter out more of the experienced component than in betas. The encoded affective-downstairs component of the memory is therefore relatively weaker and, generally speaking, extinction in alphas kicks in sooner and at a higher rate than in betas.

All this applies not only to the retrospective (past) autobiographic memories of alphas and betas, but also to their prospective memories of anticipated personal events. No wonder then that the past and future of alphas makes their 6–D far less seductive as an attention mode than their 4–D as supported by their 5–D. By contrast — and whether they like it or not — betas often gravitate to their more detailed, and emotionally colored 6–D reality.

7–D: from concrete to abstract mentation

As long as the preschooler thinks aloud in 4–D, 4–D and 5–D remain interwoven. Therefore, 5–D cannot yet serve as a platform to observe and manipulate 4–D. This only happens with internalization, when 5–D unhooks from 4–D and emerges as the child's instrument of concrete reasoning.

Notwithstanding internalization, the child's intellectual functioning still has an important limitation. Whereas elementary school children are naturally aware of their conscious stream of thought in 5–D, they cannot yet self-observe it, think in the abstract about their own thinking. Their thinking is still concrete, hooked into the visible and tangible 4–D world. For example, they do not yet grasp the idea that behind any proverb there is a general rule, an abstract meaning, as in "rolling stones gather no moss." They will explain it by saying something like: "Well, if a stone rolls there is no time for it to pick up moss," rather than "People who do not settle down go without the benefits of doing so." Another example is that when facing an intellectual challenge in 4–D they can find a solution only by trial and error. They have to act in 4–D on each and every solution that comes to mind in 5–D, rather than first in their head work through different hypothetical solutions, reason out which is the best, and only then verify this in 4–D.

The capacity for thinking in the abstract about one's concrete mentation in 5–D requires a final step in our cognitive development, namely a distinct experiential dimension that is one step removed from the concrete mentation in 5–D. This seventh and last dimension—7–D—emanates and breaks away from 5–D during adolescence. It reflects our fourth attention mode with abstract mentation or reasoning as its dominant mind-brain function.[38] Figure 3.9 presents the three non-temporal attention modes with 5–D (concrete mentation) grafted onto 4–D (perception), and 7–D (abstract mentation) in turn grafted onto 5–D (concrete mentation).

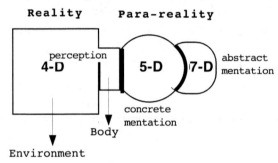

Figure 3.9: The three non-temporal attention modes: 4-D, 5-D and 7-D

In the elementary school years, 5–D becomes the medium for developing concrete models of the 4–D world. Similarly, in adolescence 7–D becomes the medium for abstracting models from, and re-imposing them onto 5–D's representative reality and, through this, onto the concrete 4–D world. This involves a progressive generalizing from specific examples in 5–D to ever more general models and rules in 7–D for use in 4–D.[39] 7–D also enables hypothetical thinking that supplements problem solving by trial and error alone.

What catalyzes this seventh dimension that emerges in adolescence? It is the span of our working memory that makes its final leap into full maturity. This is truly a crowning step, for in addition to embracing the concrete mentation in 5–D, the now fully matured working memory will henceforth encompass the novel abstract mentation in 7–D as well. No wonder that Western culture introduces a new level of education—high school—as 7–D emerges.

This new reasoning in 7–D usually starts at an intuitive and spontaneous level, but during the high school years it becomes more deliberate and intentional. For example, adolescents will eventually put the rich variety of pragmatic time concepts they have already intuitively used for years into a single unified system of time, based on a general, abstract time concept.

It is of interest to note here that, although the development of concrete reasoning in elementary school is fairly consistent across cultures and socio-economic levels, the development of abstract thinking in adolescence is not. This is in part because different cultures and social environments often provide different demands or opportunities for abstract mentation.[40] There is also the issue of intellectual endowment, of course. However, abstract mentation has its roots in a mosaic of special endowments rather than a single one. As Howard Gardner pointed out,[41] one person may be more gifted than others in mathematics, languages, logical reasoning, spatial relations, music, art, or athletics, and so on.

Even so, innate constraints on the final maturation of the working memory early in adolescence may well have across-the-board implications for one's potential level of abstract mentation in 7–D. It has been suggested, for example, that some 30% of the general population in the West have difficulties with abstract thinking.[42] This includes those who can deal with the early part of high school but are unable to cope with the later years. As a result they drop out, or move into a vocational stream.

7–D: the Inner Adult, Paraego, or Voice of Reason

I previously mentioned that our silent self-talk in 5–D reflects the internalized interactions between the nurturing, socializing adult and the six year old child. Although we experience this self-talk in 5–D simply as "I am talking to myself," the two faceless inner voices involved reflect two sides of our Self, namely the Inner Child or ego or "$Self_1$" and the Inner Parent or superego or "$Self_2$." When I say to myself "I hate myself," for example, this is shorthand for $Self_2$ saying to $Self_1$ that he or she hates $Self_1$. However, as long as we remain without 7–D, we cannot yet listen to this spontaneous self-talk in 5–D; therefore we cannot yet contemplate how we relate to ourselves.

When 7–D finally emerges to work its abstract mentation on 5–D's inner stream of consciousness, this implies an active mental complex in 7–D, a Self that does the abstract thinking and contemplates what is happening in 5–D. This acting Self in 7–D becomes sooner or later personified as the Voice of Reason, the rational and reasonable part of us, or "$Self_3$," the Inner Adult.[43] While Freudian psychoanalysis calls the Internalized Child and Internalized Parent in 5–D ego and superego, respectively, it considers one's Voice of Reason just as an expression of the maturing ego, and has no name for this Inner Adult in 7–D. In order to fill this psychoanalytic omission, "paraego" appears to be a reasonable term. Some may confuse the paraego and its Voice of Reason with the superego and its Voice of Conscience, as both are ego-modulating functions. However, the paraego in 7–D and the ego and superego in 5–D are distinctly separate from each other.[44]

The paraego's abstract thinking is initially intuitive and spontaneous, but gradually becomes more deliberate and intentional. When focusing on 5–D's representation of 4–D's public world, its role is a pragmatic one at a personal level and functions to give us a common sense understanding of the physical and social world we live in so that we may act accordingly. However, when self-reflectively focusing on the private mental experiences in 5–D, the paraego turns into a conscious and rational witness of our mental life in 5–D. The role of this rational witness is to gain some common sense understanding of the workings of its own psyche with its various emotional conflicts. In this context, the paraego in 7–D displays emotional detachment, yet also is empathetic and compassionate as it listens to the emotionally charged self-talk in 5–D between ego and superego. It may in this context begin to participate in this self-talk with its Voice of Reason. For example, when it hears "I hate myself" the paraego may exclaim: "What am I doing to myself? It does not make sense!" In other words, the Inner Adult (paraego) tries to introduce some common sense into the self-talk by interjecting: "What are you, Inner Parent, trying to do to your Inner Child?" In some psychologically sophisticated people, the Inner Adult may grow into an Inner Teacher, if not Guru. Figure 3.10 presents such tripartite self-talk schematically.

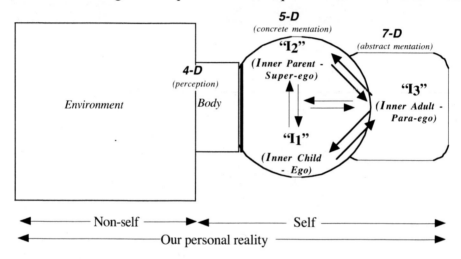

Figure 3.10: Late adolescence: three self-identities in self-talk

Naturally, the paraego may also work its abstracting magic at an academic rather than personal level—in one of the physical or social sciences, for example. Then the paraego becomes the scientist who attempts to discover ever more powerful constants, similarities or laws that underlie the confusingly heterogeneous public world in 4–D. To get to this level, the paraego must become highly schooled in working with elaborate hypotheticals, critically testing assertions, exploring various relations, and detecting discrepancies and contradictions, in other words, working step by step toward a solution of the task at hand. If present, this represents the crowning achievement of our evolution. Fortunately, the level of abstract mentation we pick up in adolescence is generally sufficient for us to get by in everyday life.

7–D and time gender

The seventh dimension is very relevant to the time gender model, and the time gender model very relevant to the way we think. People have different levels of sophistication in their abstract mentation, but there are also time gender-specific differences in how alphas and betas use their 7–D.

The idea that there exists a profound duality in our thinking has a long history which is most readily demonstrated in philosophical and scientific thinking. Scientists who are alphas tend to be more empirical, experimental and result-oriented. Their work often takes them into several unrelated areas of endeavor; they tend to be multifocal in their thinking. Beta scientists, on the other hand, tend to be more theoretical in their orientation. Their tendency is monofocal, looking more for systems rather than isolated results. In more ordinary thinking, such differences are often elusive unless one is specifically looking for them. Chapter 8 will demonstrate how the time gender model accounts succinctly for how alphas and betas think differently.

The complete time gender model

At this point, I can present the complete time gender model with its four attention modes as represented by Figure 3.11.

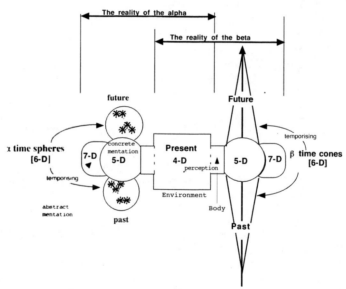

Figure 3.11: The complete time gender model and its four attention modes:
4-D, 5-D, 6-D and 7-D

Each of these four attention modes reflects a different conscious reality channel and has its own dominant mind-brain function; 4–D with perception, 5–D with concrete mentation, 6–D with temporizing, and 7–D with abstract mentation. In this time gender model of human experience and behavior, attention and memory are two fundamental concepts. Looking for a moment at 5–D with its alpha spheres in the left part of the figure and then at 5–D with its beta cones in the corresponding right side, it will be readily understood how I came to nickname alphas "round heads" and betas "cone heads."

NOTES

1   I developed the general model of the mind-body relation, or, more specifically, the mind-brain relation, in my doctoral thesis, *The Psyche-Soma Complex: Its Psychology and Logic* [Pos (1963)].

2   Brechner (1932-33), p. 204; Mowrer (1960), p. 490-494; Kristofferson (April 1966); Pos (1969).

3   Pos (1969); Edelman (1989), p. 204, 208.

4   This range of 50-500 msecs was provided by the time psychologist Michon [Michon (1975), p. 304-306].

5   Display memory reflects what others may refer to it as image memory, perceptual memory, iconic memory or immediate memory.

6   Short-term memory and working memory are commonly used interchangeably [Baddeley (1986); Goldman-Rakic (1992)].

7   M. Just and P. Carpenter quoted by Goldman-Rakic (1992), p. 111.

8   Kohut (1977), p. 97.

9   Wessman and Gorman (1977), p. 18.

10   James (1910), p.16.

11   Piaget's first sensori-motor stage of cognitive development (reflexes) (1st month) followed by his second stage (acquired adaptations and primary circular reactions) (1-4 @ 5 months) , and then his third stage (5-8 months) (secondary circular reactions) [Flavell (1963)].

12   That the baby's snapshot memory becomes operant around the age of 8 months can be demonstrated with the object-permanence task which Piaget developed [Flavell (1963)].

13   Robson and Minde (1977), quoted by Steinhauer (1980), p. 27.

14   Piaget (1952), p. 62-63, quoted by Flavell (1963), p. 133.

15   Steinhauer (1980), p. 27; Lamendella (1976), p.401.

16   Flavell (1963), p. 123.

17   This phase (18-24 months) is Piaget's sixth sensori-motor phase (the invention of new means through mental combinations). It is a transition from the sensori-motor period of cognitive functioning to his preoperational preschool period (age 2-6 @ 7), which is characterized by mental representation (5-D) which permits the child to perform mental actions (imagination, long-term memory recall, symbolization, and so on) [Green (1989), p. 171-2].

18   Flavell (1963), p. 129-130.

19   Gesell et al. (1940), p. 328; Greenspan (1985), p. 1600.

20   Jean Piaget called this pronounced characteristic of the preschooler's thought process the tendency to "center" attention on a single striking feature of the object of its reasoning, and its inability to "decenter" its attention, that is, taking simultaneously into account more than a single feature [Flavell (1963), p. 157].

21   Flavell (1963), p. 161. This lack of differentiation between 4–D and 5–D reflects the inability to distinguish between 5–D initiated fantasies and 4–D occurrences, rather than between 4–D perceptions and the short-term memories thereof in 5–D. In other words, the child can correctly declare "I saw doggie," or "I did not see doggie."

22   Although not central to my theory, someone raised the question whether a preschooler can "lie" since the child does not yet distinguish facts from fancy. If a preschooler is confronted by an adult that it ate a cookie and senses through the confrontation that it did "something bad," the child may say it did *not* eat the cookie. But since the preschooler is still in a pre-logical state, the child does not yet experience a contradiction between what it says and what it remembers. It therefore cannot be said to "lie" as "lying" involves a *logical* conclusion. Perhaps one could speak in this case of "rudimentary lying" or "proto-lying." This is contrast with an elementary school child who is able to "lie" in the sense of being able to recognize a contradiction between what it says that happened and what it remembers that actually took place. If "lying" is to include, however, self-awareness of what one is doing with a sense of causing one's own actions through volition (intentionality; Piaget's "psychological causality"), then this requires a paraego. In this sense, only adolescents can "lie."

23   Berk (1994), p. 78.

24   Flavell (1963), p. 128.

25   Piaget (1952), p. 62-63, quoted by Flavell (1963), p. 133.

26   Berk (1994), p. 78.

27   Piaget's concrete operational phase in cognitive functioning.

28   While time words as "today" appear at age two, "tomorrow" when we are thirty months old, and "yesterday" at age three, they are used indiscriminately and idiosyncratically rather than in a socially shared manner [Hallowell (1937), p. 651-652; Ames (1946)]. Early concepts -- let alone time concepts -- do not appear until the end of Piaget's pre-conceptual phase at age three.

29   Cohen (1966).

30   Cohen (1966).

31   See also Chapter 2 under "*Martha, the non-believer.*"

32   Beard, (1972), p. 67.

33   Flavell (1963), p. 158, 161-162.

34   The upstairs brain division consists of the evolutionary youngest part of the brain mantle(the neocortex) which covers the medial side, the base of the brain, and the lateral and posterior surface of the brain mantle [Pribram (1958)].

35   The downstairs division is the brain's evolutionary older part and usually is referred to as limbic and brain-stem system [Brady (1958); Edelman (1989), p. 152, 157, 162-3].

36   Jung, quoted by Jaffé (1965), p. ix-x.

37   Jaffé (1965), p. vii.

38   Piaget's formal abstract operational phase in cognitive functioning.

39   Beard (1972), p. 102-17.

40   Gardner (1985), p. 134.

41   Gardner (1985).

42   The Wechsler-Bellevue intelligence quotient (IQ) follows in the general population the normal distribution of the bell curve, with a mean value of IQ=100 and a standard deviation of 15. This means that a person of average intelligence has an IQ= 100. In this framework, persons with an IQ of 90 or less comprise approximately 30% of the population and have problems with abstract reasoning.

43   The names Inner Child, Inner Parent, and Inner Adult go back to Eric Berne (1910-1970) [Berne (1961)].

44   The paraego or Voice of Reason is inspired by adolescent and adult role models and incorporates some of their most admired features, being compassionate, willing to listen, open-minded, tolerant and creative [Vaughan (1985), pp. 42-43].

CHAPTER 4

Time Gender, Mood Regulation, And Self-esteem

Section 1: Theoretical Considerations

About mood

Our mood reflects our frame of mind which expresses itself privately in a distinct emotional state and publicly in corresponding behavior. Our mood is the key in which the Mind-Brain Symphony of the Present is being composed.

Although the English language has thousands of words for emotional feelings,[1] most find it hard to put their mood into precise words and use vague terms to do so. Witness the following conversation:

"How do you feel today?" "...

"Well...eh... not too good... I feel a bit out of sorts..."

"Can you tell me a bit more about it?"

"Hmn...I don't feel with it today... I feel kind of heavy..."

"What do you mean by 'feeling kind of heavy'?"

"Well...you know...just kind of heavy..."

Despite this common difficulty in describing the rich variety of emotional feelings, all moods fall into one of two categories: good moods to which we aspire, and bad ones we seek to avoid. Factors that affect one's mood positively or negatively include:[2]

- biological changes, such as
    - ~ normal physiological changes, such as the menstrual cycle;
    - ~ changes induced by mood-altering chemicals, legal or illicit;
    - ~ illnesses, such as the flu or a heart attack, and psychiatric conditions;
    - ~ genetic factors in temperament. One can already observe these in very young children,[3] whereas a temperament style with high responsivity, anxiety, and depression, called "general negative affectivity" or "neuroticism" is the most stable of five major personality factors;[4]
- environmental changes, such as
    - ~ the weather;[5]
    - ~ situational events, whether minor (such as losing one's keys) or major (such as the death of a loved one);

~ the proactive pursuit of self-esteem, which puts us in a good overall frame of
mind.

There are distinct differences in how these last two psychological factors (pursuing
self-esteem and reacting emotionally to situational events) affect the mood regulation
of alphas and betas. These time gender differences may be blurred by temperamental
and other already mentioned mood-influences. For example, a person's emotional
reaction to situational events is often influenced by socio-cultural expectations of
how to feel. Yet, regardless of all these variables, alphas and betas do not pursue self-
esteem or react to situational events in the same manner.

The next section clarifies this issue, first with a theoretical discussion about how
alphas and betas pursue self-esteem, and, second, about alpha-beta differences in
emotionally responding to the present, or to the past and future. The concluding
section addresses practical illustrations of these differences in mood regulation
between alphas and betas.

About self-esteem

A decade or so ago, self-esteem (pride in oneself or self-respect) was talked about
mainly by psychiatrists, psychologists and social workers. It then became the subject
of several best sellers and as a result one of the catchwords of the nineties.[6] The
following section focuses on the *proactive* pursuit of self-esteem in general and then,
more specifically, in alphas and betas. It is important to keep in mind that self-esteem
also may be *reactive* in origin, that is, secondary to any primary mood changes. For
example, there are genetic factors that influence our mood positively or negatively,
have a negative or positive influence on our self-esteem which, in turn, makes its
proactive pursuit easier or harder. Having said this, there appear to be at least three
important sources of proactive self-esteem.

- A fundamental, intra-personal source of self-esteem appears related to the
  joyful mood that follows achievement. We can already observe this when a
  four month old baby cries out from pure joy while repetitively hitting a ball
  hanging on a string over its crib. As time goes on, this basic drive for the joy of
  achievement appears in ever more varied contexts, and in progressively more
  sophisticated presentations.

- A second important source of self-esteem first appears around the age of
  eight months when the baby begins experiencing itself as separate from its
  mothering figure, and soon begins intuitively seeking her approval and avoiding
  her disapproval. While this external, inter-personal source of well being — first
  the approval of the mothering one, then of others nearby — becomes the
  major instrument in socializing the child, it continues throughout life as *the*
  interpersonal source of positive self-esteem.

- Early in the preschool years, the forerunner of a third source of self-esteem
  emerges. In their fantasy play, youngsters begin to imitate aloud approving-

rejecting scenarios involving their elders. Once successful in aping these judgmental behaviors, they joyfully repeat these games with their dolls or stuffed animals over and over again. At the beginning of elementary school children begin shifting these imaginary interaction scenarios, as well as the repetitive real ones with their nurturing adults, from 4–D into 5–D's silent self-talk.

As a result of internalization, self-esteem depends henceforth no longer entirely on what others think but on how the Inner Parent or superego judges the behavior of the Inner Child or ego. Superego development naturally does not stop at this point, but continues as the child enters the world of middle childhood and then adolescence, and selectively internalizes additional social models.

Balancing these three major sources of self-esteem (the joy of mastery, pleasing others, and pleasing one's superego) is quite a challenge. Trying to tap all three of them in the same situation is often fraught with problems, simply because meeting one need often prevents a person from meeting another. The child must therefore learn to set priorities. A balance must be struck between satisfying inner desires for empowerment on the one hand, and the need for others' approval, on the other. Arriving intuitively in a given situation at a balanced, three-fold self-ideal does not necessarily mean the child will automatically be successful in realizing its goal. A child's sense of well being depends on to what degree the child realizes its self-ideal. The more successful a child is in meeting the set situational standard, the more positive its self-esteem; the less favorable the outcome, the more negative its self-esteem.

The pursuit of self-esteem continues to function at an intuitive level until adolescence, when 7–D and the paraego emerge. At this stage, self-reflection and the Voice of Reason begin to influence one's self-esteem. Although adolescents are able to take a more compassionate and realistic look at the needs of that self-esteem, pursuing this process intentionally to its fullest potential takes considerable psychological sophistication and effort, if not professional assistance.

Let me now move beyond general considerations of self-esteem and explain specifically how alphas and betas go about pursuing self-esteem.

How alphas pursue self-esteem

Alphas pursue self-esteem in the here-and-now of 4–D. 6–D (the past, which is no longer the present, and the future which is not yet the present) plays only a marginal role. Alphas' proactive self-esteem is situational in nature, because it is directed toward their current circumstances. If they meet their current situational ambition, they are full of self-esteem. But if they are unable to find self-esteem, they can feel considerably distressed. Some alphas are innately more resilient to such situations, while others are more vulnerable. This is due to individual factors other than time gender. An optimistic temperament, for example, may for some time compensate for distressing circumstances, while a negative personality may render alphas more vulnerable. In psychological reports statements such as "this person has a weak or unstable self-esteem" might suggest some personality defect in alphas, but in reality their proactive level of self-esteem depends on the stability of their current circumstances, and how well they realize their situational self-ideal in 4–D.

Because situational self-esteem is by definition fleeting in nature, alphas have an ongoing appetite for self-esteem and constantly explore their social environs for opportunities to still this hunger. This may translate into an excessive craving for admiration or affection. The visible symbols of alphas' social position often nurture them. These include fancy clothes, an expensive car, a success in business, and having important friends. Sometimes alphas succeed in attracting great admiration by promulgating some dramatic, visionary promise for the future. I am reminded of General Douglas MacArthur, who, driven out of the Philippines by the Japanese, left behind some 30,000 of his troops. Nonetheless, against all odds, he maintained "I shall return." This he did. If they lose face, however, alphas suffer seriously.

The ongoing drive in alphas to search 4–D for supplies of interpersonal self-esteem makes them natural tacticians. In the process, however, they sometimes let immediate (tactical) advantages override long-term (strategic) considerations. When their tactics lead to unexpected success others may think: "Here is someone brilliant who dares taking chances others would not." When their tactics misfire, however, others may judge them impulsive and short-sighted, if not irresponsible, and think: "They should have known better!"

How betas pursue self-esteem

Given their timescape, betas pursue self-esteem by aligning their present goals in 4–D with their past and foreseeable future. Thus, in addition to situational elements, their self-esteem also has strong retrospective and prospective components. Since their self-esteem is enmeshed in their overall timescape, it is global in nature rather than situational.

Because the self-esteem of betas is interwoven with their extending timescape, it is rather situation-resistant. Therefore, changes in betas' global self-esteem are only incremental. This contrasts with the often dramatic changes in the self-esteem of alphas. When the going gets tough in 4–D, alphas rapidly lose any situational self-esteem they had unless there are compensating individual factors. Under similar circumstances, however, betas continue to gain emotional sustenance from preceding positive self-esteem, just as negative self-esteem will continue to drain them even when very favorable circumstances emerge in 4–D. Such favorable circumstances would in alphas dramatically replenish any previous lack of self-esteem.

Betas' preoccupation with maintaining or improving their self-esteem over time may make them forego immediate advantages, or even make great sacrifices for the sake of long-term gain. This renders betas natural strategists. Their concern with long-term planning often makes them appear deliberate and careful, if not sometimes overcautious or indecisive. Being human, however, betas at times allow immediate needs for satisfaction to interfere with their strategic judgment. Or, in their preoccupation with the future, they may overlook vitally important relationships in 4–D.

Because their self-esteem is more enduring, betas are not in need of constant praise by or admiration from others. Since their global self-esteem is inward-oriented, betas are far less concerned with appearance and showmanship than alphas. History tells us that the brilliant military strategist, General Dwight Eisenhower (1890-1969), Supreme Commander in Europe, accepted Germany's surrender in the middle of the night, without any ceremonial display. But, his colleague, the dazzling military tactician, General Douglas MacArthur (1880-1964), Supreme Commander in the Pacific, only agreed to accept Japan's surrender aboard the US Battleship Missouri in an unforgettable ceremonial extravaganza that followed days of exhaustive preparation.

As we noted earlier, some alphas are more resilient, and others more vulnerable, to loss of situational self-esteem due to factors other than time gender. The same is true of some betas with their global self-esteem. An optimistic temperament, for example, may provide betas considerable protection against developing negative self-esteem, while a negative personality may render them more vulnerable. Betas who suffer from negative self-esteem hunger inwardly as much for situational praise and admiration as alphas do all the time outwardly.

In pursuing self-esteem, all people must learn to strike a balance between the satiation or frustration of inner achievement needs, and approval by others in 4–D or in their self-talk in 5–D. This typically occurs in childhood. In this respect, both alphas and betas will rely heavily on satisfying their inner need to achieve, experiencing the joy of mastery. Beyond this, however, their priorities in pursuing self-esteem are different. In the final analysis, the preference of alphas will be to rely on situational self-esteem in 4–D (e.g., admiration by others), secondarily on approving self-talk in 5–D, and then later, perhaps, on their Voice of Reason in 7–D. For betas, however, relying on approval by others in 4–D will remain secondary. Their primary concern will be the pursuit of global self-esteem through trying to keep 4–D experiences that enter their private timescape in line with their superego (their Voice of Conscience in 5–D), later modulated by their paraego's Voice of Reason in 7–D.

Ideals that guide behavior and upbringing

Stating that self-esteem in alphas is predominantly situational and in betas primarily global may sound problematic. For if all alphas depend on their current situation for their ideals and values that guide their behavior, some may conclude that alphas must be inconsistent opportunists. This is not so, as the next chapter on identity will clarify.

Ideals that guide situational behavior form a select configuration of socializing interaction scenarios in 4–D, which the child eventually internalizes into 5–D. If these original interaction scenarios between parent and child mirror a consistent system of values and ideals, then the set of situation-bound ideals and values that guide alphas later in life will reflect the consistency in values they were taught as preschoolers. Along the same line, an early childhood marred by confusion and inconsistency of values will translate into a highly inconsistent and confusing value system later in life. Whatever the case, life experience naturally amends and extends the situational ideals and values alphas have. Inconsistencies in values across different situations may creep in and, in the absence of a timescape and without external feedback, tend to remain undetected.

When adolescence introduces 7–D with its paraego, and through it self-reflection, betas (because of their timescape) become very sensitive to contradictions—cognitive dissonance—in their time cones.[7] Even when subjected to inconsistent values during their upbringing, their ever widening timescape demonstrates blatant trans-situational inconsistencies in behavior and its underlying values. This leads to tensions that disturb their global self-esteem, and thus their peace of mind. A wave of disharmony in their cones is followed by a harmonizing counterwave, a process that is fraught with conflict and often ends in compromise rather than resolution. Betas strive intuitively toward a systematized global set of self-ideals and values. This increases their peace of mind, but does not make for an easier life.

The previous discussion stresses the vital importance of the preschool years in bringing up youngsters. This pertains especially to future alphas since they are more vulnerable to early exposure to inconsistent and confusing values. Future betas are somewhat more resilient in this respect as their later timescape allows for secondary, but painful and conflictual, corrections.

Differences in responding to the present (4–D) and the past and future (6–D)

Having reviewed how alphas and betas pursue self-esteem in order to improve and maintain their sense of well being, I now turn to how they emotionally react to both positive and negative past, present and future events.

It is probably easier to accept that betas may take up to 18 months to put behind them an intensely distressful crisis (a divorce, a job loss, or the loss of a loved one, for example) than to accept that the vast majority of alphas can turn their back on such distress once it has disappeared out of focus in 4–D. We often take for granted that people will respond to an acute psychological shock with a profound depression or a post traumatic stress disorder. We may say "No wonder he became depressed after his life's work was destroyed" or "I certainly can understand why this woman struggled for years with the trauma of her rape." We should not, however, take intensely distressing events as a valid explanation for how people respond to them.

After disturbing life events, the risk of depression is increased. However, not everybody who goes through a distributing experience becomes depressed.[8] Moreover, the prevalence of post traumatic stress disorder among people who are exposed to life threatening events, such as earthquakes, rape or torture, is much lower than one might expect.[9] Indeed, whether an event is adverse or whether it is joyful, there is no simple 1:1 relationship between the nature of an event and how people respond to it emotionally. This is because, in addition to the particular event itself and one's time gender, there are many other factors that affect the emotional response to the event (such as previous exposure, age, sex, education, intelligence, social status, social connectedness, socio-cultural expectations, belief systems, and so on).[10] Of particular importance in this regard is a person's temperament or habitual emotional response style,[11] which may be negative,[12] or positive.[13]

The following discussion focuses on how the vast majority of alphas and betas adjust differently to past, present and future distressing events and good fortunes. Pessimistic or optimistic temperaments notwithstanding, alphas and betas experience time in dissimilar fashions and therefore also relate emotionally in different ways to what happens in their present (4–D), and to what has happened in the past or will happen in their future (6–D).

As already discussed in Chapter 2, alphas experience past episodes in their life as discrete scenes that took place "once upon a time," as in mythological time. Similarly, they experience events that are likely to materialize in their futureas something that will happen "one day." As a result, alphas may walk away from past adversities or ignore opportunities for future success, unless circumstances force them to face up to deal with the past or future.

While alphas may not be distracted by past or future pain in 6–D, they are also deprived of the luxury of connecting with enjoyable foreseeable satisfactions in 6–D, which in betas can have a considerable influence on their present 4–D. Alphas enjoy or suffer the here-and-now in 4–D to the fullest. This makes their 4–D either a temporary bastion of strength, or a temporary prison. In sum, they live in the world rather than in their head; they are natural extroverts.

Once autobiographic memory encoding in 6–D begins around age 6, the contrasting response to 4–D and 6–D of alphas and betas becomes clear, since their past and future become differently structured. Betas begin to domesticate significant current events in their timescape. They assimilate, through time binding between unrelated life experiences, the 4–D flow of events in real time as a succession of events in the historic time of their timescape in 6–D. Instead of experiencing the present in its own right, they therefore experience the present in the context of their timescape, so that present adversities and good fortunes are often counterbalanced by re-living past adversities or good fortunes, or by the pre-living of futurethreats or promises. Past events are not water under the bridge but a historic reality with which they have to live.

And they cross the bridge before reaching it. Future threats and promises influence them a great deal, just as past adversities and good fortunes do. Their surrounding past or future can therefore make their present a living heaven or hell. Betas are not predominantly preoccupied with current events like alphas. Instead, their preferred attention orientation is toward the relivable and prelivable timescape in their head, and, as a result, they are natural introverts.[14]

Apart from the absence of an ongoing time-line in the past and future of alphas and the presence of a timescape in betas, there is an additional reason why alphas and betas :explanation and future. Jung's autobiography demonstrated this: the autobiographic encoding of alphas is less emotionally charged, stable and extensive than in betas (as discussed in Chapter 2).

More about the timescape of betas

With time, the emotional component of even highly memorable events fades in everyone. As time goes by, betas thus experience an incremental decrease in the emotional intensity of past positive or negative episodes until they finally matter no longer. Although beyond this "working through" period betas may recall relevant life vignettes for some reason, these no longer modulate daily life. Exceptions may occur, however, because

- prolonged consequences secondary to a distressful or fortunate event can, in betas, naturally extend the period during which life vignettes can modulate daily life; and

- some betas may preempt the re-living period by using denial (defensive inattention) or repression (defensive forgetting), mental strategies that allows one to avoid the conscious pain of natural healing.[15]

In the absence of such complications—and such is the case in the vast majority of betas—this "working through" period for past events grows with age. As mentioned already in Chapter 2, it begins at age 6-7, at which point it reaches into the preceding day. At age 12 (when a young beta's life story already reaches 6 years back) this re-living range may span one season and, at age 18 may span around 9 months. My clinical experience indicates it to be around 1 1/2 years in adulthood. Under normal circumstances, it therefore usually takes an adult beta 18 months to come to grips with the loss of a loved one or to forget about good fortunes won and lost, and get on with life.[16]

While the past timescape of betas features a *re-living* range, their future timescape features a *pre-living* range. This pre-living range stretches to where future intentions and anticipated events begin to emotionally influence a beta's present. My experience suggests that the pre-living range is similar in scope to the re-living range, that is, in grade 2, one day ahead; at age 12 a season forward; at age 18, some 9 months in the future, and in early adulthood about one year. During negotiations about student government at a university, for example, the faculty had in mind gradual changes over several years. Proposing some significant changes within a year became mandatory, or the faculty would lack credibility. In hindsight this was necessary to gain the crucial support of the beta students. A time frame of several years was too long. In adulthood, the pre-living range of betas eventually spans about 18 months, at which point, like the re-living range, it stabilizes.

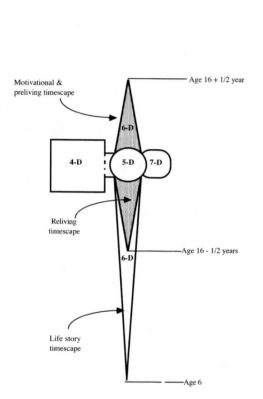

Figure 4.1: Beta timescape at around age 16
(prior to the development of
an abstract time concept)

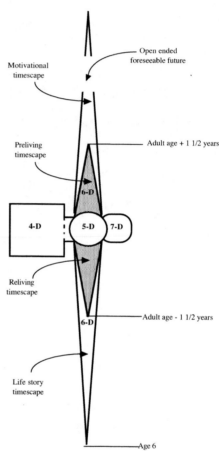

Figure 4.2: Beta timescape in adulthood

Figure 4.1 demonstrates the estimated re-living, pre-living, and motivational ranges in the beta timescape around age 16 (prior to the development of an abstract time concept), and figure 4.2 shows the same ranges in the adult beta timescape.

Section 2: Practical Illustrations

Earlier, we discussed how alphas and betas pursue self-esteem in dissimilar ways and how their emotional reactions to significant events differ. However, there often are factors that cover up these time gender differences. Nevertheless, one should not underestimate the important role time gender plays in our mood regulation, as the following examples demonstrate.

Bereavement

The popular notion about people's reactions following the loss of a loved one is that all people mourn and grieve, as if bereavement is a predictable process with predictable phases and an expected resolution.[17] Others hold that bereavement varies on a continuum between an intense, persistent yearning for the lost person to a depressive reaction with significant guilt about having failed to do certain things.[18]

In reality, grief responses vary considerably, depending, among other factors, on suddenness of loss, uncertainty about the loss (soldiers missing in action, for example), death by suicide or murder, and the preceding nature of the affected relationship. For instance, if the relationship was characterized by co-dependence on each other, rooted in fear of going it alone, the remaining partner may well destabilize. A personal loss may furthermore induce either a dramatic deterioration or an improvement in financial circumstances, which will affect the grief reaction. Grief may remain incomplete and painful, and sadness may be evoked under certain circumstances in people otherwise living complete lives.[19] On the other hand, an absence of grief may be normal.[20]

In my experience, time gender is very important in determining how people cope. Alphas, living one day at a time, can more easily walk away from a personal disaster. Rather than grieving over the past, they attempt to cope as best they can with whatever opportunities or challenges their reality provides. Betas, however, incorporate a personal disaster in their timescape and need considerable time to gain distance from their loss to feel whole again.

An alpha's ability to walk away from bereavement is one of her or his strengths. A dramatic example of this is how the world-famous American architect, Frank Lloyd Wright (1867-1959), continued without interruption his highly creative and innovative career after the tragic destruction of his home in Taliesin, Wisconsin, and the murder of the mistress to whom he had been deeply devoted.[21] Not many betas in his place would have been able to do so.

The normal bereavement process is determined by personal and cultural expectations which may range from a few days of socially appropriate depression to many months of intense emotional deprivation. If in the latter case bereavement ends too soon, the mourner may be viewed as callous.[22] To prevent being viewed as callous, some alphas conceal their non-grieving behind a public grieving persona, and only share their true feelings with someone they trust. I am reminded in this context of Shakespeare's tragedy Hamlet, more specifically of Gertrude, Queen of Denmark and the mother of Hamlet, who soon after the murder of her husband, the King, by his brother Claudius, marries the latter. In the eyes of her son, this portrayed the worst possible disloyalty to his father's memory.

Naturally, alphas and betas misinterpret each other's bereavement reactions. Alphas who witness the mourning period in betas may well view their grief as unduly protracted and wonder whether this is, perhaps, an indication of self-pity, or weakness, or something needing psychiatric attention. Betas who observe some one's short-lived grief, however, may wonder: "Did this person really love the lost one?" Even alphas, under the spell of beta-oriented pop-psychology, sometimes question their own feelings in this context. During forty years as counselor I often heard: "I should have felt something at the time, I feel bad that I didn't." For decades I assumed that these people were blocking their spontaneous emotions, hiding them deep inside. That may well have been so with some of my betas but, in the case of my alphas, it turned into a pseudo-scientific myth that I debunked in later years.

When losing a truly beloved monarch, alphas can, unlike betas, honestly exclaim: "The King is dead! Long live the (new) King!" This alpha response is a human gift, not a defect. Many betas would fervently wish they could do the same under similar circumstances.

Dying and death

Confronting death is difficult. Even physicians, notwithstanding their frequent encounter with the ultimate challenge in their practice, are not exempt from this confrontation. Not only does death highlight the inadequacy of their healing power, it reminds them of their own mortality. As a result, they frequently avoid giving their dying patients a listening ear, or delegate this to chaplains or others who are supposed to be "experts" in death and dying. But these so-called thanatologists sometimes have their own ways of maintaining their professional comfort with dying people. Rather than empathizing with the dying, they often defensively fit their 'client' into some baseless theory. For example, that dying is a clinical syndrome with five stages — denial, anger, bargaining, depression and, finally, acceptance — in which case they "diagnose" the stage the patient is in, and strive "therapeutically" toward "acceptance."[23]

Years ago , when I was Psychiatrist-in-Chief at a teaching hospital,[24] I received a referral from Medicine requesting guidance on how to inform a patient about his terminal illness. I met with the psychiatric residents to discuss this. Having told them about the referral, I asked each in turn to imagine being in the patient's position, and advise what he or she would like me to do. One resident said he, himself, should be told, but not his family; another resident said that they should tell her, and that she, herself, would like to tell her family; yet another resident said that he would not want to be told until matters got more serious. After the last one had spoken, they all looked to me for "the" expert solution. I said: "You may think you only have faced a hypothetical problem, but each of you is, indeed, suffering from an illness that has no cure. The disease that is going to kill you is Life. *Memento mori*, my friends, remember that you must die, for only if you realize you yourself live on death row, will you be sufficiently empathic to handle this consultation."

Are we all in denial of an anxiety about our mortality until we stare death in the face? In *The Denial of Death,* Ernest Becker posed two contradictory views on death anxiety. According to, what he called, the healthy-minded argument, a fear of death is not part of human nature. We may acquire such anxieties but normal development places these firmly under control of the developing ego, out of our mind. The other view, to which Becker himself subscribed, he called the morbidity-minded argument. It holds that fear of death is part of human nature and, indeed, the basic human fear influencing all other fears, and that we cope with it through denial.[25]

Either view does not invalidate the highly individualized, agonizing process of dying and facing death, of course. In my long-term dealings with alphas and betas, I have come to the conclusion that Becker's healthy-minded view of death anxiety is characteristic for alphas and his morbidity-minded one for betas. For in betas the future reality of one's personal dying and death and beyond becomes part of their timescape in their teens and, for peace of mind, needs covering up. Alphas, however, live in real time and for them death and dying and whatever follows are something that will happen "one day," in the mist of the future. They have therefore no need for denial.

An alpha client became naturally very upset when I told him his AIDS test had come back positive. Being familiar with the course of the illness—it was at that time still without hope—he was quite panicky with visions of future suffering, and dying and death. He continued, however, to feel physically quite well over the next year; his partner stayed faithfully with him, and he carried on his creative work. Soon, the original shock began fading like a bad dream. But, one day he told me: "I feel very well right now, am socially in good shape, and enjoy my work. Yet, my partner seems to think that, deep down, I feel bad all the time because I will have to suffer and die some day. I catch him looking at me with a sad face and from time to time he tries to get me to talk about death and dying. When he does, his visions of my future make me anxious and depressed. Why doesn't he leave well enough alone and let us enjoy ourselves?" I explained to him that his partner probably subscribed to the popular, beta-centric belief that my client was in denial of dying and death. But I reassured him that his behavior was perfectly well-adjusted for his time gender, indeed an alpha strength, rather than some neurotic response or personality disorder.

Some alphas may have occasional panicky visions when others anxiously focus on their future suffering. Yet, provided their 4–D is worth living, they usually return to enjoying life one day at a time with thoughts of dying and death fading out. Only when actually facing the physical threat of dying in 4–D may an anxiety of dying with its suffering and progressive isolation emerge. However, my experience as a physician tells me that the anxiety of dying should not to be confused with its future outcome, death anxiety. Suffering alphas often long for, if not actually seek, death as a welcome friend who will free them from their agony.

Betas tend to respond entirely differently to a life-threatening illness, even if they continue feeling physically well and their social circumstances remain stable. Their initial upset extends far beyond their immediate panic, unless a protective denial takes over. This permits them to gradually refocus on their previous course. Usually, they find themselves pre-living the dying reality in their timescape, experiencing waves of pervasive anxiety and obsessing over their foreshortened future and how to achieve a sense of closure. Even the future after death becomes a source of anxiety (death anxiety). For example, what will happen to their partner, or what, if any, will be the future of their soul. The outcome of the battle in their timescape may lie anywhere between a painful, anxiety-ridden disintegration of life, and a liberating peace of mind that rises above life itself. It may also have a humorous side. For example, a friend told me a story about his father, a protestant minister, who attended a Dutch farm wife in her nineties who was dying. The minister was surprised to find her constantly busy with matters other than spiritual ones. Because of her approaching death he felt that she should focus her attention on spiritual matters, such as the grace of God, the life hereafter, and so on. He initiated the conversation by saying "You are under a lot of pressure" whereupon she responded: "Yes, Reverend, but once I can feel that I have got the funeral behind me, I will be all right."[26]

Situational mood swings and mood disorders

The fact that alphas do not have to carry the weight of past failures or future threats and can get on with their current life is often their strong suit. The price they may have to pay is that they miss the mood-steadying influence of a stable past and future timescape, and do not gain strength from a promised land or the good old days. Instead, their mood is not only hypersensitive to positive vibes in 4–D, but also vulnerable to negative ones.

Given stable, favorable circumstances in 4–D, the issue of one's emotional reactivity (or resilience) to 4–D will not arise. When positive and negative vibes alternate in 4–D, however, alphas experience considerable fluctuations in their mood and, thus, in their situational self-esteem. An insightful alpha described it this way: "It is as if my mood and the way I feel about myself are always sensitized by what happens around me. When comparing myself with other people, I often feel almost naked in the face of reality, overexposed to it. It is as if I am missing a filter between myself and the world around me, something that gives other people extra protection." She was intuitively aware that there are others (betas) who look at 4–D through some kind of filter (their timescape).

More often than not alphas remain unaware that their mood is situation-driven and instead think they suffer from unpredictable mood swings. One alpha, to whom I explained how alphas and betas maintain their mood, said with some puzzlement: "You mean to say it is possible to maintain a constant mood? I wouldn't know how to!" But, once alphas recognize the problem for what it is, they can develop strategies for tackling this challenge in many situations by proactively doing something about their present situation rather than responding reactively to it. When feeling miserable, they may ask themselves: "What can I do right now to make myself feel better?"

To highlight the problem of mood swings in alphas as contrasted with betas I need only turn to my own clinical practice. Of 273 people who consulted me over a two year period, 18 (7%) came specifically because of spontaneous mood swings with 16 being alphas and only 2 betas, a statistically highly significant difference ($p=0.008$).

In alphas mood is situation-sensitive. This is readily seen when they enter a counseling session, describing — tears in their eyes — a miserable situation they are enduring. If counselors put a positive spin on what is happening in their clients' 4–D, an immediate improvement in their mood can be observed. For the positive spin disconnects these clients from the sadness they brought in with them. Leaving the office in an uplifted spirit, they soon find themselves, however, facing the misery they discussed in the first place, and will need another supportive session, and another, until they lose confidence in the counselor and stop coming. Obviously, counselors must use a different, more effective approach with these patients.

Putting a positive spin on the 4–D misery of betas does not work. The counselor soon runs into the counter-spin on 4–D that emerges from the clients' timescape. Assisting betas in amending the enduring spin of their timescape is a major, time-consuming job.

This difference between alphas and betas in responding to positive encouragement during counseling is typical. It does not mean that the emotional responses of alphas are unstable and those of betas stable, but rather shows that the mood of alphas is highly responsive to 4–D and the mood of betas depends more on how 4–D looks through their timescape in 6–D.

The story of the depressed alpha Nobel laureate

When alphas go through a discouraging period in 4–D and are unable to do anything about it, this soon may deprive them of situational self-esteem, particularly those with a pessimistic temperament. They cannot fall back on a timescape and any positive global self-esteem to be derived from it. As a result, they may slide into a simple situational depression. When one tries to comfort them by bringing attention to their past achievements, they will respond: "But what about now?" To them the past is a foreign country. When someone they trust reassures them that the clouds in their current, miserable 4–D will lift in a couple of months, their spirit will rise, but not for long. A realistic positive vision of their future does not become part of a prelivable timescape that will henceforth nurture them. It is no more than a fleeting daydream in 5–D.

My clinical experience has been that when alphas have depressed feelings, the vast majority of these depressions are situational in nature, rather than biological or rooted in past experience. The following story of a Nobel laureate of the alpha time gender exemplifies this. Upon receiving the Prize, the resulting sudden fame, publicity and admiring entourage put him on top of the world. After a few years, however, he got himself into serious financial problems through business speculations that failed. He also got himself into deep marital trouble. In short order he lost his wife, a significant group of friends, and many of his investments which, in turn, led to a great deal of negative publicity and loss of face. Unfortunately, all this coincided with a temporary but significant slow down in his work that cause him to lose his team and other admirers. Despite his optimistic disposition, his situational self-esteem crumbled and he grew depressed, calling himself a "loser."

His therapist, admittedly still rather naive at the time, tried to argue with his negative self-talk:

> "Well, you know, you cannot be that much of a loser. After all, a few years ago you did get the Nobel Prize."

> "...But, doctor, that was years ago. What about now? I have nothing left. No money, no wife, no friends, no staff, nothing. Nothing is going right for me. And never mind the Nobel Prize; everybody is laughing at me now! People get a kick out of it when a man falls flat on his face."

> "Listen, right now your life does not look so great, but you told me yourself that three months hence your staff will reassemble and your new project will get underway."

> "...Three months down the road?! How is that going to help me now?

Only his dismal 4–D reality counted. As time went on the news media lost interest in his misery, and his new project proposal received major funding support. This not only reestablished a more stable, personal financial situation, but also enabled him to reassemble his professional entourage. As a result, his 4–D began turning positive so that his situational self-esteem was no longer a problem and, as he lost himself in his new exciting project, his depression evaporated.

In sum, the Nobel Prize provided this alpha laureate with an overabundance of situational self-esteem until his 4–D went sour. He developed a simple situational depression which was resistant to past achievements and future promise, but which lifted as soon as his 4–D turned positive again.

Troubled alphas often look to the past for answers, troubled beta often look to the present

Situational circumstances in 4–D that cause alphas emotional problems are usually far more subtle than the obvious ones in the life of the depressed alpha Nobel laureate. They may seem trivial as a cause of depressed feelings, particularly in the eyes of betas. Therapists often miss the point that a depressed patient is extraordinarily sensitive to persistent negative vibes in 4–D and pursue other explanations for these rather volatile, depressed moods. They may ask: is this an affective disorder rooted in the metabolism of some neurotransmitter which requires antidepressants? Or is there some underlying unresolved conflict or trauma in early childhood that requires counseling? Current pop-psychology which has childhood conflicts and abuse high on the list of causes for emotional problems (and is therefore strongly beta-oriented) reinforces the latter thinking. Some popular talk shows on TV have reinforced this trend by promiscuously exploring a person's intimate background and then parading genuine or alleged childhood traumas as explanations for present difficulties.

Alphas often buy readily into the quasi-wisdom of the pop psychology of our media culture. They often remain unaware of the role of time gender in their current problem. They feel their emotional problems *must* originate in some unresolved childhood problem with a parent or sibling or in some early traumatic events. They accept that these alleged experiences were so painful that they had to repress them, leading to unconscious motivations behind their problematic behaviors.

This way of thinking relieves alphas of any direct responsibility for their problems. To "uncover" and "get in touch with" their forgotten painful past, they may turn to a therapist who uses hypnosis or dream analysis or primal therapy. These approaches not only feed into the intrinsic curiosity of alphas, but also place them in the temporarily rewarding centre of their therapist's attention. Yet, when all this has been attended to, the client often finds he or she is not really much further ahead. Disappointed, he or she may well lose interest in the past and, instead, end up demanding assistance in the here-and-now: "We have gone through my past over and over again. Now I need help handling my problem."

I recall a woman in her thirties who suffered from depressive mood swings. About three years earlier, she had gone to her general practitioner with her problem. When she told him that between the ages of 9 and 11 her father had sexually abused her, he concluded this probably had a lot to do with her depressive moods and sent her to a psychiatrist. This specialist worked with her for some considerable time, but when they got nowhere, he referred her to a women's center for victims of sexual abuse. There she participated for many months in group therapy and saw several women going through the re-living of their past traumas. She herself however, could not get into this, so she and the others finally concluded that significant aspects of her traumatic experiences were so deeply repressed that she needed depth therapy by someone like myself.

After a few sessions in which we broadly explored her life it became clear she was an alpha. At that point I told her that her depressive mood swings had nothing to do with her history of sexual abuse which she had not repressed in the first place. She was one of those people who can walk away from past traumas. Her mood swings had to be related to the circumstances in which she had been living during the last years. I explained the time gender model to her, stressing various strengths and weaknesses alphas and betas have, especially in alphas the sensitivity of situational self-esteem toward a negative 4–D. We went over the consistently negative circumstances she had encountered over the last years. It became clear that her depressive moods were related to her job which was boring and unchallenging given her intelligence, ambition, and energy. This new insight drove her to look elsewhere for a job and, being the gifted person she was, she was soon offered a more stimulating and better paying job. This really thrilled her. We kept in touch intermittently for another year. She remained just fine.

The client in this case fortunately was not totally committed to the assumption that her depressive moods could be explained by her past sexual abuse. Often this is not the case. In similar circumstances, many alphas cannot easily give up the belief that some past abuse accounts for their problem. This would make them lose face in the eyes of others. It may take months of work and much patience in helping them free themselves from this myth before they can begin tackling the actual cause of their problem.

The story of the depressed beta Nobel laureate

In the following story a beta Nobel laureate became depressed *because* he received the Nobel Prize. This demonstrates the role his timescape played in triggering his depressed state.

This scientist had devoted himself completely to a particular project for over a decade. Indeed, it became all he lived for. One day when he walked into his laboratory, he made a serendipitous observation which had nothing to do with what he had been searching. Yet in due course this chance observation created a major breakthrough in his field that eventually brought him the Nobel Prize.

Becoming famous overnight came to him as a shock. It brought an abundance of situational self-esteem which elated him initially. Once the storm of excitement died down, however, his timescape with its global self-esteem produced second thoughts. Had he received the Nobel Prize because of his devoted research over all these past years? No! His chance discovery had just been a "fluke." Looking back, his past research had really led to naught. Looking forward, he wondered whether his future research would suffer a similar fate. Thus, the Nobel Prize gradually started eating away at his global self-esteem. The more people applauded him, the more he began feeling an impostor and a failure. "I have fooled everybody," he told himself. He became increasingly depressed and began to avoid people.

Eventually, he decided to avoid people altogether and to spend time alone in an effort to regain composure. For a considerable period of time, he struggled to put the Nobel Prize and its overwhelming impact on his global self-esteem behind him, and recommit himself to his life's work. Yet even after he became able to do so, he continued avoiding the limelight and avoided talking about his Nobel Prize.

This story demonstrates how a beta's positive global self-esteem can ironically be shattered by a positive 4–D experience.

The important emotional role of a beta's future

Interestingly enough, young adult betas often erroneously explain emotional troubles they experience as situational problems. They may say they are unhappy because their job is not stimulating, or because they do not have an intimate relationship, or because their living conditions are depressing, or because it is just genetic. Naturally, a persisting shame or guilt in a beta's timescape, rooted in some past experience, can have a very negative influence on a beta's enjoyment of the present. On close scrutiny, however, their problem often does not lie in their genes, or in 4–D, or in their posterior time cone, but rather in not having a concrete idea what they want to do with their future. Their frontal cone does not supply them with the much needed emotional sustenance that a positive outlook on the future provides. An important chunk of their future timescape is missing. It is not their past timescape that needs care, but their future timescape.

A future threat can also be a source of beta trouble. Consider a beta in favorable circumstances who suddenly learns he or she has to pay a large sum of money three months hence, but lacks the funds. The first realization of this will upset alphas and betas alike. Alphas soon put such future adversity in the back of their mind, and refocus on their day to day life. Betas, on the other hand, will feel threatened and worry for the entire three months, constantly thinking of finding a way out, or worrying about what will happen when they cannot pay. The future threat spoils their enjoyment of an otherwise pleasing present. They may attempt to lose themselves in their work, or keep busy in some other way. Yet, as soon as they relax they are again anxiously worrying in their future time cone. No wonder alphas often view betas as a bit neurotic, and that betas frequently think of alphas as having nerves of steel or being irresponsible.

Far more serious to betas than some future threat is when they have their future taken away, their anterior time cone amputated, so to speak. In that case, we have a very depressed, sometimes suicidal beta on our hands, as in the following example.

A highly successful beta executive in his early fifties was expecting a promotion to one of the vice-presidencies of a large corporation. Restructuring began, however, and his career ground to a sudden unexpected halt. In short order, he was bypassed twice, and then demoted from his high position without any explanation. Although his considerable salary stayed the same, the perks he had been enjoying for years began disappearing. First, he lost his parking spot, then a club membership, then his office with its executive washroom. His situational self-esteem received a daily beating, and his 4–D became a continuous hell. More important, however, was that the promising futurama in his anterior time cone was obviously being destroyed. He lost confidence in any future for himself. Instead, he began dwelling in the past, trying to figure out where he had gone wrong. There was no answer, of course, for it was the restructuring that had amputated his future with the corporation he had served so successfully for so many years.

Without his future, life lost meaning and he came dangerously close to a "balance suicide." A balance suicide is the result of balancing the hell of today's future against death, as in the case of the rampant balance suicides that followed Black Friday in 1929, the day of the great stock market crash.

From a therapeutic point of view, two steps were vital to prevent suicide. The first was to extract him from his present humiliating, traumatizing situation. The second step was even more fundamental, namely to help him realize he, a beta, had to create a new futurama in his anterior time cone. While people understandably tend to focus on the traumatizing present, they should not forget that a reasonably meaningful futurama is to a beta as vitally important as a reasonably meaningful 4–D is to an alpha.

This two-step strategy absorbed our beta in an intense inner struggle. He had to block his posterior cone, and found this very difficult. The corporation had been his life and pride. He felt more equal to the task of battling his corporate superiors in the hope of obtaining some satisfaction. He first succeeded in negotiating a reasonable settlement, thus extricating himself from his poisonous work environment. It was not a glorious victory but a victory that, at least, restored a measure of his dignity, his global self-esteem. He then began making the rounds in search of a new occupational future and eventually found it. This restored his global self-esteem. Looking back into his posterior cone, he realized he had overcome the most serious threat to his integrity he had ever experienced and, as a result, felt himself a much more confident person.

How would a top alphaexecutive with comparable skills and gifts have fared under similar circumstances? At the time of the shameful job demotion, this executive's situational self-esteem also would have hit a very low level, in this case because of a situational depression. Being an alpha, however, and living in the world rather than in his head, this executive likely would have sensed the imminent threat to his position much earlier than the beta. And he or she would not have had to face a loss of futurama and, as a result, a loss of meaning. Nor would there have been be a preoccupation with past devotion to the corporation and with self. Alphas tend to be more flexible in their occupational crisis responses, including changing their occupational niche. They already would have scanned their network for alternatives, if they had not already quit by the time of their projected demotion. If alphas do not get back on their feet right away, however, they run the risk of slipping into the quicksand of a more lasting and disabling situational depression.

Summing up

Many variables, notably an optimistic or pessimistic temperament, determine one's current mood. In the pursuit of self-esteem—the main psychological handle on positively influencing one's mood—time gender plays a significant role in mood regulation. Alphas pursue situational self-esteem in 4–D, and betas pursue global self-esteem in 6–D.

In addition, time gender also influences how people cope with rewarding or distressing events in the present, as opposed to the past and future. Alphas focus on the good and bad that happens in the present while turning their back on the pastand future, whereas betas continue to experience the motivating force of past and future events, as well as how these events, within certain time limits, emotionally color the present.

In sum, time gender plays an important role in our emotional coping style. Alphas and betas have complimentary strengths and weaknesses in this regard. To gain a fuller understanding of these emotional coping strategies, we must realize we are not all cut from the same cloth and acknowledge these time gender differences. Furthermore, for mental health professionals to know a client's time gender will allow for a more rational approach to separating what is normal and natural in the client's current emotional state from what is genuinely pathologic and in need of therapeutic help.

NOTES

1   Whissell, Fournier, Pelland, Weir & Makarec (1986).
2   Cowdry, Gardner, O'Leary, Leibenluft & Rubinow (1991), p. 1505.
3   Thomas et al, (1963, 1968); Thomas & Chess (1977); Escalona and Leitch (1953); Escalona and Heider (1959); Murphy et al., (1962); Escalona (1968); Murphy and Moriarty (1976).
4   McCrae and Costa (1987).
5   Merritt (1993).
6   Safran (1993), p. 50-57.
7   I borrowed the term 'cognitive dissonance' from Festinger (1957).
8   Paykel (1978).
9   Choy and de Bosset (1992).
10   Bowman (1999), p. 22-23.
11   Block (1995); Kagan (1994).
12   Tellegen, Lykken, Bouchard, Wilcox, Segal, Rich (1988).
13   Argyle (1987); Myers (1993).
14   The concepts of "extroversion" and "introversion" were introduced by Jung, and share significant aspects with the alpha and beta time gender, respectively. Differences between his and my views are discussed in Chapter 6 under *The alpha time gender is extroverted, the beta time gender introverted.*
15   That betas are no longer bothered by what happened may make them seem like an alpha. Yet while alphas can, if need be, recall a distressful event with some emotion but without significant emotional turmoil, betas who intuitively block conscious recall, experience a great deal of emotional turmoil if they regain conscious access.
16   This period of 18 months may have a wider significance. It may represent the time required for any major reprogramming of the brain. For example, it takes in my experience an addict around 18 months to begin wondering what the need for the booze, the cigarette, the drug, was all about. It also takes around 18 months of long-term reconstructive psychotherapy to achieve any significant personality change.
17   Carr (1985), p. 1286.
18   Prigerson et al. (1995)
19   Viederman (1995).
20   Worman and Silver (1989); Viederman (1989); Paykel (1978).

21   Twombly (1973).
22   Weisman (1975), p. 1754.
23   Kübler-Ross (1969).
24   The Toronto General Hospital, presently The Toronto Hospital, General Division.
25   Becker (1973), p. 13-15.
26   Aris (2000).

CHAPTER 5

Time Gender And Identity

Inner Child (ego), Inner Parent (supereg o), and Inner Adult (paraego)

Most contemporary humans experience and treat their minds and bodies as a single unit and so the singular nature of one's individual identity appears self-evident.

"This self...regards itself as one, others treat it as one, it is addressed as one, by a name to which it answers. The Law and the State schedule it as one. It and they identify it with a body which is considered by it and them to belong to it integrally. In short, unchallenged and unargued conviction assumes it to be one. The logic of grammar endorses this by a pronoun in the singular. All its diversity is merged into oneness."[1]

Yet, one's individual identity is not necessarily singular in nature.

> "...Most of us have probably, at some time, found ourselves talking or acting as if we were two people rather than one. We talk sometimes of being of "two minds" about something, part of one wanting to do one thing and part wanting to do something else. Quite often we hear people talk of having to "battle" with themselves, as if one aspect of themselves was in conflict with another."[2]

Although self-talk in 5–D only uses "I," there are at least two sides to our identity: first, an encouraging or dissuading, but authoritarian Inner Parent (superego or Voice of Conscience) and, second, a submitting, cooperating or rebelling Inner Child (ego). Consider this exchange with one of my clients:

> "Doctor, I need your help. I am so unhappy with myself. I feel inadequate all the time. This makes life miserable. Do you think I can change?"

> "Give me an example of what you mean by 'inadequate.'"

> "Well, when it comes to important personal matters, I seem to have no judgment."

> "Are you sure you have no judgment?"

> "Doctor, I am absolutely sure."

It is ironic that he was confident in his judgment about himself yet maintained that he had no judgment in personal matters. This is because the singular pronoun I/me is often used as a figure of speech for one's ego and then again as a metaphor for his superego. Once recognized, his externalized self-talk can be paraphrased to make the apparent contradiction disappear:

> *"Doctor, I (Inner Parent, superego) feel all the time that I (Inner Child, ego) have been inadequate since I was a child. This makes life miserable. I (Inner Parent) would like to find out whether I (Inner Child) can change."*

> "Give me an example of what you (Inner Parent) mean by [you (Inner Child) being] 'inadequate'."

> *"Well, when it comes to important personal matters, I (Inner Child) seem to have no judgment at all."*

> "Are you (Inner Parent) sure you (Inner Child) have no judgment at all?"

> *"Doctor, I (Inner Parent) am absolutely sure."*

The personification of this client's superego reflected an impatient, inflexible, domineering character that never seemed to shut up. His ego, on the other hand, came across as an overdependent, oversensitive yet passive character who submitted to this chronic abuse in silent suffering. The relationship between these subidentities reveals itself to be one of severe codependence, reflecting an internalized script of habitual early parent-child interaction.

Listening to ego-superego duets in my office often evoked in me alternating visual images of a parent and child. I listened to or addressed one, then the other, trying to understand each and make peace between them. This is difficult given their adversarial relationship.

Fritz Perls, who created Gestalt Therapy, also attended to the conflict in people's self-talk. He called it the "self-torture game" between the Underdog (Inner Child) and Top Dog (Inner Parent). He considered the Underdog to be the dependent crybaby who is apologetic and compliant by being passively manipulative whereas the Top Dog was the bullying, authoritarian, self-righteous self who knows best. When a client would speak on behalf of the Underdog, Perls had her or him sit in one chair. When giving voice to the Top Dog, the client had to move over to another. The two self-talk players would then encounter and identify each other. [3]

Both Perls and I implicitly reinforced and educated our clients' Inner Adult or paraego with its Voice of Reason, instead of aligning ourselves with the Inner Child/ego or Inner Parent/superego. Eventually, our clients would be expected to internalize relevant aspects of our paraego. Then their self-talk would no longer include only the repetitive dialog of their Inner Child/ego and Inner Parent/superego but would become more creative by also involving their Inner Adult/paraego as a built-in counselor.

The role of Freud and Jung in this Chapter

Jung was an alpha and Freud a beta, and since their theories were grafted on their self-analyses, their personality models contain an implicit model of their personal identity. Because neither used the term "identity" as we are using it here, namely individual ("I") or self-identity, the model of their personal identity was not explicit.

Instead, Freud and Jung used the term "identity" only to denote group or collective ("we") identity.[4] Using "identity" in the sense of individual identity is only possible through reasonably reinterpreting what Freud and Jung wrote or using interpretations of qualified followers.

Freud's individual identity was un-partitioned and monofocal. He viewed himself as a singular personality. The theory of Freud therefore infers that a person's identity is singular and that experiencing multiple personalities is pathological. By contrast, Jung saw his psyche as consisting of a plurality of personalities, with his identity partitioned and multifocal. As a result, the theory of Jung claims there are within each of us many potential personalities, each with their own identity, and their own self-talk between Inner Child and Inner Parent. Displaying a singular personality or identity is a pathological fixation. In the time gender model, Freud is a beta and Jung an alpha. The theoretical challenge is to show how these contradictory personality models both can be accommodated in the time gender model.

Freud's model of the mind

Freud's monofocal identity model considers the "ego" and "superego" as the prevailing structures in one's conscious psyche. Following internalization of 4-D, one's silent self-talk in 5-D represents the relationship between the ego (inner child) and the superego (inner parent). Freud introduced the "id" as a third, mainly unconscious complex of antisocial impulses. Prior to internalization, one learns to repudiate and disown this repressed counter-part of the ego through socially induced, external pressures, and after internalization through the superego. Occasionally, the id participates in the self-talk between ego and superego through a conscious fantasy of forbidden temptation. When the id's temptation wins out over the ego's impulse control and the forbidden act is exposed, the ego may disown responsibility by claiming "the devil made me do it."

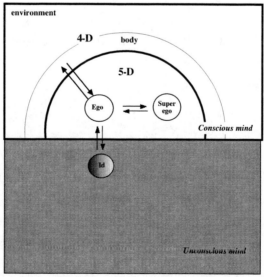

Figure 5.1: Pos' elaboration of Freud's model of the mind

These three, interacting sub-selves—ego, superego and id—are like three actors in a play called *An ego-state,* in which the ego is not only the director, but also the carrier of one's personal identity which conveys a sense of singular self, and which in the time gender model is reflected by a beta's timescape in 6-D. Figure 5.1 depicts Freud's model of the mind in the context of the 4–D-5–D model and accounts for the self-talk between ego and superego as well as for the participation of the voice of evil (or the voice of the devil) that represents the id. Because Freud was a beta, this figure depicts the structure of the beta mind with its implicit singular, contextually unified, monofocal identity.

Beyond self-talk as an ego-superego duet: from monofocal to multifocal identity

Historicly, psychiatry taught that having more than one coherent personality indicates abnormality. Any current standard text testifies to the historic dominance of this viewpoint.[5] Yet not everyone experiences one's silent self-talk as an ego-superego duet. Some experience a group session of several egos, if not superegos. I have discovered that group self-talk is characteristic of alphas and duet self-talk of betas.

"Mona," for example, a young, intelligent woman, explained that she got into an argument with herself when she saw her own image in a shop window:

> *"You idiot, why don't you diet? Look how fat you are!"*

> "Dammit, don't give her such a rough time; get off her back!"

> *"There we go again. Please, stop this boring argument! Haven't you got something more pleasant to think about? What is so bad with the way you look anyhow? Haven't you got a boyfriend who is in love with you? In any case, you are on your way to see your mother. Why not think about that?"*

> "Mom is a real bitch and doesn't care about me."

Then a voice defended mother, and another voice stated that mom did not matter one way or the other. Mona said this could go on for hours and that she wished she could stop all of the voices.

"Cory," a 17-year-old woman, said:

> *"One day I am a punk rocker, another day a very churchly person, no lipstick or anything, etc. Then I can be the poor daughter who grieves over her mother's recent death. I can also be a real cry-baby. Then there is the one who is like the lady living in a big, expensive townhouse in a conservative neighborhood. It all depends on who I am with, or what I am at. My sister says she never knows who the real Cory is. Neither do I."*

And "Jane," a woman in her mid-thirties, with several university degrees, stated:

> *"Sometimes I wonder who I really am. There is a philosopher inside of me, but also a vegetable who just likes reading novels and eating chocolates, or*

just hanging out. Then there is the analytic scientist, the nurse, the mother, the athlete, the musician, the politician, the sexy woman who knows how to live, and the religious nun who has absconded from the world and lives in solitude to serve God. I can invest myself in any one of them, I can be any of them."

Jane then drew on a sheet of paper a large circle with little circles surrounding it (see figure 5.2) and said that each little circle represented one of the people, and, in effect, they sit around the table.

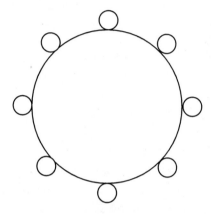

Figure 5.2: Jane's illustration of her psyche as eight different identities
sitting around a table that may represent her "real self"

She thought the table might be the real her, her Self, the one who could move into the clothes of any of the people at the table. She could not give it an identity of its own. She did not know who coordinated the different types.

"Maybe this unknown Self does the coordination, or maybe the philosopher or the analytical scientist who sit at the table? I am not sure … I cannot analyze it by myself. That's why I need you. I am going around in circles wondering who the real me is."

Mona's, Cory's and Jane's personified voices in self-talk in 5–D did not fit Freud's ego-superego model of self-talk. I have learned that others have observed a similar self-talk not only in clients but in themselves. One therapist had a 23-year-old female client with an eating disorder and discussed what she experienced just before going on a binge and vomiting bout. She described a confusing cacophony of voices in her head and, to her amazement and that of her counselor, could readily identify several of these voices. One was highly critical of her, particularly of how she looked. Another came to her defense, making her parents responsible for her difficulties. Another voice made her feel sad, despondent and inadequate, with yet another one ordering her to binge. Not only had this therapist heard similar statements before made by others who suffered from bulimia, but also became aware of having personally experienced similar silent multiple inner voices.[6] Another counselor stated:

> "It was during a time of painful conflict that I first began to experience myself as more than one. It was as though I sat in the midst of many selves. Some urged me down one path and some another. Each presented a different claim and no self gave another self an opportunity to be fully heard."[7]

Accordingly, one of Pearls' Gestalt therapists found it necessary to use several chairs instead of only one for the underdog (ego) and one for the top dog (superego), noting that "I know something about where they are inside as I see where they sit."[8]

The viewpoint that some people (alphas) have access to several distinct, discontinuous ego-states and personalities, and have therefore a partitioned, multifocal identity, in contrast with the unified, monofocal identity in betas, is not new. The French novelist Marcel Proust (1871-1922) felt personality does not mirror a single ego but a succession of egos. He was obviously an alpha. So was Carl Jung, who in the 1920s led a movement to counterbalance the dominant Freudian assumptions that a contextually unified, monofocal identity is normal and a contextually partitioned, multifocal identity pathologic. Jung held that normal people have a multifocal identity and a monofocal identity indicates pathologic rigidity.[9] After World War II, this stream of thought representing a contextually partitioned, multifocal identity saw a number of alternative psychotherapies that implicitly, if not explicitly, backed the identity proposed by Jung. Now, in addition to the dominant stream of opinions favoring a monofocal identity, there are ever widening streams of opinion in support of multifocal identity. These two currents indicate that multifocal Jungian alphas and monofocal Freudian betas are not just interesting hypothetical creatures (or a mere polarity) but are real people who co-exist side-by-side, as they have for tens of thousands of years.

Meet Carl Jung No. 1 and No. 2, and the three George Bernard Shaws

The singular ego-state represented by Freud's model (see figure 5.1) clearly did not fit Jung's partitioned, multifocal identity. Demonstrating his plurality of personalities Jung stressed, for example, in his biography the importance in his life of Jung No. 1 and Jung No. 2.[10] Jung No. 1 was the son of his parents, the schoolboy who was "less intelligent, attentive, hard-working and clean" than many others. The "other," Jung No. 2, felt grown up and old, "skeptical, mistrustful, remote from the world of men, but close to nature, the earth, the sun, the moon, the weather, all living creatures, and above all close to the night, to dreams." As soon as he was by himself he could become Jung No. 2, which was like visiting a temple "in which anyone who entered was transformed and suddenly overpowered by a vision of the whole cosmos... Here nothing separated man from God..."[11] He did not consider this pair polar opposites (as in Jekyll and Hyde) or as personifying his ego and superego. He considered them alter-personalities,[12] as different as apples and oranges.

The famous Irish dramatist, critic and Nobel Prize winner, George Bernard Shaw, was asked at the age of 70 to review and preface two unpublished volumes of fiction written in his early 20s. Shaw gave a detailed analysis of a young Shaw.[13] This enabled the Freudian theoretician on identity, Erik Erikson, to identify three distinct identities of Shaw: the Snob, the Noisemaker, and the Diabolic One.[14] Shaw himself noticed:

> "...I had to become an actor, and create for myself a fantastic personality fit and apt for dealing with men, and adaptable to the various parts I had to play as author, journalist, orator, politician, committee man, man of the world, and so forth."[15]

Each of these egos or self-identities was associated with a characteristic role, a recurrent behavioral script, with consistent attitudes, hopes, fears and goals, and each far more encompassing than the mere roles. Shaw recognized himself in each character.[16]

The public often invests a great deal of emotion in a seemingly monofocal image of certain popular personages who actually have a contextually partitioned, multifocal identity. Consider, for example, Simone de Beauvoir, the Doyenne of the feminist movement, or John Kennedy as the Camelot president. Many of their supporters refused to believe that they had private alternative identities which were dramatically out of step with their public images.

Jung's model of the mind

Jung believed that the ongoing stream of consciousness in the mind consists of separate, identifiable mental states (which he referred to as "functional complexes"), each with their own behavior, emotions, ideas, memories, and dreams or fantasies, and which operate as independent personalities. When a functional complex temporarily takes over from the current one, it presents itself as an actual alternative personality with its own alternative identity.[17] Jung included in this multitude of personalities in one's psyche the Freudian three-some of ego/superego/id although, eventually, he replaced the name "superego" by "morality complex," and the name "id" by "shadow personality." But, he allowed for many more functional complexes or personalities or identities. Among these I came to make a distinction between "contextual" complexes and "elemental" complexes. "Contextual" complexes are defined by a particular person with whom one interacts (such as the father complex, or mother complex), or by a distinct major life event (such as the marriage complex, or birth complex). There are as many contextual complexes as there are typical situations in life.[18] One can, however, always recognize in each context a group of six "elemental" complexes which, according to Jung, together define in each context the basic structure of the psyche, as follows: 1) The ego or master function; 2) The morality complex or superego; 3) The shadow personality or id; 4) The persona or outward personality (representing one's interpersonal identity); 5) The soul image or inward personality (the medium for inner adaptation to the Collective Unconscious); 6) The anima through which men apprehend the nature of women, or the animus through which women apprehend the nature of men.[19]

Jung's word association experiments convinced him that each personality or functional complex (whether contextual or elemental) consists of a central theme or nucleus with associations clustered around it (all with an upstairs descriptive brain component and a downstairs emotional brain component as described in Chapter 3). These central themes or nuclei he called "archetypes," which are genetic in nature, acquired over the course of evolution. All humans share the combined endowment of archetypes, which represents the entire potential of the human psyche, and which Jung called the "Collective Unconscious" or "Collective Self." Early in life, suitable events trigger an archetype in one's Collective Unconscious to release a corresponding central theme into one's Personal Unconscious. This enables relevant perceptions, emotions, ideas, dreams and fantasies to crystallize around it, constituting a corresponding functional complex or personality or identity. For example, the antisocial shadow personality emerges from the archetype of the devil and becomes fleshed out with personality qualities rejected as bad by the parents.[20] During these developments, life experience may be contrary to the realization of a functional complex's full potential. But the Self continues to pressure each functional complex toward its full potential, to self-realize,[21] which makes Jung's Self an omniscient, goal-directing omnipresence in the psyche. Figure 5.3 depicts in 4-D and 5-D Jung's multifocal, contextually partitioned model of the (alpha) mind. In each personality or ego-state, the ego is the bearer of the particular contextual identity (as reflected by 6-D) and has its own ego-management style, public presentation by the persona, morality of the superego, antisocial tendencies in the shadow, and comprehension of femininity or masculinity through the anima or animus.

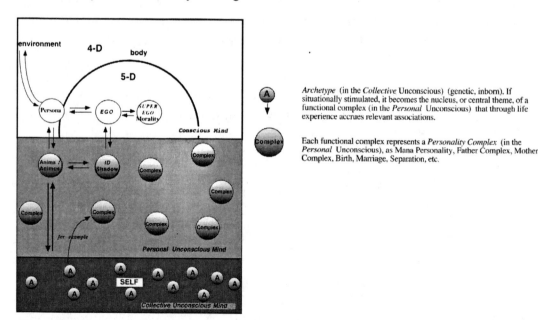

Figure 5.3: Pos' elaboration of Jung's model of the mind

One of Jung's followers concluded that people no longer represent a singular being in the image of a single God. An individual is made up of an abundance of figures: the mischievous child, the heroic one, the controlling judge, the asocial one, and so on. The idea of multiple personality need no longer threaten people. It is quite normal to see visions and hear voices and one should feel free to talk with them, and they with each other, without this meaning that one is insane.[22]

Compare the multifocal identity of an alpha to the following statement from one of my monofocal beta clients:

> "I am a scientist, sometimes lost in the brain, sometimes in the psyche, sometimes in evolution, sometimes in history. But there is also a spiritual priest in me who longs for solitude. Not only a primary care physician, also a neurosurgeon, and also an empathetic long-term therapist. Then again someone who is really good in emergencies. Then there is the artist who is, at heart, a pianist-composer-conductor, but also a bit of a poet and painter, if not a budding architect. Then there is the child feeling sorry for himself, or, at other times, overwhelmed by a fear of being abandoned."

When asked who the real "me" was, he looked puzzled and responded:

> "What do you mean? I have just told you in great detail!"

He did not speak, as alphas may do, about experiencing himself in different contexts as different personalities that are discontinuous with each other. He clearly believed that he experienced his different gifts, moods, or roles as the same singular personality with a monofocal identity which transcends different affective contexts.

Accommodating the models of Freud and Jung in the time gender model

To date there has been no unifying theory other than the time gender model that recognizes, and accommodates in a common framework, the contextually portioned, multifocal identity of Jungian alphas and the fused, monofocal identity of Freudian betas. With some minor amendments, Freud's and Jung's personality models (as represented in figures 5.1 and 5.3, respectively) can be comfortably brought in line with each other to fit in the time gender model.

Both models do not allow for "the voice of the devil's advocate" that sometimes may be heard in one's self-talk. This voice in support of the id's attempts to seduce the ego comes from the counter-part of the superego and represents a permissive sub-self which I called "superid." In this light one can translate "I really want to do this unacceptable thing, but I know it is bad and I should control myself. But why not do it only once when no one is around?" into "Id really wants the ego to do this unacceptable thing, but superego knows it would be bad so that ego should control id. But why not doing it only once when no one is around (says superid in support of id)?"

A second point is that both Freud and Jung were aware of a person's "voice of reason" but considered it an expression of a mature ego [in 5-D]. They did not realize that the voice of reason comes from the paraego [in 7–D] which is independent from the ego in 5-D and represents therefore a sub-self in its own right.

A third point to be made is that Jung's persona complex is notoriously absent in Freud's model. This sub-self, mediated through verbal activity and body language in 4-D, is important because it represents one's "interpersonal" rather than "intrapersonal" identity. Because of Freud's intuitive preoccupation with a singular identity, he would have implicitly viewed the persona as expressing this singular ego identity. He would therefore not have viewed it worthwhile to consider the persona separately from the ego. Yet, the "interpersonal" persona in the body box of 4-D is not identical with, or part of the ego in 5-D who is the carrier of one's "intrapersonal" identity.

A fourth, more complicated point concerns the role of the anima/animus complex in Jung's model. On the one hand, Jung thought of this anima-animus complex as active when dealing with a member of the opposite sex. This means that men and women must also harbor an iso-sexual complex for dealing with same sex members. Since both are affectively contextual complexes, they need not be part of Jung's elemental model of the alpha psyche, as depicted in figure 5.3. On the other hand, Jung viewed the anima/animus complex as one's counter-persona (or "inward personality"), namely the *persona non grata* one avoids to be at all costs. If it is valid that most people do not want to behave like a member of the opposite sex then, in someone with a multifocal identity, this counter-persona (anima/animus) should remain the same for every identity. Yet Jung argued that one's various personae ("outward" personalities) demonstrated one's multifocal identity, which automatically means that one's counter-personae (or "inward" personalities) should also differ from one identity to another. Thus the *elemental* counter-persona complex cannot be identical with the *contextual* anima/animus complex, and should therefore be considered a sub-self in one's personality structure which deserves a place in the elemental model of the alpha psyche. What may explain this confusion is that Jung used the terms "anima/animus" and "soul image" (or "inward" personality) interchangeably. When speaking of the counter-persona (which represents one's inward personality), he may implicitly have been referring to the soul image, rather than to the anima/animus complex.

Finally, the time gender model holds that the multitude of human situations (affectively motivating contexts) is genetically determined with each context producing its own ego state or identity or personality, at least prior to internalization. My description of the involved developmental process does not make use of Jungian concepts as "archetypes," "collective unconscious," "goal-directed self" (which, Jung said, are genetically determined), or "personal unconscious" (which, Jung said, life experience grafts on this genetic basis). Hence, I need not represent these concepts in the elemental model of the alpha psyche.

THE GENDER BEYOND SEX: TWO DISTINCT WAYS OF LIVING IN TIME   91

Amending figure 5.1 (Pos' elaboration of Freud's model of the mind) and figure 5.3 (Pos' elaboration of Jung's model of the mind) according to these five points makes clear that Jung's multifocal identity model that represents alphas (figure 5.4) and Freud's monofocal identity model that represents betas (figure 5.5) comfortably fit in the time gendermodel.

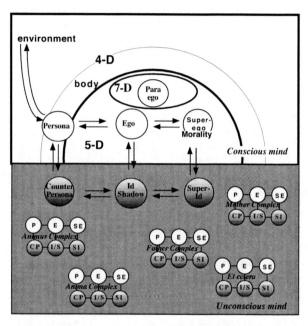

Figure 5.4: Pos' contextually partitioned, multifocal identity model of Jungian alphas

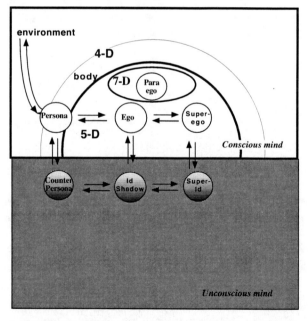

Figure 5.5: Pos' contextually unified, monofocal identity model of Freudian betas

Figures 5.4 and 5.5 show that the self-talk within each personality (whether singular as in the Freudian model, or reflecting a plurality of personalities as in the Jungian model) involves seven interacting sub-selves: 1) the executive ego or inner child (in 5-D) which is the bearer of ones identity (in 6-D); 2) the superego, inner parent, or morality complex, with its voice of conscience (in 5-D); 3) the id or shadow personality, with its voice of evil (in the unconscious, occasionally emerging in 5-D); 4) the superid, with the voice of the devil's advocate (in the unconscious, occasionally emerging in 5-D; 5) the persona or outward personality (in the body box of 4-D); 6) the counter-persona, inward personality or soul image (in the unconscious); and 7) the paraego or inner adult, with its voice of reason (in 7-D).

Table 5.1 lists various synonyms for these seven elemental complexes.

In 5-D:		
Persona (Jung)	**Ego (Freud)**	**Superego (Freud)**
Social mask (Jung)	Inner Child (Berne)	Morality Complex (Jung)
Outward personality (Jung)	Voice of the Executive ego (Pos)	Inner Parent (Berne)
External attitude (Jung)	Master complex (Jung)	Voice of Conscience (Pos)
Public identity (Pos)		
Interpersonal identity (Pos)		
In the uncsoncious mind:		
Counter-persona (Pos)	**Id (Freud)**	**Superid (Pos)**
Persona non grata (Pos)	Shadow (Jung)	Counter-superego (Pos)
	Counter-ego (Pos)	Voice of the Devil's Advocate (Pos)
	Voice of (the D) evil (Pos)	Quasi-conscience (Pos)
In 7-D:		
Paraego (Pos)		
Inner Adult (Berne)		
Voice of Reason (Pos)		
Transpersonal Self (Vaughan) (*23)		

Table 5.1: Synonyms for the elemental complexes of the psyche

(*23)=Endnote[23]

The origin of multifocal and monofocal identity: about motivational contexts

As during the adualistic phase the newborn's reality unfolds first in 4–D alone, the baby's upstairs brain processes the repetitive sensory input from interacting parts of its body, its parents, its bottle and so on, while an amalgam of biological needs and drives and emotions originating in the baby's downstairs brain energizes each unique motivational context. These affectively colored motivational contexts include experiencing an intensifying appetite with a desire for pleasing sounds that brings cooing and babbling, a craving for movement that provokes trampling and swinging arms, the enjoyment of being cuddled, and yielding to an urge to bang or suck on a toy. Once one emotional-motivating context deflates, another takes over. Growth, experience and parental focusing induce for each motivational context an increasingly differentiated and familiar 4–D. In other words, each state of mind of the baby unfolds in its own emotional-motivational context. The baby's reality is multifocal or multilayered in nature.

This remains so as the adualistic phase melts into the bonding phase, and the separation between the baby's body and surroundings has become a fact of life. Progressive brain mapping renders each of the baby's affect-specific editions of 4–D increasingly more structured and objectified. Each affect-specific edition of its 4–D reality features its own distinct displays or conscious personifications which remain unfused with those of other affect-specific states.

The core of affect-specific, motivational contexts is inborn and vested in the need/drive systems of the downstairs brain. Life experience gradually elaborates these motivational states into more complex contexts with more refined, affectively colored 4–D imagery and increasingly efficient behavior. On the other hand, a mosaic of inborn personality traits puts restraints on these developments. They determine, for example, whether the baby's general energy output will be high or low, whether its mood will be pleasant, whether its sleeping will be regular, how much stimulation is required before a response, and how flexible or rigid its newly learned patterns will be.

There is no general consensus on a detailed list of nuclear needs and drives and their incrementally evolving derivatives. This is not immediately clear when focusing on the primary level of vital needs and drives that the immediate predecessors of mammals, reptiles, already possess and that are concerned with individual survival (e.g., hunger) and survival of the species (e.g., sex). Our inability to adequately catalog motivational contexts may not even be self-evident when it comes to the secondary level of needs and drives that mammals add to the human inventory, such as the drive to mimic, to play or to explore. At the human level we are not only facing primary and secondary drives, but also the additional variety of tertiary human needs and drives that have arisen. These include self-esteem, self-realization, power, recreation, creativity and so on. This open-ended collection of overlapping, instinctive-emotional themes is difficult to sort out and often puts limits on discussions about specific motivational contexts. Nonetheless, motivational contexts play a fundamental role in how we experience reality and how a newborn's reality unfolds.

The preschooler's interwoven 4–D and 5–D realities remain multilayered

We noticed that, at the end of the bonding phase, long-term knowledge memory displays begin entering 5–D independent from what happens in 4–D. If someone drops out of the picture, the child can recall them in 5–D. This is especially meaningful because the child experiences 4–D and 5–D as interwoven, as the same. The child can now keep a representation of the mother, for example, in a particular affective context in 5–D, even if she is not looked at or manipulated in 4–D.

A dominant view among traditional Freudians holds that, when this object permanency becomes stabilized between 24 and 36 months, it renders the emotional variety of affectively contextual mother personifications not only independent from 4–D but fuses them into a single personification. They consider this fusion the basis for the child's maintaining stable feelings towards the mother despite changes in her behavior.[24] They assume that this and other fusions are the basis of the normal identity development which they consider to be contextually unified and monofocal. They judge this development, however, vulnerable to various factors, including flaws in the relationship with the mothering one. These may result in failure to achieve the fusion of personifications, thus leading to a pathological splitting of the child's reality with a resulting abnormal identity that is contextually partitionedAn argument in favor of such fusion early in childhood is based on the power of language. It claims that the learning of language fuses various personifications into a single one. The high pressure acculturation makes one person "mama" and another person "sister," so that individual personifications do not survive for long.[25] However, there are good reasons why this argument does not hold. For example, behind the pronoun "I" is hidden a variety of self-personifications. Furthermore, although a baby begins using the word "mama" around 15 months of age, until the age of 3 words have a variable and idiosyncratic rather than stable meaning. If a pet dog is called "Audrey," a two-year-old child may call all animals by that name. Until the age of 3, the youngster cannot grasp words such as "large" or "small," for example. One should understand that, even when the youngster moves beyond this pre-conceptual phase and simple concept formation becomes possible with the meaning of words becoming more stable, language is not simply based on a relationship between objects and sustainable memories of these objects. Word meanings always remain relative to a particular context. As a result, language by itself does not fuse various conscious displays or personifications into a single one.

Despite language development, the 4–D reality of preschoolers does not become automatically fused into a single display. Objects and persons remain unfused as they have appeared and continue to appear in separate affective-motivational contexts, so that the entire reality of preschoolers remains contextually multilayered. For example, the preschooler cannot sort out the multiple facets of its emotionally charged relationship with the mothering one. The child who cries upon facing an angry mother cannot realize that she can be also loving. The mother's various, affectively colored personifications remain functionally separate and unfused. She does not obtain a single personality in the eyes of the child, so that the preschooler does not respond to fluctuations in maternal behavior based on a stable image of the mothering one it developed in early childhood. Instead, it responds to these fluctuations with corresponding stable interaction schemata it gradually generates in specific motivational contexts.

This applies to all interaction schemata the preschooler establishes in the rich variety of affective-emotional contexts he or she has to become familiar with. Thus the preschooler intuitively learns to master various contexts in all their perceptual dimensions and symbolic meanings. Daily rhythms, such as eating, sleeping, and playing are specific interaction schemata. No matter how complex this process is, it proceeds without integrating these interaction schemata into a single overall scheme of behavior and without fusing multiple personifications into single persons, and multiple displays of objects (where personality does not enter the equation) into single objects. In other words, 4–D's physical and social reality of future alphas and future betas is, at this point in their development, still partitioned by affective context and therefore contextually multilayered or multifocal.

The preschooler's body self

Prior to internalization and the time gender differentiation of multifocal alphas and monofocal betas, 5–D is still interwoven with 4–D, so that preschoolers, apart from communicating, still think aloud, and display their fantasies and emotions publicly in 4–D. All their actions in 4–D are still intuitive, rather than plotted in 5–D with forethought. They cannot at this point deliberately manipulate their bodily persona. At 15 months, babies appear to develop a dawning prehension of the pronoun "I" and "mine."[26] Two year olds know their name, although using their name and various personal pronouns correctly will take considerable time. [27] Once preschoolers have learned to use the pronoun "I" and "mine" correctly, how do they respond to the question "who are you?" They respond: "I am Max," and when asked "but who is Max?" they point to their chest, claiming "this is me!" It is their body in 4–D interwoven with associated imagery in 5–D that intuitively personifies who they are. Preschoolers do not yet distinguish between 4–D and 5–D. It takes internalization of 4–D into 5–D to crystallize the sharp border between the 4–D world and the autonomous para-reality in 5–D, and for the executive ego (the Internalized Child in 5–D) to take over as the mental carrier of their identity from their body box in 4–D. Only then can they say "I have a toothache" instead of "my tooth hurts."

From preschooler to alpha or beta

In the preceding section, I explained that the entire 4–D reality of preschoolers (including their body imagery) remains affectively context-bound and unfused (or multilayered). What happens when internalization of 4–D into 5–D occurs and, more specifically, when significant, unique personal 4–D memories (needing only a single exposure) begin to get stored in the emerging autobiographic memory with displays in 6-D which, therefore, soon is to become the medium of one's life story and the implicit foundation of one's identity?

Although, with internalization, children begin to separate "foreground" and "background," thus considering objects and persons as single perceptual images in their own right (that is without any perceptual background contamination), this does not mean that objects and persons that have remained partitioned by and unfused in various *affective-motivational* contexts become automatically fused into a single display with various affective meanings.

Earlier, we discussed that, during internalization, the appearance of autobiographic knowledge memory (which functions differently in alphas and betas) introduces the differentiation between the time genders. In alphas, the autobiographic memory becomes like a network of intertwining memory islets that are perceptually and cognitively bound to their affective context. Since serialized time-binding between these affective contexts does not spontaneously occur, the autobiographic memory of alphas remains, in terms of affective contexts, partitioned (or multilayered or multifocal). This process I called "alphacization." Each motivational context has its own ego-state (or personality or self-identity) with its own ego (Inner Child), superego (Inner Parent), id superid, persona and counter-persona, and also develops its own past and future (as depicted in figure 5.6). Each contextual ego-state contains its own unfused, partitioned personifications of self, others, and objects. As a result, trans contextual inconsistencies in the behavior toward, and thinking and feeling about self and others occur. These tend to remain undetected by alpha children. It is as if when mother is angry, she is always angry, and when she is nice she always is. She does not have a single personality.

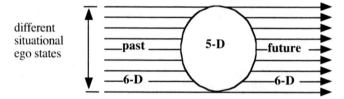

Figure 5.6: Multiple, partitioned, situational ego-state in alphas,
each with its own past and future connections

In young betas, a spontaneous, before-after time-binding is gradually superimposed on the intertwining, context-bound memory complexes that are formed in their autobiographicmemory. This time-binding consecutively serializes personal events that occur in unrelated affective-motivational contexts and results in a slowly extending timescape in 6–D with selective, personally significant life events as its milestones as depicted in figure 5.7 ("betacization").

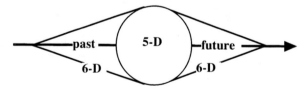

Figure 5.7: Singular, contextually unified ego-state in betas
with its singular past-future timescape

Since this timescapein 6–D reflects a singular, enduring personal past and future, it goes beyond motivational contexts which are biologically, emotionally, or socially different from one another. As the timescape slowly extends in size, it gradually merges the multitude of contextually partitioned ego-states into a unified ego-state with a singular ego and superego, id and superid, persona and counter-persona. The identity of young betas gradually becomes untied from each current context in 4–D and changes from multifocal to monofocal. Personifications of self and others become fused.

Betas cannot complete this process to a significant extent until their paraego emerges in adolescence, and becomes exposed to blatant discrepancies between various past or present motivational contexts. This triggers deliberate efforts at harmonizing their 6–D which may continue, often at the cost of considerable emotional suffering, throughout life. The ideal of a conflict-free 6–D, however, is never completely reached. Life is too complex. There are always unresolved dilemmas. If not in the open, these dilemmas are covered by denial or repression or other mental tricks that help the beta avoid facing up to reality.

The betacization or time-binding[28] or domestication of time[29] in betas is part of their genetic endowment which originated as an evolutionary genetic variation on how alphas store autobiographic events.

Concluding remarks

Once children internalize 4–D into 5–D, they become aware of self-talk between ego and superego. Sometimes the voice of evil, if not of the devil (id), may be heard, less often the voice of the devil's advocate (superid). In alpha children this self-talk may be different from one motivational context to another, while in beta children it becomes progressively similar, despite different contexts. Although rare, the self-talk can be like a quintet; recognizing the nature and roles of its players is, upon analysis, no different from describing the personalities and the roles of five people in a group session.

In adolescence, the emergence of the paraego and its voice of reason changes things. The paraego permits both alphas and betas to self reflect on their self-talk and superego, are consistent with each other in different contexts. But the paraego of alphas enables them for the first time to contemplate various faceless voices from *different* ego-states. It might seem as if they are in group session. Alphas find a silent cacophony of arguing voices shifting from one context to another. This melting pot of silent voices from different motivational contexts makes it difficult to analyze who plays which elemental role in what context.

Given the six sub-identities in any given ego-state, a fair question at this point is: how many faceless personifications may alphas experience in their self-talk in 5–D? It is generally accepted among group therapists that a group of eight is probably the upper limit for effective interaction of all participants. With a larger group the interaction may be too great for members or the therapist to follow.[30] In terms of individual clients, one clinician found that 4-8 sub-personalities is the "normal" range; that 9 and above suggests duplication; but that some people do not fit this model [betas no doubt].[31] In line with these findings, a Gestalt therapist found that she used up to ten chairs with individual clients; and that sometimes she needed only one or two chairs [with monofocal betas, no doubt], but that four to nine were the rule [multifocal alphas, for sure].[32]

Apparently, our brain can only handle the individual two-way communication of up to eight members. When moving beyond this maximum capacity, one begins to create subgroups treating, for example, "the two classy women," or "the three Italians" as single communication units. Similarly, once an alpha's self-talk goes beyond eight personifications the brain may automatically combine some that share similarities into hybrid ones, thus keeping their total number within manageable proportions.

NOTES
1   Sherrington (1947), p. xvii, quoted by Galin (1977), p. 404.
2   Mair (1977), p. 130.
3   Perls (1969).
4   Erikson (1960), p. 37 quoting Freud (1926); Jung (1977], p. 441-442.
5   Rowan (1990), p. 175.
6   Schwartz (1987), p. 26 quoted by Rowan (1990), p. 55.
7   O'Connor (1971), p. 3, quoted by Rowan (1990), p. 27.
8   Baumgartner and Perls (1975): p. 64-65.
9   Jung (1977), p. 466-468.
10 Jung (1977), 44-45, 57, 59-63, 65-69, 72-83.
11 Jung (1965), p. 44-45.
12 A term derived from Beahrs (1982).
13 Shaw (1952).
14 Erikson (1960), p. 42-44.
15 Shaw (1952), quoted by Erikson (1960), p. 44.
16 McAdams (1985), p. 116.
17 Jung (1936), quoted by Rowan (1990), p. 64; Groesbeck (1985), p. 434.
18 Stevens (1990), 28, 36-37.
19 Jung (1970); Jung (1977) 469
20 Stevens (1990), 28, 45, 84.
21 Jung (1970), 200.
22 Hillman (1985), p. 24, quoted by Rowan (1990), p. 35-36.
23 Vaughan (1985), p. 42-43.
24 Mahler et al. (1975), p. 110, quoted by Jacoby (1990), p. 60-61.
25 Sullivan (1953], p. 180.
26 Greenspan (1985), p. 1600.
27 Allport (1961), p. 113-122, quoted by Rappoport (1972), p. 166-7.
28 Buss (1966) introduced the concept of time binding, thinking its absence characterized psychopaths, rather than a difference between alphas and betas, but not all psychopaths are alphas; some are betas.
29 Kastenbaum (1975).
30 Frank and Powdermaker (1959), p. 1365; Sadock (1985), p. 1407.
31 Reason and Rowan (1981); Rowan (1990), p. 47.
32 Shapiro (1976), p. 13-14, quoted by Rowan (1990), p. 85.

CHAPTER 6

Time Gender And Social Behavior

Living in society requires social behavior. Social contexts (occupational, educational, political or religious, and so on) define one's interpersonal behavior. Social interactions on a one-to-one basis are usually determined by assigned social roles (such as strangers and friends, boss and employee, teacher and student, doctor and patient, lawyer and client, man and woman). A social setting of an intimate nature (a couple or nuclear family, for example) has its own facilitating and inhibiting influences on the social interaction of its participants.

Time gender is an additional factor that puts its stamp on one's interpersonal behavior. Keep in mind that time gender is only one among many factors that mold social behavior. While the social needs and behavior of alphas and betas stand in sharp contrast with one another, these other factors often lead to social behavior that lies somewhere on the continuum between the pure time gender profiles.

Chapter 7 deals with the impact of time gender on sexuality, choosing a partner, marriage and the nuclear family. This chapter focuses on the wider social milieu.

- Section 1 presents a general discussion of how alphas and betas differ in balancing the social needs for solitude and social interaction, and for individuality and group membership; the impact of this difference on how alphas and betas relate to significant groups and their institutional rules and goals; and a review of how alphas and betas differ in their attitudes toward social value systems (internalized rules).

- Section 2 discusses three aspects of social behavior in which time gender plays a significant role: 1) the extroverted versus introverted style of interpersonal relating; 2) the authoritarian-competitive, as opposed to egalitarian-cooperative styles of interpersonal relating; and 3) the nature of a person's curiosity and response to familiar situations.

- Section 3 focuses on how alphas and betas respond to ongoing interaction with each other (time gender interfacing), which is more frequent than alpha-alpha or beta-beta interactions.

- Section 4 considers how alphas and betas use language, and how time gender linguistics complicate their already existing time gender bias (alphacizing or betacizing)) toward each other.

Section 1: time gender and social needs

Balancing solitude and interaction

There is a fine balance between people's individual need for solitude and their social need to interact with others. When the need to interact with others becomes satiated, people feel crowded and crave solitude. Yet when their need to be alone is over, they begin to feel lonely and long to be with others. This balance varies a great deal from person to person. Some people prefer living alone and some prefer a roommate. Others fancy group living, as in a convent or monastery, aboard a ship, or in the armed forces.

Many factors influence the balance between one's need for social interaction versus solitude:

- age (generally speaking, the more mature and further into the life cycle, the less the need for interpersonal interaction).
- personality factors (such as an engaging versus avoidant trait or, more generally, one's overall level of comfort or discomfort in being with others);
- individual life experience; some people seem never to want to be alone or, by contrast, always appear to avoid others, but this is not the norm and usually means that solitude or interacting with others has become an emotionally threatening life experience;
- cultural life experience (World War II showed that the Japanese culture prepared soldiers quite well for long-lasting operations in solitude, in contrast with Asian Indians whose strength lay in operating in groups);
- circumstances (most people prefer to be alone when they have work to do, but prefer company for after hours relaxation).

Time gender also plays an important role in balancing the needs for social involvement and solitude. To begin with, alphas are socially inclined (extroverted) but they also depend for their outward-directed, situational self-esteem on social interaction. Betas, on the other hand, are inward directed (introverted) while their self-esteem is timescape-oriented and thus global.

Experiencing individuality versus group membership

There is another set of opposing social needs intersecting with the balance between the need for social interaction and the need for solitude. There are the need to experience oneself as an individual and the need to experience oneself as being part of a significant group. Although nowadays there is great emphasis on the need to experience oneself as a unique individual with individual rights, one should not underestimate the importance of the need to belong to a meaningful social network. For if this tribal need remains chronically unfulfilled, one becomes alienated. Since modern society is one of transition with the disintegration of many traditional social groupings, alienation is widespread. As a result, many socially regressive, closely knit, isolationist sub-cultures—from street gangs to religious or political sects—have emerged to substitute for lost social connections.

Let me now explore the role time gender plays in this balance between the need to be an individual and the need to belong to an emotionally significant group.

Alphas have a partitioned multifocal, contextual identity and value system, and a situational, outward-oriented self-esteem. Betas have a unified monofocal identity, a value system rooted in their timescape, and an inward-oriented, global self-esteem. The need to belong to an emotionally significant group with which they can identify is for alphas of primary importance while the need to be seen and behave as an individual remains secondary. For betas it is the other way around.

This modulates how alphas and betas relate to various institutions to which they belong. Since alphas experience their individuality as situational and discontinuous (their central existential problem may be: "Who is the real me?"), a social institution such as a firm of high prestige, the army, a religious or political sect, may readily provide them with an institution-derived identity. The institutional value system sets them apart from, and naturally holds precedence over, the value system of "outsiders." Thus the institution is their "tribe" and becomes their major source of self-esteem.

Because the value system of alphas is contextual, they identify more readily than betas with institutional values and expectations. They find comfort in identifying with externalized institutional goals because their forward planning and deliberate goal setting is not their strong suit. They tend to find comfort in explicitly stated institutional values or ethics and in the written rules their social environment offers. Sanctions placed on breaking these rules make for a more predictable environment.

Although betas may be very proud of the institution they belong to, they experience themselves (and by extension others) as individually unique and want to act and be treated as such. Individual initiative and success are more important to their self-esteem and identity than belonging to the institution. In group settings the individualism of betas often outweighs their need to belong and sets them apart from the others. It also renders their relationship to their institutions more calculated and less tribal in nature than in alphas. In the case of betas, institutional hierarchies should not be taken for granted but viewed as an arrangement that benefits all concerned.[1]

The attitude of betas toward institutional goals is quite different than of alphas. Betas often develop in their timescape their own ideas as to which direction the institution should move. Considering themselves (and hence everyone else) as individuals, they believe that people should express their personal opinions, even if deviating from stated institutional goals. They prefer personal over institutional positions. Since they already live with a rigid set of internalized rules (values), they favor as few additional prescriptive rules to adhere to as possible. Rather than having to break rules, they feel the rules should be changed. Furthermore, for betas value systems should not be selective but apply both to insiders and to outsiders. In sum, betas generally find it harder to identify with, and integrate smoothly into, institutional structures than alphas do. Public institutions will have less potential for fulfilling the tribal need of betas. Betas usually attempt to satisfy this need through more private, traditional ties within their community, such as church, clubs, friends and neighbors.

Time gender and social value systems

Sharing the same value system—a set of internalized rules about the desirability or undesirability of certain behaviors—is an important precondition for optimal social interaction. It reflects the internalization of the collective judgments of the culture or sub-culture to which one belongs.

I pointed out in Chapter 4, that in alphas self-esteem, as well as the value systems used in pursuing self-ideals, are predominantly contextual; in betas these are primarily rooted in their timescape and thus global. Because of their contextually partitioned, multifocal identity, the contextual value systems of alphas are, as a rule, not subject to self-reflecting scrutiny for trans contextual consistency by their singular paraego. Even when their paraego sometimes self-reflects on their trans contextual inconsistency in behavior and feeling, its apparent tolerance for such contradictions usually does not create undue discomfort. But sometimes, self-reflection on, or criticism by others of their situational flexibility in values becomes a problem. These alphas begin to feel confused. They may find an answer to this problem by adopting the outspoken value system of an influential elder they work with. Or they may find a solution in joining a group with a clear value system, a particular religion, for example. Upon adopting the value system of their newly found tribe they will feel reborn.

In this regard betas develop differently. Once self-reflection sets in during adolescence, they develop a certain intolerance for inconsistency in their overall value system and try to correct for this. This produces a more singular, consistent set of internalized rules. When facing environs with values that conflict with their own global values betas therefore exhibit a certain rigidity. For example, an alpha and a beta got at their workplace into a serious battle. This caused the beta to leave his job. Months later, when the two accidentally met in an entirely different context, the alpha pleasantly approached the beta, but the beta did not want to socialize with him and turned his back.

It is ironic that, while alphas are generally more flexible and betas more rigid in their overall value system, alphas tend to be more intolerant, and betas more tolerant toward others with different values. For example, when a value conflict between an alpha and beta occurs, the alpha is often inclined to attack the beta's ethics, rather than the other way around. Because alphas are inclined to view their particular contextual values as self-evident, they tend to take deviating values in that context as a personal threat. Although betas enjoy the security of assuming that their own value system is written in stone (in their timescape) they tend to appreciate individuality and, as long as they themselves remain free of a value conflict, can afford to be tolerant of others who hold different values. Note that I speak here of *tendencies,* not of matters that are written in stone.

Section 2: Time gender and interpersonal style

Prologue

Social behavior depends on the interaction of the social context and the personality of a participant, including one's time gender. Time gender by itself has many ways of impacting social behavior, depending on

- how alphas and betas differ in relating to time;
- how they contrast in regulating their mood and self-esteem;
- how they are dissimilar in experiencing their identity;
- how they differ in balancing interaction and solitude, and in individuality and group membership;
- how they differ in language use;
- how they differ in sexuality, partnering and parenting (chapter 7);
- how they differ in thinking (chapter 8); and
- how they have dissimilar inclinations in educational and occupational contexts (chapters 9 and 10).

Nevertheless, the impact of all these time gender features on social behavior is rarely clearly evident. The reason is that other variables often function as a curtain that covers them up. For example, an alpha with an avoidant trait, tends to avoid social contacts which, in turn, hides that person's natural social inclination. Or, if a beta has an engaging-exploring trait, that can make her or him appear to live in the present in 4–D rather than in the timescape in 6–D.

The relation between time gender and social behavior can be broken down into three major aspects: 1) the extroverted versus introverted style of interpersonal relating; 2) the authoritarian-competitive, as opposed to egalitarian-cooperative styles of interpersonal relating, and 3) the nature of a person's need for stimulation and response to familiar situations.

The alpha time gender is extroverted, the beta time gender introverted

I previously noted that alphas live in the world—their focus is on the here-and-now of 4–D—and they become natural extroverts as their time gender unfolds, just as betas, who prefer to live in their head—their timescape in 6–D—become natural introverts. In my terms, extroversion reflects that a person's preferred attention mode is 4–D, and introversion that a person's preferred attention mode is 6–D.

Jung made the terms "extroversion" and "introversion" popular.[2] He said that these types are so contrasting that even a layperson who has been made aware of them can recognize them.[3] Jung furthermore pointed already to the genetic nature of these two basic personality profiles by stating that they occur in all classes in society; that sexual gender does not play a role; and that their random distribution suggests a biological underpinning.[4]

Jung and I differ, however, significantly in our view on extroversion and introversion. To begin with, Jung did not account for extroversion and introversion as expressing a duality in how people relate to time. Instead, he seemed to have ascribed extroversion and introversion to what we now know to be the opposing, genetic traits of engaging, as opposed to avoiding, new stimulation, respectively. He wrote, for example, that when facing a situation, introverts at first draw back as if communicating an unvoiced "No," while extroverts immediately engage the situation, confident that their behavior is right. "But not all extroverts (alphas) have an engaging trait; many are avoidant; and not all introverts (betas) are avoidant; many have an engaging trait.

Furthermore, Jung claimed that extroversion and introversion were already noticeable shortly after birth.[5] But, according to the time gender model, introversion is not an option until time gender differentiation occurs in middle childhood. During the preceding 5-6 years, 4-D and 5-D are interwoven and constantly alternate, with 4-D playing an important role in cognition, thinking and fantasy, so that introversion is not yet an option for preschoolers. They do not yet experience their external stream of consciousness in 4-D and their inner stream of consciousness in 5-D as distinctly separate. What is noticeable shortly after birth is not whether the baby is extroverted or introverted, but whether the genetic personality trait of engaging or of avoiding dominates.[6] Jung's view is understandable because an adult extrovert (alpha) with an avoidant trait may be easily misidentified as introvert, just as an adult introvert (beta) with an engaging trait may be readily thought of as an extrovert.

Much research on the genetics of Jung's extroversion/introversion was done by the German-born British psychologist Hans J. Eysenck (1916-1997). Like Jung,[7] Eysenck considered that the structure of personality consists of dimensions or traits (such as extroversion-introversion) which can be scored and quantified through a personality questionnaire. Jung and Eysenck viewed "pure" extroversion and "pure" introversion as opposite poles on a continuum on which one may occupy any position—from extreme extroversion on the one end, to extreme introversion on the other, but with a higher probability of a middle position ("ambiversion").[8] Jung felt that, although a middle position is the ideal one, frequently one attitude is developed and the other remains unconscious, or is manifested in an inferior way.[9]

However, any single issue of major psychological and psychiatric journals testifies to a lack of precision in defining personality traits by featuring competing models of personality which do not overlap.[10] This means that, although "extroversion" is a central concept in virtually all theories and measures of personality,[11] the results of research that use personality questionnaires which define "extroversion" differently are not compatible.[12] It is therefore no surprise that Eysenck found that introverts appear to be more prone to fear and anxiety than extroverts,[13] whereas I found in my clinical practice that anxiety disorders neither favor extroverts (alphas) nor introverts (betas); or that Eysenck found that males tend to have higher extroversion scores than females,[14] whereas I showed that females outnumber males among extroverts (alphas);[15] or that Eysenck reaffirmed the correlation between extroverts and a short, rotund (pyknic) body build[16] (which the German psychiatrist Ernst Kretschmer (1888-1964) had proposed),[17] while I could not demonstrate any connection between such body build and being extroverted (alpha).

Jung's view that extroversion/introversion is a personality *trait* or *dimension* (variously defined by and measured through different personality inventories) clearly differs from my view that being alpha and extroverted personality type or class, on the one hand, and being beta and introverted on the other, reflect two mutually exclusive *classes* or *types* of people (such as female or male); someone is either alpha or beta. While personality inventories that measure extroversion/introversion may be used to assign a *probability* of someone being alpha and extroverted or beta and introverted, Eysenck's work demonstrated that the results of these personnel questionnaires may be contaminated by various other variables. In sum, the extrovert/introvert distinction as proclaimed by Jung cannot explain many differences between alphas and betas as described in this book.

This is not to say that Jung did not list correctly many characteristics of extraverts (the alpha time gender) and of introverts (the beta time gender). [18] He stated, for example, that the "objective" environment [4-D], rather than a "subjective" view [6-D] dominates the consciousness of extroverts, [19] so that extroverts' decisions and deeds are determined by situational factors rather than by "subjective" ones.[20] He was right also in assuming that the inner life of extroverts remains secondary to external pressure [from 4-D], and that introverts interpose a "subjective" view between perceiving the environment and acting in it [because introverts look at the world in 4-D through their timescape in 6-D].[21]

Authoritarian-competitive versus egalitarian-cooperative interpersonal style

Humans were certainly not the first to evolve social behavior with social needs as its underpinning. Social needs first appeared when egg-yielding reptiles evolved into breast-feeding mammals perhaps some 300 million years ago.[22] Mammals began living in groups with a hierarchy in which each mammal establishes its place through dominance-submission fights, resulting in a social role division, including leadership, fighting to death to protect the young or the herd, food gathering, and so on, an arrangement serving the survival of the individual animals as well as of that of the group.

The mammalian hierarchical power structure based on dominance-submission fights is readily recognizable in human groups whether, for example, economic, political, or occupational in nature. When this dominance-submission theme expresses itself at an interpersonal level, we may call the relationship authoritarian-competitive. Both participants compete as to who shall be the author of the rules and who will submit to those rules. Having won the dominance-submission fight the authoritarian one is no longer accountable, but the submissive one remains accountable at all times.

The classical model of the authoritarian relationship is the one between parent and child in which parental authority is normally used to protect, socialize and educate the child. Any authoritarian relationship, therefore, can be said to reflect a kind of parent-child relationship, whether involving business partners, romantic partners, friends, doctor and patient, lawyer and client, or pastors and their congregation. Options open to the dominated one include unconditional submission, proactive cooperation, passive resistance, open rebellion, or mustering enough courage to leave.

There is, however, a uniquely human alternative to the authoritarian interpersonal style of the parent-child relationship. This alternative has its roots in the peer relationship between children that emerges during the later elementary school years. When with peers, a child may suddenly realize that saying "No!" no longer means disobedience to parental authority, but rather a disagreement between friends. Reaching agreement is no longer yielding to a quasi-parental authority with one winning and the other losing, but rather reaching a compromise between two equals. This is the beginning of the egalitarian-cooperative interpersonal style of relating.

Whether one is dealing with such an egalitarian-cooperative relationship at a personal or (far less frequently) at an institutional level, cooperation and negotiation based on mutuality and reciprocity replace competitive authoritarianism. One-party-control is replaced by a committee of participants in which all parties have equal status in fulfilling their needs, equal accountability for their actions, and an equal stake in decision making.

The spontaneous alpha style is authoritarian-competitive

For alphas the territory for the pursuit of happiness and peace of mind is the here-and-now. As a result, they are forever vigilant in scanning 4–D for opportunities to fulfill their needs and avoid dangers. Without pre-living their future and re-living their past, however, each new day feels like an inherently unpredictable, new beginning. As a consequence, alphas typically believe that one should leave as little as possible to chance, and their best insurance policies against surprises are 1) to have as much structure in 4–D as possible through institutional goals, rules, and stated ethics; and 2) to have as much control in and over their 4–D as possible, making 4–D not only an arena for pursuing self-esteem, but also for securing the best possible position in the relevant hierarchy.

Even when around the age of nine or ten, young alphas begin to experience other children as peers, they intuit this as their playing field for dominance-submission fights as opposed to one of equal opportunity. Which sibling or friend can out-negotiate or out-perform the other? Whose needs will dominate? Who will have a higher standing in class? This rivalry continues into adulthood. Among equals, alphas try to be more equal than others. Alphacizing everybody, they assume that everyone considers all interpersonal relationships, including those between peers, as competitive and authoritarian. As a result, they confront others with their needs as they arise. The exception to this is those alphas who previously learned, as in an optimal parent-child relationship, to adjust their impulse control for their own personal growth.

In enhancing control over their 4–D through their competitive approach, alphas intuitively rely on certain qualities in out-maneuvering not only alphas who are intellectually less endowed, but also betas. This makes their behavior generally predictable in a number of ways.

- Being extroverted, alphas live in the world and derive from their multitude of relationships various degrees of expertise and comfort in dealing with others. This exceeds what introverted betas derive from their more limited number of relationships.

- Living in 4–D alphas are not distracted by past and future implications. Hence, they develop an ability to assess a here-and-now situation and the people involved. This leaves them socially and situationally more perceptive, and makes them better interpersonal tacticians than betas in as much as interpersonal relationships are viewed as confrontations.

- Their partitioned, multifocal identity makes alphas natural actors in picking and performing the most effective role to control the situation at hand. They may take a humble approach; appear helpless; play the unhappy victim with an irresistible appeal for help; be helpful and ingratiating; act attractive, appealing and charming; or, by contrast, tough as nails, if not overpowering.

- Alphas display various levels of skill in adjusting their contextual use of language (as opposed to the more generalized language use of betas) to their particular audience and circumstance. They find the exact words to fit the occasion. For example, they are good at promoting their own values while making the values of their opponents sound unattractive.

In a personal context, alphas practice their dominance-submission challenge in every relationship. Think about doctors who do not like to be questioned by their patients, or lawyers who want to control their cases rather than function as counselor to their clients. Their time gender forces them to relentlessly try to gain, or maintain, or regain control over their 4–D. Believing that others share this attitude, they assume that trusting others without strings attached is a sign of weakness and will lead to being taken advantage of. Trusting someone is possible only with appropriate control mechanisms in place.

At work, in the community, or in a political party a typical dream of alphas is to reach the top of that hierarchy. Short of this, they strive to gain as much ascendancy in the pecking order as their wit and intelligence permit. In order to protect and reinforce their current position, they keep their superiors as happy as possible, while exercising firm control over their subordinates. It is not unknown for them to use explicitly stated codes of ethics to justify their actions while criticizing the actions of others. Knowing intuitively that in institutional settings knowledge is power, they are possessive of, if not secretive about their own data base, while rigidly controlling the flow of information between those above and below them. Notwithstanding statements to the opposite, their spontaneous, unguarded institutional behavior tends to reflect an implicit value system that accepts a natural order in the world in which everyone has their place. They believe that in this hierarchy power is a basic given which needs no justifications and entitles the powerful to privileges. Furthermore, mistakes are blamed on underlings. This may seem like the individual who looks up and kicks down. But there is more to the alpha than that. In order to climb the hierarchical ladder and feel more secure (and who does not want to?) one must look for opportunities to dethrone the one above. As a result, alphas assume a latent, yet unavoidable power struggle throughout the hierarchical structure. The more powerful can never trust those with less power. They must exhibit their own power as much as possible, and, where feasible, divide and rule.[23]

Pursuing control in their interpersonal or institutional 4–D does not mean that alphas are always driven by selfish motives. As parent, spouse, physician or lawyer, for example, their motives remain basically mammalian in character, meaning they may be just as often altruistic — as in protecting the herd or their offspring with their life, — as selfish as in being the first to eat and taking the choicest pieces of food.

Despite potential advantages in their competitive jousts, among alphas there are more losers than winners. All being winners would result in social disintegration rather than in social hierarchies with role division. Furthermore, alphas do not only have to compete among each other, but also with betas, some of whom are highly skilled and motivated in turning their future timescape into a reality.

Despite their competitive-authoritarian attitude alphas may establish small, cooperative alliances in which the struggle for one-sided control is replaced by a more cooperative style between peers of equal value and importance. In this case, power as a tool for control in 4–D is abandoned and replaced by negotiation with compromise so that nobody wins or loses.

Egalitarian-cooperative relating is a natural beta optionn

Rather than being preoccupied with controlling their present in 4–D, betas are more concerned with controlling the future in 6–D which holds the key toward their global self-esteem. Just as alphas take for granted that everyone experiences the social reality in 4–D as a constant dominance-submission challenge, so betas assume that everyone pursues their own future in 6–D and is entitled to do so without interference. In this regard betas prefer cooperation over confrontation.

As previously mentioned, the seed for this egalitarian-cooperative option is planted when, around age eight or nine, children experience their first peer relationships. At this point the time cones of young betas have already been developing for a few years. These young betas are already learning to negotiate a compromise between future-oriented pressures from their timescape in 6–D and here-and-now demands from the social reality and their own impulses in 4–D. During adolescence, the personal future of these young betas gradually gains in depth and stability while self-reflection is added. Egalitarian cooperation becomes progressively more desirable as opposed to the authoritarian style of relating to others.

One should remember, however, that like alphas, betas are driven by their self-talk which reflects the authoritarian relationship they once had with their parents. The egalitarian-cooperative attitude young betas start to display is still driven by their authoritarian automatic self-talk in 5–D. As a result the authoritarian relationship toward themselves in 5–D can readily spill over into 4–D. What may begin as an egalitarian-cooperative attitude may unwittingly slip into an authoritarian-competitive one as they project their parent-child experience into an emotionally charged relationship, such as a troubled marriage. In due course, the present relationship becomes the same as those they experienced in childhood.[24] When displaying a cooperative-egalitarian attitude, betas do not transcend the prototypical authoritarian relationship with their parents unless their paraego in 7–D matures. Developing a strong mature paraego, however, may often require considerable professional assistance.

In an emotionally charged marital situation between an alpha and a beta, the latter is preoccupied with what has to be done for the future, while the alpha is concerned with the present. Neither understands where the other is coming from.

The beta belief that the future should somehow fall in line with their expectations explains why they have frequently explode suddenly like a volcano. Betas often defer confronting bothersome interpersonal issues until their accumulating frustration eventually reaches its limit. This results in a delayed explosive confrontation with much angry berating of the other's past performance. If the other is an alpha, he or she may well respond in genuine puzzlement: "But why didn't you tell me how much I was upsetting you when it first started?"

Two specific genetic traits should not be confused with time gender. 1) Both alphas and betas may be strongly competitive in a way unrelated to time gender. When facing a particular challenge, these people just want to win, despite the fact that in interpersonal relationships such competitive betas may be very inclined toward an egalitarian-cooperative approach; and 2) Some alphas and betas have an inborn leadership drive. Often this is already noticeable by middle childhood. For alphas with their built-in drive to control 4–D becoming a leader is not a particular challenge. Betas must learn, however, that the road toward leadership often requires maneuvering for power in and control over 4–D. But for betas, achieving power over 4–D does not translate into emotional security and self-esteem as it does for alphas. Rather, it gives betas the means to achieve the goals they have set for their group, corporation, army, or country.

Curiosity, resilience to boredom, and time gender

Being curious engenders a broader variety in one's overall knowledge base. Inquisitive people easily get bored in familiar situations. On the other hand, those who are less curious are less likely to be bored with familiar situations. As a result, their reservoir of information is less varied and less broad, but will have greater depth because their experience has been more focused.

For betas, the past and future are part of a stable, familiar timescape in 6–D. As we know, they are introverted and live a great deal in their familiar timescape. This makes them more resilient to boredom in habitual, familiar situations in 4–D than alphas. Indeed they prefer 4–D input with a familiar ring to it (it is in line with their timescape) over a variety of input that is new and unrelated to their 6–D. The preoccupation of betas with their timescape tends to put a brake on their appetite for stimulation in 4–D.

Alphas of course live in the world rather than in their head. Their 6–D is without a stable past or future timescape. They lack a brake on their appetite for stimulation in 4–D, nor do they have preferential restrictions on their 4–D input. Alphas are by nature more curious, have a greater stimulus appetite, and get more readily bored by the familiar aspects of life than betas. They are interested in new and varied input. They are much more concerned with avoiding boredom than betas. For example, recreational activities that break the daily routine, like going out for dinner or a movie, are more sought after by alphas than betas. Indeed, betas often avoid much of the stimulation alphas seek, which might distract, if not over stimulate them.

When alphas find themselves in a monotonous environment — say, on the subway or alone at a restaurant — they readily turn to reading something. Most of them are, indeed, voracious readers of diverse materials, rather than pursuing a set of limited areas of interest. It is not unusual to find a pile of unrelated books or journals at their bedside. They often are informed about a broad range of subjects. When betas, whose interest in 4–D is less driven, find themselves in monotonous environment, they more likely contemplate their timescape, or read the newspaper to keep up to date, or study a paper or book related to their occupation. Their reading habits tend to be more selective and, as a result, their knowledge available for conversation more restricted. Alphas tend to be more entertaining and since they are also more sociable, they are genuinely curious about people and often come out of a transient encounter with a stranger with all kinds of personal information. Habitual interpersonal relations, however, soon tend to become boring to alphas, which is why they seek to establish and maintain a broad range of interpersonal involvements. Betas, on the other hand, are more low key and reserved. They usually tend to restrict the range of their interpersonal relations. It usually takes them time to get personally interested in someone they encounter, and it takes others time to get to know them.

Alphas not only seek a variety of interpersonal relations, they also like a change of scene. They enjoy traveling too. Alphas are also more inclined to get bored with where they live, and change residence with greater ease, and more frequency than betas. Betas travel because holidays are part of their timescape, or provide a culturally prescribed excuse to get away from what they are doing without having to feel guilty. They tend to change residence less frequently than alphas. It is in this context easy to speculate that once Europeans landed on the East Coast of North America, there were more alphas than betas among those who began drifting westward. As a result, I would hypothesize that the current culture of the West Coast of North America is more alpha-oriented, and the one of the East Coast more beta-oriented.

Section 3: Time gender interfacing

My Vancouver sample of 405 subjects contained 60% alphas (38% females, 22% males) and 40% betas (16% females and 24% males).[25] I argue elsewhere that his alpha-beta distribution is more or less representative of the general population of Greater Vancouver, B.C., Canada.[26] This distribution may not be applicable to other populations, However, my sample suggests that interaction with one's opposite time gender—time gender interfacing—is a frequent, if not daily, occurrence. It often involves spouses, and therefore the resulting children and siblings. But time gender interfacing occurs between friends, teacher and pupil, doctor and patient, lawyer and client, and employer and employee. Given the frequency of time gender interfacing, it is worthwhile knowing how alphas and betas respond to one another.

There are two fundamental problems in time gender interfacing. The first has to do with the fact that alphas and betas are unable to be spontaneously empathic with each other. A few words about the concept of empathy are in order here. The central meaning of the term is the process of feeling oneself into the entire conscious state of others, of knowing what they are aware of,[27] including their mood, needs, motives and intentions, how they think, grasping their psychic life.[28] Some consider one's empathic capacity an innate human endowment,[29] just as basic as vision, hearing, touch, taste, and smell.[30] In any case, the empathic capacity to know the psychological state of others is far from infallible, particularly in time gender interfacing, Alphas do not understand what people with a timescape are all about, while betas do not comprehend what it is like to live in the here-and-now. Because their interpretations are wrong, their empathic understanding is off. This problem is far from insurmountable. My clinical experience tells me that, when people of opposite time genders gain adequate knowledge of the time gender model, they develop a mutual, more realistic empathic insight into one another.

A second fundamental problem in time gender interfacing is the opposite ways in which alphas and betas spontaneously tend to assign blame. In attempting to account for the source of conflict, alphas, looking around in 4–D, tend to blame the other. This is not helpful because by blaming someone else, they deprive themselves of any control over their part. By contrast, when betas try to explain an interpersonal problem they usually start searching their timescape in 6–D for the answer, ending up blaming themselves. This is not helpful either. By accepting responsibility for the other's behavior — and therefore all responsibility — they pretend to be more powerful than they are.

Assuming there is shared blame and given how alphas and betas tend to assign blame, one can easily imagine what happens when two people of the opposite time gender run into trouble with each other. The alpha tends to blame the beta, who tends to accept responsibility and tries in vain to make the problem disappear. But only a fundamental change in attitude on both sides can produce a solution. The alpha has to learn to retrieve half of the blame from the beta, and the beta must learn to allow the alpha to accept half. One of my female clients was an alpha whose husband was a beta. After she got familiar with the time gender model, she became exasperated with her husband's continued tendency to hold himself responsible for whatever went wrong, exclaiming: "Where do I come in? You are diminishing me!"

Rationalizing behavior of the opposite time gender

How do people who are unknowingly involved in time gender interfacing deal with behavior that is out of line with their own time gender? Since the involved behaviors may be subtle to begin with, they may well allow for a temporary quasi-understanding of the other time gender with each putting their spin on what happens. In these cases one's "understanding" is simply based on pseudo-empathy and amounts to saying: "If I were in that position then I would behave that way too."

Selective denial may work for a long time. Usually it fails because there is a tolerance threshold. Although both alphas and betas may begin with common sense reasoning, alpha common sense is not the same as beta common sense. In the end, trying to reason things out frustrates both parties while each tries to convert the other to their point of view, a sense of polarity emerges and conflict ensues. Short of converting the other, the best one now can expect is a skewed harmony with one person dominating the other, revolt resulting in a trade-off, stalemate, if not complete relationship breakdown. No matter what the eventual outcome of the conflict, one still needs to answer why the other behaved the way he or she did. Once alpha- and beta-spinning, selective denial, and common sense reasoning have run their course, people usually find some other way to rationalize the behavior of the opposite time gender.

Some simply replace their hidden time gender bias with a sexual gender bias as in "only a woman would do this kind of thing; women are just that way, you know..." or "only a man would do this; that is the way men are." However, when men and women try to establish a creative partnership by mistaking time gender behavior for female or male behavior, this locks them into a counterproductive view of the opposite sex. The fact remains that there is not one kind of man and not one kind of woman, but alpha men and beta men, and alpha women and beta women. Confusing sexual gender and time gender goes back a long way. Early Chinese philosophy introduced 2,500 years ago the Yin and Yang symbols as representing femaleness and maleness, respectively. This symbolic meaning still is current, not only in modern Chinese thinking, but also in Western thinking. Jung, for example, compared the feminine Yin with the mother archetype and the masculine Yang with the father archetype.[31] Elsewhere, however, Jung spoke of the Yin person as "the man of the earth, whose attitude is permeated by the earth under his feet," and of the Yang person as the one "whose chief characteristic is an attitude conditioned by ideas."[32] This suggests that Jung not only used the Yang and Yin symbols as explicitly referring to the sexual gender duality but implicitly also to the time gender duality, with Yin the representing the earthbound alpha and Yang representing the idealistically oriented beta.

Another popular way of making sense of behavior which is out of step with one's own time gender is to fall back on fashionable quasi-psychological explanations, such as some alleged or real trauma suffered in one's past. Talk shows are full of this. Others "explain" such behavior through a host of religious, class, or racial biases. Mental health professionals have been blatant in defining one time gender behavior as "normal," and the other as "disordered," "sick," and in need of treatment. Freud and Jung gave the lead in this, for Freud interpreted alpha behavior as pathologic, while Jung interpreted beta behavior that way. The response of an interfacing alpha and beta may well be for either one to say to the other: "I think you have a problem. Maybe you should seek some professional help..."

Section 4: Time gender linguistics

This chapter concludes with focusing on language because shared language is an essential prerequisite for any meaningful social interaction. People have put their faith in shared language as the royal road toward greater, mutual understanding and peaceful cooperation since the days of Confucius (551-479 BCE). Language is, however, more than just a medium through which people exchange information about their private conscious experience. It also structures how we experience reality in that there is a circular feedback between language and the way we experience reality (see figure 6.1 next page).

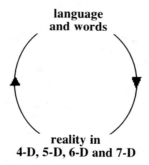

**language
and words**

**reality in
4-D, 5-D, 6-D and 7-D**

Figure 6.1: The circular feedback between language and reality

English is rich in the areas involving individuality and democracy. Chinese languages are deficient in this regard.[33] They stress groups, rather than individuals.[34] Instead of having only a single word for "we" as in English, Mandarin Chinese has two: one inclusive we, "zamen" (this includes the addressed person), the other an exclusive we, "women" (referring to the speaker and one or more others, but excluding the person being addressed). On the other hand, Chinese languages have unlike English an abundance of words for various relatives.[35] Mandarin does not have a word that fully corresponds to the Western "guilt," (a painful individual emotion that is unrelated to being in the presence of others). Instead, they verbalize something akin to the Western "shame" (a painful emotion related to the actual, or imagined, presence of others). This makes it nearly impossible to translate the works of Freud, which speak a great deal about guilt, into Mandarin. Such translation was made, but turned out grossly deficient and earned only ridicule.

Another example of the relationship between language and the structure of reality is that Western languages have a clear, built-in discrimination of tenses in their verbs, which express an action as either having occurred in the past, or occurring in the present or future. This "common sense" concept of time in the West reflects a continually changing 4–D reality with a linear arrow of time extending from the past through the present into the future, and consisting of an orderly sequence of quantitative durations. The languages of the Indian subcontinent, however—both ancient (Sanskrit) and modern—structure time very differently. For example, in Hindustani the same word, "kal," means both "yesterday" and "tomorrow"; the word "parson" means the "day after tomorrow" as well as the "day before yesterday." Their "common sense" of time is circular and static, without beginning and end.[36]

To give further examples of this feedback between language and reality experience, the Zulu language has a word for "red cow," and a completely unrelated word for "white cow," but not a single word for "cow."[37] Similarly, there is in Western languages a complete conceptual separation between the word "space" and the word "time." There is no single word that embraces space and time as a single concept. " The language of the North American Hopi Indians, on the other hand, apparently always indicates both where (3-D) and when (4th-D) an action occurs and has therefore a built-in time-space grid, which in my model I refer to as 4–D. One linguist claimed that if the Hopi would have reached a level of Western scientific sophistication, they would have arrived automatically at the relativity theory of Einstein, who had to abandon his mother tongue and find rescue in the language of mathematics in order to develop his famous theory of relativity.[38]

While different languages structure the same reality differently, this also happens when different populations use the same language.[39] Winston Churchill was quoted as saying that "England and the US are two nations divided by a common language."[40] But even within the same nation, the language and reality of various age groups is quite dissimilar,[41] just as male language is often inadequate in describing female feelings, as is female language in describing male feelings.[42] The lingo of the legal, medical, civil service, police and military professions each create within a given language their own view of reality. Since alphas and betas experience reality quite differently, one can expect each time gender to occasionally use language that expresses these differences. For instance, "Out of sight, out of mind" was coined by alphas and resonates more with alphas. The same applies to Sir William Osler's statement: "Live for the day only, and for the day's work...The chief worries of life arise from the foolish habit of looking before and after." [43] On the other hand, "Absence makes the heart grow fonder" was coined by betas and resonates more with betas, just as Galsworthy's statement: "If you do not think about the future, you cannot have one."[44]

There are, however, far more subtle differences in how alphas and betas use language. For example, let us say there is an alpha and a beta each of whom is of the same age, sex, intelligence, ethnic origin, religion, socio-economic class, education, occupation, and so on. Now, if each person uses the same word, they still may convey profoundly different meanings. When time gender differences start to crystallize during middle childhood, time gender linguistics enters the picture. The crux of time gender linguistics is that words, which for alphas may have a rather flexible, situational connotation, have for betas a more fixed meaning. This naturally adds to the rife mutual misunderstanding that already exists in time gender interfacing, which is based on the fact that alphas alphacize, and betas betacize each other.

Some examples

Words like "guilt" or "anxiety" mean different things to alphas and to betas. A female alpha client, very conversant with the time gender model, told me one day:

> *"Last weekend my father made me feel really guilty because I didn't want to help him out."*

"Are you still feeling bad right now?"

> *"No, not really."*

"Well, if you would still have felt bad right now, it would have been a typical example of what a beta experiences as guilt. In the eyes of a beta, your father made you feel bad last weekend, not guilty. For betas, guilt refers to bad feelings that continue to nag them for some time. Only when a guilt-provoking event moves deeper and deeper in their posterior cone and, eventually, out of reach of their time-distance-perception, do they get rid of it."

Along similar lines, alphas and betas give different meanings to the word "anxiety." When alphas have a vision of a feared future image, they experience a momentary fear, which they call anxiety, but in betas anxiety means a persistent negative emotion in response to a threatening event in their future timescape.

The word "goal" is another example. An alpha shared with me his enthusiastic vision on the future: "I want to become a social worker!" However, in short order he became distracted by alternative options and never followed through on becoming a social worker. Alphas only achieve a goal they envision at one point if their feedback from 4–D continuously reinforces their vision of the future; their endowment is quite up to the challenge; and they like the work involved. When a beta emphatically states: "I want to become a social worker," this represents a goal which is built into her or his future timescape, and is therefore more likely to evoke relevant goal-directed action, whether 4–D is favorable or not; whether the effort involved comes easy to them or not; or whether they particularly enjoy it or not.

A final example: Years ago, a beta told me that, prior to his taking a senior position in an organization, he seriously worried about potential problems that might be involved. He therefore discussed his concerns with the man who was to be his superior, an alpha. At the time, the other man was strongly supportive and reassuring, so he took the job. A few months later the anticipated problems materialized, yet his superior was not supportive at all. The beta then went over their previous "agreement." The boss seemed genuinely puzzled: "Did I say that?" Nonetheless, the beta came away feeling he had once more convinced his superior of the righteousness of his position. In fact, this time he made, in fact, sure their understanding was put on paper and signed by both of them. Yet, six months later the story repeated itself. This time his superior was not only unsupportive but outright antagonistic. The beta then showed him their written agreement. His superior seemed puzzled and exclaimed: "But, my dear fellow, this was six months ago! The present situation is entirely different. Things change, you know!" Had a beta been in the position of the superior, he would have gone to his subordinate ahead of time and have said: "Listen, we have to renegotiate our agreement, for circumstances are changing."

About learning alpha speak and beta speak

At some stage of evolution, language evolved and then, with the betacization of some members of a tribes, the time gender duality emerged. Alphas continued to orient themselves to the here-and-now, while betas began to orient themselves to their new timescape with its coherent, stable past and future. One may reasonably assume that, depending on one's time perspective, certain words implicitly acquired a different connotation, such as the word "goal" or "agreement" in modern language. The new betas also began to reflect in the language they used the trans contextual nature of their novel timescape. If, for example, prior to betacization, the meaning of the same word had varied across different contexts, betas began to restrict the use of this word to a specific context, or replace it with a new, context-specific word. They also began to add new words with a fixed meaning across several contexts. These gradual language changes became a challenge to the alphas in the tribe. They had to learn to interpret the language which betas used in a situationally meaningful way. This evolutionary story repeats itself during the development of children.

During the preschool years, fixing the meaning of words is not yet a high priority; what is important is perceptually structuring the 4–D reality. Once the perceptual world in 4–D has become sufficiently stabilized, however — this happens around age 5 — the child discovers it can mentally manipulate objects in 5–D by using the words for these objects, and soon becomes enamored with this magic power of words.[45] Thus, children's interest in the precise, stable, socially agreed upon meaning of words becomes a major focus. Nevertheless, at this stage the child does not yet understand abstract concepts, such as: "Love is the profoundly passionate, tender affection for another person." Instead, children must explain the meaning of love by saying something like: "Love is what Mommy and Daddy feel for each other." Even so, children do not usually learn the meaning of words by giving them concrete examples. Instead, they intuitively figure out their meaning from the context in which adults use them.

At this point young betas are just beginning to experience their budding timescape. Mastering timescape attitudes is for them just another instance of intuitively zeroing in on the meaning of words. Because young alphas are unfamiliar with a timescape, responding to how a beta expresses her or his attitudes through language is more than a challenge to figure out the contextual meaning of words. Young alphas are in this regard like congenitally blind children who intuitively learn to use visual language in a situationally meaningful way, as: "I see what you mean," "Yes, that looks good," "Can I see you for a moment?" A young alpha becomes an expert in intuitively figuring out in a particular context, the appropriate word that will satisfy a timescape-oriented beta for whom that word has a fixed meaning. In this process, they naturally pick up a lot from at least one alpha parent, or alpha teachers, or older alpha siblings who have already mastered situational beta semantics. This helps the young alphas to associate timescape language with their own relevant experiences.

In this light, it is worthwhile remembering that alphas are extroverts. As a result, their language is far more oriented toward making sense to others than the language of the introverted betas, for whom making sense to themselves comes first. Since alphas have to learn flexibility in using timescapelanguage under a variety of circumstances by trial and error, they become good at using *all* language situationally, reaching for the right word at the right time. They soon learn that appealing to the heart and emotions is, as a rule, far more effective than appealing to logic. They are good at persuading other people.

Walesa and Mazowiecki

A perfect example of the contrast between alpha and beta speak played out in the fall of 1990, during the presidential elections in Poland. The two main contenders were a charismatic alpha, Lech Walesa, the Chairman of the Solidarity union which had pioneered the way out of Communist rule, and a rather uninspiring, aloof and removed beta, Tadeusz Mazowiecki, the Prime Minister of Poland. Mazowiecki had responded to his country's economic crisis by courageously planning Poland's economic future with meticulous thoroughness, and imposing on hi country his daring and radical economic program for a rapid transition from communist principles to a free market economy.[46]

Walesa invoked, with ringing proclamations of nationhood and professions of Catholic faith, the stubborn national spirit that allowed Poland to survive partitions over many centuries. Although a highly intelligent man, he did not elaborate in great detail on the issues he talked about. He was therefore easily understood, and this had a powerful appeal. Mazowiecki, on the other hand, preached tolerance for national minorities, instead of responding to prevailing contemporary emotional themes. He asked Poles to vote with their heads rather than with their hearts, and contemplate how the country of tomorrow should be and how to get there. Being obsessionally driven by the orderly unfolding economic plan in his future timescape, he felt that as long as he knew where to take the country, it was not all that important for others to understand exactly how this would work. All that mattered was that they believed in him. Instead of using simple, emotionally colored, highly communicative language, he tended to use complex correct formulations which failed to set those around him afire, except for those who thought at his level and shared his perception of the future. In the end, he missed popular appeal and lost the election.

NOTES

1   Hofstede (1980), quoted by Aris (1998a)
2   Jung (1977), p. 3.
3   Jung (1977), p. 330.
4   Jung (1977), p. 331.
5   Jung (1977), p. 332.
6   Thomas, Chess & Birch (1968). Another way of looking at engaging versus avoiding is to define same quantitatively by high or low scores on one of the five domains of the Five-factor-model's personality questionnaire, the NEO-PI-R, namely "openness to experience (O)" [Costa and McCrae (1992)]. Avoidant and engaging traits can already be recognized in many animals. I know in this respect of two cats, Chester who hastily avoids any contact with unfamiliar people, and Keith who readily explores such contents for whatever possibilities they may contain. They clearly demonstrate that these traits are distinct from introversion and extroversion which cannot possibly be attributed to them.
7   Jung (1977), p. 333.
8   Eysenck (1968), p. 165-166.
9   Fordham (1978), p.31.

10 Jang, Vernon and Livesley (2001), p. 236.
11 Jang, Vernon and Livesley (2001), p. 236.
12 Depue and Collins (1999) quoted by Jang et al. (2001), p. 236; (2001), p. 223.
13 Eysenck (1977), Gilbert et al. (1994).
14 Eysenck and Eysenck (1985); Eysenck (1987), p. 50.
15 See Chapter 1 under *The inversed female : male ratio among alphas and betas.*
16 Eysenck (1968), p. 170; Eysenck (1960).
17 Kretschmer (1936).
18 Jung (1977).
19 Jung (1970), p. 54.
20 Jung (1977), p. 333-334, 373-374.
21 Jung (1977), p. 333, 373-374.
22 Ross et al. (2005).
23 This section reflects "power renunciation" (strong acceptance of differences in personal power), as quoted from Hofstede (1980) by Aris (1998a).
24 In psychoanalytic psychotherapy this phenomenon is referred to as "transference." The transference in alphas and betas differs in that transference in alphas is re-living situational 4-D experiences, while transference in betas is re-living earlier overall patterns of parent-child interaction.
25 See Figure 1.1.
26 See Appendix 1 *(The research sample)*.
27 Wispé (1987), p. 34. The term "empathy" was coined by Tichener (1909)."
28 Stein (1964), p. 11.
29 Stein (1964), p. 34.
30 Kohut (1977), p. 144.
31 Jung (1964), p. 35).
32 Jung (1964), p. 484.
33 Kristof (1991).
34 Barmé, quoted by Kristof (1991), p. 10.
35 Kristof (1991).
36 Nakamura (1964), p. 79-81.
37 Jesperson (1964), p. 429.
38 Whorf (1956).
39 Yamamoto (1975), p. 235.
40 Coles (2000).
41 For example, if a four year old enters a building on one set of stairs to exit via another, it may call the former "the going-up stairs" and the latter" the going-down stairs." The child only wants to re-enter the building by way of the going-up stairs and leave again via the going-down stairs. The eight year old calls both stairs just stairs, and feels free to enter and leave the building by either set.
42 Orasanu et al. (1979).
43 Osler (1913).
44 Galsworthy (1928)
45 Piaget (1929).
46 Engelberg (1990).

CHAPTER 7

Time Gender And Sexuality, Partnering, And Parenting

This chapter will rely on statistical data I obtained from 273 successive clients seen during 1987-1989. This sample is approximately representative of the corresponding general population of Greater Vancouver, BC, Canada.[1] Findings based on these data should therefore be more or less valid for the Vancouver general population which, in turn, may give these findings a wider validity. Other researchers will have to confirm or deny this, but none of the conclusions about how alphas and betas behave sexually, as intimate partners, or as parents, will be mutually exclusive. These conclusions only point out that among alphas the tendency to behave in a certain way is stronger or weaker than among betas, or that time gender plays no role. This is consistent with the fact that behavior usually is the product of several interactive determinants.

A person's age influences one's sexual behavior, partnering, and parenting. The age of my subjects at the time of data collection is therefore relevant to this chapter. Figure 7.1 highlights the age distribution in my research cohort and shows that 64% were between the ages of 25 and 44. While this indicates that the majority of the subjects were of prime child-bearing age, it also indicates the generation to which they belong.

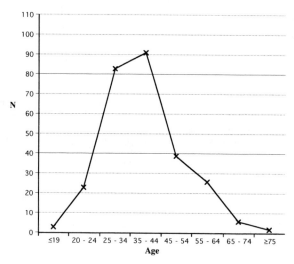

Figure 7.1: Age distribution of subjects in the 1987-1989 data sample (N=273)

Figure 7.2 shows that just under 2/3 of the subjects were born between 1946 and 1965 and thus belong to the baby boom generation, while 1/3 fitted into the generation that precedes, and only 6% into the one that follows the baby boomers.

However, despite the potential role of age and generation, this chapter will demonstrate that alphas and betas show distinctly different trends in some specific aspects of their sexuality and partnering and parenting.

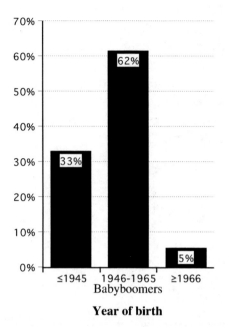

Figure 7.2: Birth year distribution of subjects in the 1987-1989 data sample (N=273)

In measuring the quantitative difference in the responses of men and women to any variable one may be testing, up until now the alpha-beta duality within each sex remained a masked and unaccounted for variable. Whether from a statistical point of view a difference in values between the sexes is significant or not, men and women are not homogenous groups, for I found that the values of responses of alpha and beta men frequently differ significantly, as do the responses of alpha and beta women. Often there is, by contrast, a statistically significant difference between how alphas and betas respond to such a variable, with the difference between alpha men and alpha women, and between beta men and beta women not being significant. Once the time gender duality is known in behavioral research, one should therefore, where possible, compare not only the sexual genders, but also the time genders.

- Section 1 on sexuality discusses the relation between time gender and sexual orientation, the age of first sexual intercourse, the incidence of engaging in casual sex and the occurrence of abortion.

- Section 2 on partnering discusses first whether time gender plays a role in remaining single as opposed to partnering; and how it influences choosing one's partner, and the prevalence of the four time gender combinations in marriage (alpha-alpha, beta-beta, alpha-beta, and beta-alpha).

- Section 3 first reviews statistical data about alphas and betas as intimate partners and parents; then discusses identical time gender marriages (alpha-

alpha and beta-beta marriages) and, finally, time gender interfacing marriages (marriages between an alpha and a beta).

Section 1: time gender and sexuality

Sexual orientation

Most people choose a partner of the opposite sex, some choose a partner of the same sex. Bisexuals find satisfaction with partners of either sexual gender. Table 7.1 shows the sexual orientation (self-identified) of my cohort of 273 subjects, broken down by sexual gender and time gender. The sample did not include exclusively lesbian women. As a result, heterosexual women were slightly over-represented and the total group of homosexuals under-represented.

Sexual orientation N	<-----ALPHA----->			<-----BETA----->			<------TOTAL------>		
	male	female	total	male	female	total	male	female	total
Heterosexual	43	99	142	60	45	105	103	144	247
Homosexual	10	0	10	7	0	7	17	0	17
Bisexual	4	4	8	0	0	0	4	4	8
Un known	1	0	1	0	0	0	1	0	1
Total (N)	58	103	161	67	45	112	125	148	273

Sexual orientation %-age	<-----ALPHA----->			<-----BETA----->			<------TOTAL------>		
	male	female	total	male	female	total	male	female	total
Heterosexual	74% (.69-.74)*	96%	88%	90% (.87-.92)*	100%	94%	82% (.80-.85)*	97%	90%
Homosexual	17% (.14-.21)*	0%	6%	10% (.08-.13)*	0%	6%	14% (.12-.16)*	0%	6%
Bisexual	7% (.05-.09)*	4%	5%	0%	0%	0%	3% (.03-.04)*	3%	3%
Un known	2%	0%	1%	0%	0%	0%	1%	0%	0%
Total (N)	100%	100%	100%	100%	100%	100%	100%	100%	100%

* indicates 95% Confidence level and is only indicated for men
as no information was available for Lesbian women [see text]

Table 7.1: Sexual orientation in my research sample (N=273),
broken down by sexual gender and time gender

When discussing sexual orientation, a fundamental issue is whether one's sexual orientation is genetic in nature or due to the environment one grows up in, or both. Even if the time gender model does not provide any insight into this matter, the relation between sexual choice and time gender still remains relevant. For, if the distribution of alphas and betas in any sexual orientation would be the same as in the general population, this would indicate the absence of a linkage between that sexual orientation and time gender. On the other hand, any significant difference in distribution would suggest a linkage between sexual orientation and time gender.

Unfortunately, the sample of 273 subjects contained only eight bisexuals (four men and four women, all alphas), too few to draw conclusions from. In the absence of lesbian females I also could not compare the time gender distribution among hetero- and homosexual women with that among the 215 women in my sample of Greater Vancouver, BC. But I had sufficient data to compare the time gender distribution among the 103 heterosexual and 17 homosexual males with that among the 190 males in my sample of Greater Vancouver, BC. Figure 7.3 presents the results.

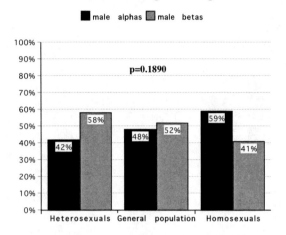

Figure 7.3:
Time gender distributions among heterosexual and homosexual males in the 1987-1989 sample (N=273), compared with time gender distributions among all males in the 1997-1991 sample ("General Population") (N=405)

The center portion of figure 7.3 shows that the time gender distribution among males in my general population sample was alphas 48% and betas 52%. The left side of the figure shows that this distribution among the male heterosexuals of my sample appeared to favor betas a bit (alphas 42% and betas 58%); and on the right, that among the male homosexuals it favored alphas somewhat (alphas 59% and betas 41%). These deviations from the Greater Vancouver, BC sample were, however, statistically insignificant. Such findings could be expected in one out of every five probes (p=0.1890). These data lead to the conclusion that there is no evidence of a connection between time gender and male heterosexuality or male homosexuality. I am confident that the same conclusion will eventually be found to pertain to female heterosexuality and female homosexuality.

The age at first sexual intercourse 208[2]

The age at which sexual intercourse first takes place has been studied rather extensively over the last two decades. Since the early 1930s, this age has been steadily declining. In the U.S. men and women born between 1933-1942 had their first sex at an average age of about 18; those born about twenty years later (1953-1962) at about 17.5; and those born between 1963-1967 showed a further drop.[3] By 1998 the average age for boys had come down to age 16 and for girls to age 17.[4] However, most recent indicators suggest a turning point with an incipient increase in the average age of first sex. In

2001 self-reported data from more than 10,000 high school students in the U.S. found that high school virgins outnumbered those who had engaged in sexual intercourse, 54% to 46%.[5]

I obtained data about the first age of sexual intercourse in 195 out of the 247 heterosexual subjects (close to 80%) in my cohort of 273. The results are shown in figure 7.4.

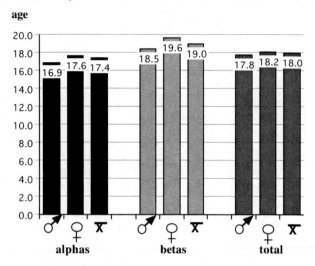

Figure 7.4: Average age at first sexual intercourse,
broken down by sexual gender and time gender (N=195 heterosexual subjects)

It is evident that the time gender model cannot account for the progressive decline or increase in the age of first sex over time. But it predicts that alphas tend to get sexually involved earlier than betas.

The total on the right side of figure 7.4 shows that my adult Vancouver subjects had their first sexual intercourse at an average age of 18.0 with men and women not significantly differing in this regard (p=0.498). However, alphas had their first sex at an average age of 17.4 years and betas at 19.0, a statistically highly significant difference (p=0.004). There was no significant difference between alpha men and alpha women (p=0.270) or between beta men and beta women (p=0.243).

Casual sex

Recent sex surveys in North America and Europe were concerned with the spread and prevention of AIDS and emphasized therefore not only the age at which sexual intercourse first occurs but also issues such as the total number of sexual partners people have had. This number depends on three factors.

• A social trend in sexual behavior since the 1960s in that people tend to experience an increased number of consecutive steady sexual relationships. This because they begin having sex earlier; have live-in partnerships preceding marriage more often. These, in turn, frequently break up and induce a new cycle of sexual activity. As a result, marriages and new live-in relationships are being entered later in life.[6]

• Unfaithfulness during a committed sexual partnership. This occurs with some regularity, but, according to recent sex surveys,[7] appears not to have substantially increased since the 1960s.

• Casual sex — a social euphemism for sexual promiscuity — referring to sexual activity without any personal commitment to the sexual partner. In my Vancouver cohort of 247 heterosexuals, I obtained relevant data in 84% (207) subjects, the results of which are shown in figure 7.5 (the prevalence of casual sex), and figure 7.6 (the average age at which casual sex first occurred, broken down by time gender and sexual gender).

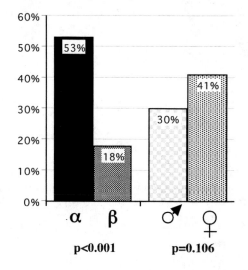

Figure 7.5: Prevalence of self-reported casual sex in 207 heterosexuals,
broken down by sexual gender and time gender

The left side of figure 7.5 shows that around 30% of the men and 40% of the women had at some point in their life been involved in casual sex but this difference was statistically insignificant (p=0.106). Since the average for all subjects was 36% one may assume that approximately a third of men and women had experience with casual sex.

I predicted, however, that among men and women alphas had had a greater tendency toward casual sex than their beta counterparts. This because alphas have a more intense curiosity drive; are living today without having to relive yesterday or pre-live tomorrow; and in different situations experience different identities and values. Betas, on the other hand, are less curious and since they have to live with their timescape and global values they experience themselves as a single continuous identity. The right side of figure 7.5 demonstrates this prediction to be valid. While there was no significant difference between alpha men and women (p=0.658), or beta men and women (p=0.958), it was highly significant that 53% of the alphas, but only 18% of the betas reported they had been involved in casual sex (p<0.001).

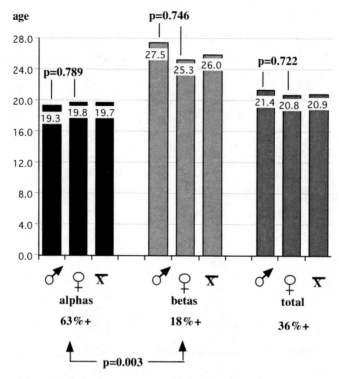

Figure 7.6: Average age at which casual sex first occurred,
broken down by sexual gender and time gender (N=59)

Figure 7.6 demonstrates that, in addition to being less often involved in casual sex than alphas, those betas who had casual sex did so on the average 6.3 years later than alphas. For alphas the average age of first casual sex was 19.7 years, for betas 26.0 years, a statistically highly significant difference (p=0.003) with, again, no significant difference between alpha men and women p=0.789), or beta men and women (p=0.746), or, for that matter, all men together and all women together (p=0.722).

Abortion

I predicted that alpha females, particularly during their teens, tend to engage more readily in sexual intercourse without giving forethought to an unwanted pregnancy. Because of their situational values and ability to walk away from a trauma, alpha teenagers also resort more readily to abortion as the solution to an unwanted pregnancy than betas do.

In my cohort of 273 subjects I had relevant information in 145 of the 149 women (97%). 17% had experienced at least one abortion. Figure 7.7 shows that 22% of alpha women, but only 4% of beta women had been so involved, a highly significant difference (p=0.009).

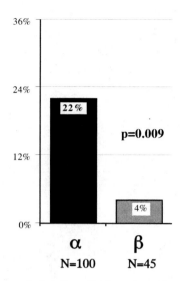

Figure 7.7: Prevalence of abortion, broken down by time gender (N=145)

This and the fact that among the 145 women in my cohort, some alpha women (unlike beta women) had more than one abortion, produced a highly significant time gender difference in the average number of abortions per woman (p=0.021), namely 0.32 abortions per alpha female, compared to 0.04 per beta female. This contrasts with the average number of live childbirths per woman, which was 0.79 per alpha female and 1.24 per beta female (p=0.04), as figure 7.8 demonstrates.

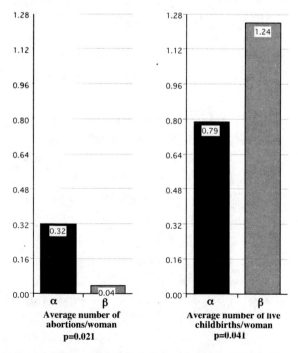

Figure 7.8: Average number of abortions and live childbirths per woman, broken down by time gender (N=145)

These figures resulted in an abortion prevalence in alpha women of 405 abortions per 1000 live births and of 35 abortions per 1000 live births in beta women, with an overall prevalence of 252 abortions/1000 live births. This appears to be in line with similar statistics for the Province of British Columbia, Canada or, for that matter, for the U.S.[8]

Section 2: time gender and partnering

Table 7.2 shows the relevant data on the 247 heterosexuals in the cohort used in this section.

HETEROSEXUALS N=247	alpha			beta			total		
	male	female	total	male	female	total	male	female	total
Currently married	7	29	36	31	19	50	38	48	86
Currently common law	3	18	21	2	4	6	5	22	27
Currently cohabitating	10	47	57	33	23	56	43	70	113
Separated	7	11	18	9	4	13	16	15	31
Divorced	2	12	14	6	5	11	8	17	25
Widowed	1	2	3	1	6	7	2	8	10
Previously cohabitating	10	25	35	16	15	31	26	40	66
Past/present cohabitation	20	72	92	49	38	87	69	110	179
Single throughout	23	27	50	11	7	18	34	34	68
Total heterosexual cohort	43	99	142	60	45	105	103	144	247

Table 7.2: Cohabital status in 247 heterosexual subjects

The sample of 17 homosexual men was too small to draw conclusions. However, since the time gender distribution among heterosexual and homosexual men was the same, I assume that conclusions drawn from the 247 heterosexual men and women hold also for homosexual men, if not for homosexual women. This does not necessarily apply to the sample of 8 bisexual men and women, because bisexuals are, as I will point out shortly, quite dissimilar from heterosexuals and homosexuals, so that different rules may apply.

Concerning the role of time gender in remaining single or getting into a marriage or live-in relationship, I hypothesized that a marital attitude—the tendency toward sexual bonding with a live-in relation or marriage—is stronger among betas than alphas as betas are more inclined to long-term commitments and are less inclined toward casual sex (sexual involvement without sexual bonding).

Figure 7.9 illustrates the prevalence of a marital attitude as compared with being single by conjoint gender. It shows, as predicted, a dramatic difference in the prevalence of a marital attitude among alphas (65%) and betas (83%) (p=0.002), but also something unexpected. There was a significant difference in the prevalence of a marital attitude among alpha men (47%) and alpha women (27%) (p=0.003), but not among beta men (82%) and beta women (84%) (p=0.709). With the benefit of hindsight, I concluded that more alpha men than women stay single, probably because alpha women of childbearing age are more likely to look for the stability of a marital-type union than alpha men.

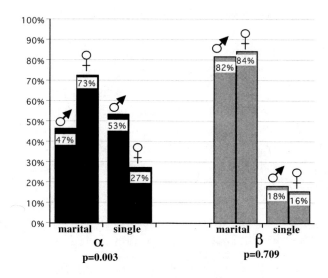

Figure 7.9: Prevalence of a marital attitude versus being single among 247 heterosexual subjects, broken down by conjoint gender

About legal and common-law marriages

Since the 1960s there has been a considerable increase in heterosexual couples living together without getting legally married. In my group of 113 heterosexual subjects who were living with their sexual partner, three quarters were legally married, and one quarter were living common-law. In many jurisdictions common-law marriages have achieved the same rights as legally married couples. This has made the distinction between common-law and legal marriages rather fussy, so that I often group them together as marital-type unions. Even so, I predicted that betas are more inclined than alphas to choose legal marriage over a live-in arrangement because of their concern with cementing long-term arrangements.

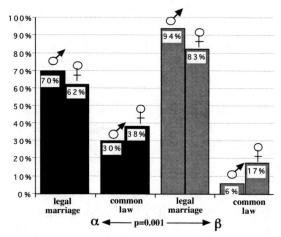

Figure 7.10: Preference for legal versus common-law marriage in 113 subjects, broken down by conjoint gender (p=0.008)

Figure 7.10 compares the incidence of legal marriages with live-in relationships by conjoint gender. It confirms, first of all, that betas were, indeed, far more inclined to prefer marriage over a live-in relationship than were alphas (p=0.001), but it also indicates something I had not predicted, namely that the men, whether alpha or beta, tended to have a stronger preference for legal marriage than the women (p=0.017). This may suggest that, despite the increasing popularity of live-in relationships, contemporary men still tend to be more concerned with social appearance and contemporary women more with the long-term protection of their freedom than with any long-term security implied in a legal commitment by their male partner. I recall a female lawyer who told me: "I lived with him for a couple of years, but I finally had to leave because he kept pestering me to get married." While in the West it is still very usual for the man to pop the question, the option of refusal and of delaying the answer through a trial union has become a female privilege.

To prefer legal marriage over live-in relationships is certainly not because legal marriage is more enduring. 40% of the legal marriages in my series had ended in separation or divorce, and this was unrelated to sexual gender, time gender, or conjoint gender. The divorce statistics did not appear to differ greatly from those in the U.S.[9]

Choosing a partner (1): dependency versus autonomy

Early in my career as a long-term psychotherapist, a businessman brought his wife to see me. He told me his "little girl" (his wife) was so phobic about going outdoors and about being alone that she was virtually incarcerated in her home and needed a "babysitter" to keep her comfortable. Soon he left with the words: "Look, doc, see what you can do for her, and if there is anything I can do, just tell me!"

By following my advice, the young woman greatly improved. First, she fired her "babysitter," then began attending a health club and, ultimately, returned to university to finish the degree she had abandoned because of her marriage. Then one day, when I was busy with someone else, there was loud knocking on my office door. Annoyed at being rudely interrupted, I opened the door and saw the businessman standing there. He looked very upset. I excused myself to my client and took the businessman aside. In an angry voice, he demanded:

> "What did you do to my little girl? She now insists I come home for supper and spend time with her! She wants to accompany me on my business trips! Does she not understand I have a million things to look after? I want her to lay off, you understand?"

> "Well, I guess you will have to make up your mind whether you want a phobic infantile wife or an adult autonomous partner with needs of her own."

He obviously felt I was siding with his wife and left in disgust.

As it turned out, he began frequently phoning his wife at home, asking her how she was doing but in reality checking out whether she was at home and, if she was going out, where she was going, and with whom she would be spending time. He began overindulging in alcohol and soon was accusing her of being interested in other men. Her growing independence exposed *his* hidden conflict. Although he was a capable executive, deep down he was convinced that no woman could love him for who he was and be faithful to him. That is why he had married a woman with a built-in jail. To make a long story short, she eventually divorced him and engaged in a promising career, whereas he went through a profound crisis.

For me this was a profound experience, happening long before I developed the time gender model. It introduced the idea that people often stabilize a hidden problem by marrying their polarized opposite, as symbolized in figure 7.11.

To check this out, I began working with troubled couples which reinforced the idea that people often marry their own hidden conflict. Interlocking dependency needs which remain hidden in one partner but are overt in the other are common in partners who seek marital counseling. When first meeting, each partner senses the manifest personality of the other as complementing their own. This means that the overt personality of one represents the unrealized side of the other. As a result, each feels as if the other fully realizes them and therefore makes them a whole person, and they fall in love with each other.

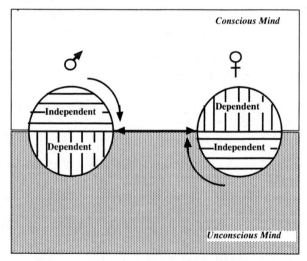

Figure 7.11: Polarization in marital-type situations:
"People often marry their own hidden conflict"

As long as they still live apart, each usually remains the desired fulfillment of the other. Once they start to live together, however, each gradually turns into the actual symbol of what the other consistently has been unable to realize. As a result, the partners become more and more irritating to each other. They begin alienating one another and, to avoid this, each begins to force the other to behave like her or himself, first subtly and then more and more overtly. Efforts to reform the other remain unsuccessful so that, eventually, the relationship becomes a chronic frustration. This was why the business executive eventually brought his wife to me.

Such adults have not outgrown their normal childhood craving to depend on one or both parents. In adulthood they transfer this need onto others. This may be caused by previous parental overindulgence, excessive frustration of the child's emotional needs, a lack of properly weaning the child's from its dependency on parents, and genetic factors. Living without a committed sexual mate leaves these people feeling incomplete and longing for a partner to fill this void. Their dependency needs override their need for self-esteem and integrity so that they unknowingly lower their standards in looking for a mate. Although their eventual marriage partner may turn out to constantly deflate their self-esteem, their deep-seated separation anxiety keeps them attached, no matter what the emotional price. Consciously rationalizing this they tell themselves they "really love" the other person, or that they feel too guilty to leave, or that the children would suffer, or that they can't afford to leave.

Since the dependency needs of these couples are complementary one is dealing with an almost unconditional togetherness, a co-dependence. No matter how problematic the relationship, each partner's deep-rooted fear of going it alone continues to hold the two together. Co-dependent individuals sometimes escape this attachment jail by exchanging their hurtful partner for another one who seems more understanding to begin with, but in reality fits their dependency needs just the same. Thus the whole cycle repeats itself. Sometimes one partner may realize eventually that

separating and dealing with one's separation anxiety cannot possibly be worse than the emotional pain in their relationship.

To make my point about the role of dependency needs in matchmaking, I have painted them in the strongest of colors. In reality extreme dependency needs reflects one pole of a continuum with the other pole representing those who have mastered the fear of going it alone and thus have reached emotional autonomy. Autonomous people prefer living alone in peace over living together in constant turmoil. The Romans used to say: "If you want peace, be prepared to go to war."[10] Applying this as a metaphor to autonomy in marriage one might say: "If you want a peaceful marriage, you must be prepared to walk out."

Resolving marital problems between partners who appear to have married their own hidden conflict requires from both partners considerable mutual commitment and goodwill. Rather than defensively keeping the focus on the other as "the problem" by constantly sending the message "Why can't you be more like me?" each must learn to shift the focus to oneself and recognize one's own complimentary problem, and then begin to work on it.

Choosing a partner (2): the role of time gender

Because the strengths of an alpha represent the weaknesses of a beta, and the other way around, the personalities of an alpha and a beta are complementary. One might therefore expect that this complimentarity plays an important role in people choosing a partner.

Jung thought that in choosing one's partner the complimentarity between being extroverted and introverted (which in my model reflects being alpha or beta) plays a role.[11] He concluded that either type tended to marry its opposite, with the extrovert taking the initiative toward practical action and the introvert doing the reflecting. He thought of such marriages as ideal "symbioses" as long as both partners are busy with the external pressures of their new life. But because each speaks a different language, they eventually find out that mutual understanding is completely lacking. At this point the spouses become involved in a bitter, abusive marital conflict.[12] Jung felt that mutual understanding can be reached , however, if each marital partner has the urge to grow and the couple has sufficient time to work things out.[13] If Jung was right then marriages between an extroverted alpha and an introverted beta should be far more frequent than between two alphas or two betas.

Table 7.3 shows what I actually found based on 100 subjects in whom I could identify the time gender of their partner. While a substantial minority of marriages (30%) was between same-time gender couples (13% of the alpha-alpha, and 17% of the beta-beta type), 70% of the marital unions indeed involved time gender interfacing. Yet, 63% were between a beta man and an alpha women, and only 7% between an alpha man and beta woman. Did this mean that beta men had a strong tendency to be attracted to alpha women, but that beta women tended to avoid alpha men?

	α female	β female	
α male	αα 13%	αβ 7%	20%
β male	βα 63%	ββ 17%	80%
	76%	24%	100%

αα –Marital union between alpha male and alpha female	13%
ββ – Marital union between beta male and beta female	17%
Marital unions without time gender interfacing	30%
αβ – Marital union between alpha male and beta female	7%
βα – Marital union between beta male and alpha female	63%
Marital unions with time gender interfacing	70%

Table 7.3:
Distribution of the four time gender combinations in marital-type unions (N=100)

These assumptions could be valid only if the pool of eligible partners contained an equal number of alpha and beta men, and of alpha and beta women. However, the distribution of the four conjoint genders in my subjects was very uneven as was the tendency among them to start a legal or common-law marriage (their marital attitude). As a result, the pool of men contained 80% betas and only 20% alphas, and the pool of women 76% alphas but only 24% betas. In the final analysis this distribution of the four time gender combinations in marital type unions turned out to be simply a matter of chance. For as table 7.4 demonstrates, the numbers based on chance alone produced a distribution which was virtually identical with the one I found (p=0.892). In the mating game, love seems to be blind to time gender.

p=0.892	My findings	Chance occurrence
αα – marriages	13%	15%
ββ – marriages	17%	19%
αβ – marriages	7%	5%
βα – marriages	63%	61%

Table 7.4: Actual findings compared with chance occurrence regarding the frequency of the four time gender combinations in marital-type unions (N=100)

The fact that I found that a significant majority (63%) of marital-type unions are between an alpha female and beta male has led many to the naive conclusion that all men are betas and all women alphas (or, in my terms, that all marriages are of the male beta-female alpha variety). One popular metaphor has it that men are from Mars and women from Venus.[14] Such people confuse their hidden time gender bias with an explicit sexual gender bias, as in "Women are this way, and men that way." This is not so, of course, for "many men come from Venus and many women from Mars." Table 7.5 shows the chances of becoming involved with someone of the same or opposite time gender, based on the distribution of conjoint genders in the mating pool and their chance merger into combinations.

Chance for	to match	with
	alpha female	beta female
alpha male	65%	35%
beta male	79%	21%
Chance for	to match	with
	alpha male	beta male
alpha female	17%	83%
beta female	29%	71%

Table 7.5: The chance of a match between a man or woman of a given time gender with a partner of the same or opposite time gender

Section 3: marriage and the nuclear family

The main discussion in this section is about the nature of identical time gender marriages (apha-alpha and beta-beta marriages) and time gender interfacing marriages (alpha-beta and beta-alpha marriages). However, to place this discussion in perspective, I will first summarize my statistical data on alphas and betas as intimate partners and parents.

Alphas and betas as intimate partners: statistical data

I had statistical data on alphas and betas as intimate partners, based on 177 heterosexual subjects with a marital attitude. I compared 1) their tendency to import a certain kind of sexual experience into their first marriage; 2) their tendency to remain faithful to their current marital partner; and 3) their tendency to stay married to the same person as opposed to entering into more than one marital union.

Previously I found 1) that when getting married for the first time, alphas were likely to be sexually more experienced than betas since alphas tended to begin their sexual activity earlier (age 17.5) than betas (age 19.7) (p=0.001); and 2) that alphas tended to gravitate considerably more to casual sex (48%) than betas (14%) (p<0.001). In both instances (age of first sexual experience and tendency toward casual sex) there was no statistical evidence of a difference between females and males (respectively p=0.713 and p=0.290).

The fact that prior to marriage alphas tended to gravitate considerably more to casual sex t led me to assume that they also might be more inclined to extramarital sex. However, this hypothesis was invalid. Among the 16% who had experienced extramarital involvement, there was no statistically significant difference between alphas and betas (p=0.274) nor, for that matter, between men and women (p=0.724). Marriage, whether legal or common-law, is a social institution that apparently provides strong protection against infidelity. This is in line with several American surveys.[15]

The fact that the great majority of legal and common-law marriages remain sexually exclusive is no guarantee, however, that most of these unions endure. Although in my sample 40% of legal marriages had ended in separation or divorce, this is not a valid indicator of marital endurance since it does not indicate whether people have been involved in more than one marriage. I therefore used the total number of successive marital partners as a more realistic indicator of marital endurance. Since in my cohort marriage ending with the death of a partner accounted for only 4% of the sample, one can assume that the higher the number of successive marital unions, the more marital breakups occurred. About the endurance of marriage I entertained two hypotheses.

- I predicted that men are more inclined to stay in a marital union than women The reason is that men in my sample tended to feel stronger than women about legal marriage as opposed to a live-in relationship, suggesting they are more concerned with social appearance than women.

- I predicted that betas, with their timescape and global values, tend to stick more to the long-term commitment implied in a legal or common-law marriage than alphas, since the latter live in the here-and-now with a situational value system.

Figure 7.12 supports both hypotheses. The average number of previous unions was the highest among alpha women (1.24 with 30% still in their first marriage), somewhat lower in beta women (0.95 with 37% still in their first marriage), again lower in alpha men (0.75 with 40% still in their first marriage), and the lowest in beta men (0.69 with 54% of them still in their first marriage).

One may speculate that adultery plays a major role in marital breakup. This was not the case since extramarital affairs appeared as frequently in men as in women, and in alphas as in betas and was therefore unrelated to conjoint gender and hence to marital endurance. Marital breakup is apparently more an expression of an incompatibility of personality and its ensuing marital dysfunctionality.

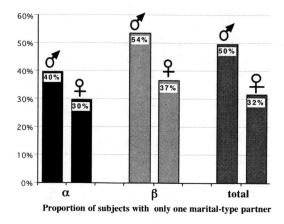

Proportion of subjects with only one marital-type partner

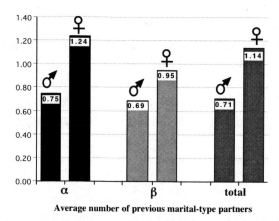

Average number of previous marital-type partners

Figure 7.12: Two indicators of marital endurance,
broken down by sexual gender and time gender (N=177)

Alphas and betas as parents: statistical data

This section focuses on the willingness of 179 heterosexual alpha and beta men and women with a marital attitude to assume a parental role, as indicated by having children of their own, stepchildren, or adopting children instead of remaining childless. The 67% of subjects in figure 7.13 together had 234 natural children, 14 adopted children, and 41 stepchildren, while 33% remained childless, with alphas being far more likely to remain childless than betas (p=0.002). It was somewhat surprising that women were more likely to be part of a childless marital union than men (p=0.028).

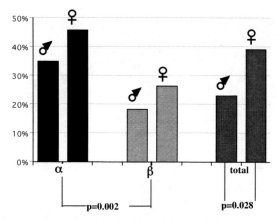

Figure 7.13: Proportion of marital-type subjects without any type of children,
broken down by sexual gender and time gender (N=179)

I predicted that time gender plays no role in someone's willingness to have natural children or to adopt children, for these parents feel, at least in principle, entitled to equal control of their offspring and often have an equal stake in their future. Stepchildren are, however, an entirely different matter. Here one partner must accept children of the other as a precondition for marriage. Even if the natural parent and stepparent have worked out paraental control rules, the fact remains that the children's natural parent remains the primary emotional bond and thus controller of the children, with the stepparent exercising control only through the natural parent. Since controlling the here-and-now and attaining an appropriate position in the hierarchy of the nuclear family is far more essential to alphas than to betas, I predicted that alphas are less inclined to get involved with stepchildren than betas.

Figure 7.14 reveals that for the 67% of subjects with one or more children these two predictions were valid. There was no statistically significant difference between alphas and betas in having natural children (p=0.590) or in adopting children (p=0.303), or between men and women in these regards (respectively p=0.724 and p=0.109). But accepting a potential partner's offspring by a previous marriage was quite another matter. As predicted, betas were far more willing—in fact ten times more willing—to accept stepchildren than alphas (20% to 2%; p<001). What came as a surprise, however, was that sexual gender also played a role; men were three times more likely to become a stepfather than women a stepmother (17% to 6%; p=0.020).

This may be due to the fact that on marital breakup women are far more likely to be awarded custody of the children. Another factor, perhaps, may be that women are more keen on rearing the fruit of their own body than looking after someone else's offspring. As a result, only 1% of alpha women

and 5% of alpha men had stepchildren, as opposed to 16% of beta women and 22% of beta men.

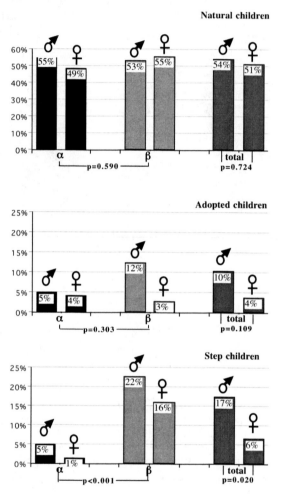

Figure 7.14: Proportion of marital-type subjects with natural children only, with adopted children, and with step children, broken down by sexual gender and time gender (N=179)

Identical time gender marriages

Identical time gender marriages (alpha male/alpha female—marriages and beta male/beta female-marriages) constituted 30% of the marriages among my subjects. When two partners share the same time gender, this does not override personality differences which are non related to time gender. Yet these people do not have to cope as couples with the many differences between alphas and betas or to engage in defensive maneuvers involved in time gender interfacing, as I mentioned in the chapter on social behavior.

I will now separately discuss alpha male/alpha female-marriages and beta male/beta female — marriages.

About alpha male/alpha female marriages

In my cohort alpha-alpha marital unions represent 13% of all marriages. Both alpha men and alpha women tend to begin their sexual activity earlier in life than betas and, in adolescence and young adulthood, gravitate considerably more, and earlier, to casual sex. When entering a marital-type union both are therefore likely to be sexually more experienced than betas. When having to choose at this point between a legal marriage or live-in relationship alphas, especially alpha women, tend to be more willing to engage in a live-in relation than betas. But, once legally married or living together, alpha men and women are just as likely as betas to stay faithful (84%).

An alpha-alpha marriage can be most exciting, at least for quite some time as both spouses live in the here-and-now, are extroverted or outgoing, and socially perceptive, and prefer social interaction over being by themselves. In addition, both possess an attractive, broad-based curiosity, socially, recreationally, as well as intellectually, and thus look constantly for variety. Does the Camelot myth surrounding the marriage of John Kennedy and Jackie Kennedy-Onassis suggest that their marriage is a famous example of an alpha-alpha combination? [16]

Keeping a realistic eye on the future is, however, a potential problem in these marriages. If one or both are preoccupied with the future, they do not follow a well thought-through internal travel plan, but only do so in a visionary manner, depending on external reinforcement — following the Star of Bethlehem, so to speak.

The mood regulation of both partners in an alpha-alpha marriage is situational; each consequently pursues situational self-esteem, craving social status and praise from others. Hence, both partners' motivations are predominantly present-oriented, so that each tries to control their 4–D. They will be mutually supportive, if their immediate goals coincide, or are complementary, but if their goals are antagonistic — and this frequently is the case — competitive friction ensues. This may be hurtful to either one or both and, when publicly displayed, may be rather embarrassing as, for example, when one criticizes the other in public for behaving in a way one deems socially improper.

Because the identity of alphas is context-sensitive and therefore partitioned or multifocal, each spouse rotates within and outside their marriage through their own particular set of discontinuous personality presentations (each with its own persona and contextual value system). These personality shifts may be subtle or dramatic. Whatever the case, spouses are seldom familiar with all the part-identities of the other. One parent may, for example, make a child occasionally mislead the other parent, or one may fit into a particular social context outside the marriage which remains virtually unknown to the other, as in "angel abroad, devil at home." Or, it could be the other way around: ruthless and willful in public life, but good-natured, mild and compliant at home.

Both spouses, being alphas, experience the world as basically unstable and unpredictable, because their present intra-psychic structure—their self-esteem, identities, value systems, and so on—is not continuous with their past and future, but instead contextual and changeable. This is why alphas view external social structures as stabilizing factors, and why they therefore usually fit so well into corporations, the army, political or religious cults, or even gangs. No wonder, then, that both alpha spouses usually attempt to introduce a structure of set rules and expectations, if not routines, in their marriage and family.

Nevertheless, alphas are intolerant of boredom and they therefore tend to compensate for the routine of marital bliss through varied activities and engagements in their extramarital social network. Their actual source of emotional support is thus not necessarily derived from the marriage itself, but often comes from these outside interests and involvements. In any case, their intolerance of boredom makes it important for both husband and wife not to get bored with their life in general. While each tends to be relatively immune to painful or rewarding past and future events, both are rather vulnerable to longer lasting existential boredom. This may lead to a situational depression which, because one partner forms a large part of the environment of the other, one may emotionally contaminate the other. External circumstances play a major role in alpha spouses' marital contentment.

Alpha-alpha-marriages appear far less stable than beta-beta-marriages, the average number of previous marital unions being the indicator of the endurance of these marriages ($p=0.012$). Alpha-alpha couples live in the here-and-now and are therefore situation-reactive, without any strong emotional connection to the future. They are unable to envision a long-term commitment to each other. As a result, external circumstances often play an important role in keeping such marriages together. These include the expectations of a closed social class or religious sect; living in a highly visible social position—the lives of a television evangelist couple, for example, or a President of the United States and his First Lady; or more down to earth conditions, such as sharing a business, getting a welfare check, or even belonging to a gang.

When invoking their past, alphas usually do so by associating their present state of mind with concordant, emotionally-cognitively related personal memories, rather than placing their present in the perspective of their historic past. In other words, they unwittingly use their past to reinforce the way they feel in the present. When both alpha spouses are together and feel well, they may use their past to reinforce their present agreeable state of mind. If quarreling with each other, however, they both not only blame each other rather than looking inside, but also recall only those memories which reinforce their current hostile view of the other. Add to this that both have the gift of the gab, and are able to use language flexibly and fitting the situation. Furthermore, the thinking of both shows a certain tolerance for logical inconsistencies. An argument between two alpha spouses is therefore not settled on logical points, but on emotional grounds, in line with whoever holds the upper hand in their authoritarian-competitive relationship.

I have encountered a particular scenario in dysfunctional alpha-alpha marriages that are kept together by a mutually complementary dependency problem. These marriages often reach a seemingly decisive emotional crisis in which one, or both, feel so wronged that they separate. While both genuinely believe this will be "it," they are, however, only aware of the emotional pain of the present, and do not emotionally connect with the future of having to go it alone. Yet when they actually enter this future and do find themselves alone, then their dependency problem with its accompanying depressive and anxious feelings pops up again. Meanwhile they already are de-emotionalizing the painful crisis which brought the breakup. So, in due course, the separated spouses begin exchanging mutual promises of better behavior and sharing a vision of a new beginning, whereupon—both being future-blind—they reunite once more until the cycle repeats itself. They usually rationalize this scenario quite easily. One woman reported, for example, that while her husband served her divorce papers, he also kept telling her that he could not live without her. In the hope that he had changed she "gave it one more shot." Those who work in shelters for abused women will be familiar with a far more dramatic example of this scenario, in that some women who arrive there, beaten black and blue, repeatedly return to the very source of their agony.

Both alpha men and women are as likely as betas to become natural parents or adopt children. That both alpha parents have a here-and-now orientation rather than being preoccupied with the future affects the way they raise their children who, in case of daughters, have the same time perspective, but in terms of sons may be either alphas or betas (see table 11.1 in Chapter 11). Raising children on the basis of the idea that "as long as the day ends well, all is well" is, generally speaking, not a problem in a homogenous culture. In these circumstances, expectations of long-term goals and of value systems about social behavior and education are built into the culture and shared by nearly everyone. Introducing such long-term goals and value systems are therefore not specifically parental tasks. But, in transitional, mixed cultures—a progressively spreading phenomenon in the West, if not elsewhere—children are constantly exposed to the confusion of fragmented value systems during their socialization and education phase. Under these circumstances female and male alpha children need structure and firm consistent guidance at home (more so than any beta sons who are more resilient to these circumstances; see Chapter 9). However, alpha parents are likely to respond with a day-to-day, crisis-oriented management of their youngsters which increases, rather than diminishes, the existential confusion of their alpha daughters and sons and frequently results in behaviors, including scholastic failure, that are at variance with the vision the parents held for their children's future. Despite these difficulties, later in life some troubled alpha children may become surprisingly successful, as many charismatic leaders in politics and business have demonstrated.

About beta male/beta female marriages

Beta-beta marriages represented 17% of marriages in my cohort. When entering a marital-type union a beta man and beta woman are equally likely to be sexually less experienced than alphas. If having to choose between a legal marriage and a live-in relationship betas, especially beta men, tend to be more inclined to a legal marriage than alphas. Once legally married or living together beta men and women are just as likely as alphas to stay faithful (84%).

Usually, beta-beta marriages tend to be less flamboyant and more private than alpha-alpha marriages. Since both spouses are introverted or inward looking they tend to be more private and socially less broadly involved than alphas. Being by themselves, or spending time with each other or their family is more important than interacting with outsiders. Their intellectual and social curiosity tends to be more focused and in depth, rather than being wide ranging. In terms of recreation, they often tend to prefer quiet enjoyment over variety and excitement.

Because of their global, unified monofocal identity, both spouses tend to see each other as rather unchanging, although both may be subjected to individual mood changes. But their intra-psychic structure—their self-esteem, identity, value system, and so on—is rather constant. They both sense a continuity with their past and future and usually experience their reality as more stable and predictable than alphas do. Hence, both tend to find external social structures somewhat restrictive and inhibiting to their individuality, rather than providing a sense of security. They therefore tend to accommodate individual differences in their marriage more readily than alphas do.

Outside interests and involvements of these beta spouses are less important for their emotional well-being than their timescape, their careers, their marriage, and their family. Generally speaking, external circumstances do not play a major role in whether a beta-beta marriage is happy or in keeping the marriage together. Indeed, both spouses are relatively resilient to longer lasting, unfavorable circumstances, provided they can draw on a positive past and, in particular, can see hope for the future. If they share an unhappy past, or have little to look forward to, then beta-beta couples are in for an emotionally difficult time.

The strength of the future orientation of beta partners is that they tend to work persistently toward the particular future timescape they have in mind, following a well thought-through internal travel plan to which they stick even in the absence of external reinforcement, and which often involves current sacrifices. Both are far more interested in controlling their future than their present. That beta couples constantly cross the bridge before reaching it can, however, turn this preoccupation with the future into a liability. It may make them people who have a hard time fully enjoying their married life when all is well.

A beta-beta marriage is a mutually supportive source of strength if the individual ambitions of the spouses do not conflict. If, however, the ambitions of the partners diverge significantly then their inflexible adherence to their conflicting timescapes turns the marriage into an ongoing battle. Initially, they often fight in silence. One reason for this is that both tend to look in their own timescape, ending up silently holding themselves responsible for both halves of their troubled equation. Another reason is that what these two introverted betas have in their head often stays there. In other words, these spouses tend to communicate insufficiently with each other about how and what they feel, particularly when facing marital problems. As a result, the interpersonal problems are kept in their respective timescapes to fester, and explode into the open only much later.

Yet, whatever problems there are in a beta-beta marriage, both spouses find it hard to give up on the commitment to their marital union since two stable, interdependent, if not co-dependent timescapes are involved. In addition, two beta spouses have the potential for a cooperative-egalitarian relationship and may therefore negotiate a compromise when facing a marital problem. However, if their fight takes an authoritarian-competitive turn with one partner winning out, they will eventually separate. Since neither is likely to want confronting their painful past again, such a breakup will be permanent.

Despite the fact that breakups are possible in beta-beta marriages, they appear to be the most stable of the four time gender combinations. The measure of marital endurance expressed as the average number of previous marital unions tends to support this conclusion, but further research involving a larger number of marriages is needed.

Two beta parents have a future orientation toward raising their children. Since their natural children are also betas (see table 11.1, Chapter 11) they, too, are future-oriented. This parental attitude and that of their beta teenagers is particularly helpful in a transitional, mixed social environment. At home the parents' consistent long-term strategies toward achieving social behavior and an adequate education will serve as an effective counterbalance against the potpourri of fragmented value systems outside of their home. Beta teenagers, in turn, tend to mold their future timescape in line with their parents' expectations. This further facilitates their pro-social behavior and educational goals. Indeed, beta children usually end up contributing considerably to the global self-esteem of their parents.

About time gender interfacing marriages

Marriages between spouses of different time gender in my series were determined only by availability and chance and constituted 70%, with apha male/beta female-marriages accounting for 7% and beta male/alpha female—marriages for 63%.

I mentioned that the alpha partner (whether female or male) is usually sexually more experienced than the beta partner and tends to be far more willing to engage in a live-in relationship than a beta partner, who generally favors a legal marriage; and that once legally married or living together, both partners are equally likely to stay faithful.

An alpha and a beta in an intimate relationship are not unlike the two Greek deities, Dionysus and Apollo. According to the German philosopher Nietzsche, they symbolize a powerful polarity in the Ancient Greek world, as each was energized by opposite impulses. The Dionysian and Apollonian represented a warring antagonism between, on the one hand, the Dionysian outward bound vision, living out oneself and unconcerned with the individuality of others and, on the other, the Apollonian inward vision whose individuality is the cornerstone of existence.[17]

Although picking a partner is not determined by a complimentarity of time gender, the time gender difference does carry hidden seeds of a love-hate affair. On the one hand, each spouse admires and loves the other's strengths for which he or she has no natural endowment. On the other hand, time gender interfacing constantly exposes her or his weaknesses. This makes each partner feel inadequate and incomplete, so that jealousy and its accompanying hostility are never far away. Both spouses may end up saying "Gee, I wish I could be that way" as frequently as "I never, never would want to be like that."

Initially, however, and often for quite some time, alpha and betas spouses may use selective denial of the other's time gender-specific behaviors. Or they proclaim empathy for and understanding of the other's behavior by putting their own time gender spin on it, superimposing their view of reality on the other. While using the same words, they give these words different meanings. In this context I asked a beta husband and alpha wife of 28 years standing to apply a long list of personality characteristics to both themselves and the other. It turned out that their judgments coincided in about 70-80% of the listed personality traits. In terms of the rest, they were diametrically opposed: the beta husband judged himself, for example, as sensitive, caring, flexible, sympathetic and serious, while his alpha wife thought of him as insensitive, uncaring, inflexible, unsympathetic and not serious. Discussing these differences they found that she defined these traits in terms of how she experienced his reactions in the here-and-now, while he viewed himself in terms of his overall behavior towards her over time. Given their different time frames, they were both right.

In most cases, the alpha and beta spouse eventually sense a vague polarity in their relationship and become aware that the other is surprisingly different from what they originally had in mind. Usually, attempts are made to press the other to change and, if unsuccessful, conflicts become rationalized in personal terms. They eventually may end up explaining the other's behavior by saying "this is because this is how men — or women — behave," or by coming up with some pseudo-psychological formulation: it must be their early youth, or the class or culture they grew up in, or they are mentally ill and need help, and so on.

A fundamental concern in time gender interfacing marriages is that the alpha spouse constantly puts the blame for any problems on the other, while the beta spouse tends to assume responsibility for both sides of the relationship. By doing this, the alpha abandons control over her or his own contribution to the problem, while the beta unrealistically attempts to assume control over the other's life. Betas tend to have a Messiah Complex in interpersonal relationships, as if they can be responsible for someone else's happiness. However, when they pick a seemingly needy marital partner, they usually end up frustrated Messiahs who get crucified. I remember instances of highly capable and successful beta men who married twice or even three times the same type of overtly needy alpha women who, instead of becoming happily satisfied, felt misunderstood and were soon looking for another Messiah. Or the case of a very capable female beta who assumed that marrying a depressed, alcoholic alpha would cure him of his problems.

Another frequent concern is how these spouses relate differently to time. The alpha spouse is preoccupied with, and tries to control the here-and-now, while the beta spouse tries to control the future. The beta usually gives in to the here-and-now demands of the alpha, provided this does not interfere with future concerns. This often becomes a source of friction. For example:

> The alpha: *"How can you keep working on and on? Where do I come in? Why do I always have to compete with tomorrow?"*
>
> The beta: *"Why do you always bother me at the wrong moment? How will I ever be able to get us where we want to be if you keep interrupting me?"*
>
> The alpha: *"Even when you are with me, you are not there!"*
>
> The beta: *"Am I not even allowed to think?"*

Shifts in the persona and identity of the alpha usually are subtle and may, throughout the entire marriage, completely escape the attention of the beta spouse. After all, betas betacize their partner and therefore assume a consistency in their partner's identity which is non-existent. Yet shifts in persona and identity which become so dramatic that the beta spouse can no longer deny them can turn into a serious threat to the marriage. The alpha partner not only becomes unpredictable in the eyes of the beta, but such personality shifts can become very anxiety provoking. "Why do you behave totally out of character? How can you be so inconsistent?" the beta spouse may exclaim. To the alpha partner, slick words will likely come across as unprovoked accusations, if not as an over controlling, persecutory attitude. Yet the alpha's behavior may drive the beta to the breaking point: "I will lose it if I have to continue living with two realities! I don't know what's is what any longer! If I want to keep my sanity I have to get away from this!"

Whatever alpha and beta spouses may argue about, the beta initially tries to approach the argument with an egalitarian-cooperative attitude, and in a somewhat intellectual, logical manner, supported by time-ordered memories from the period under consideration. The alpha spouse, however, falls back on a more emotional, authoritarian-competitive style, and senses the approach of the other as a weakness. Readily demonstrating the gift of the gab, which the beta rarely has, the alpha uses lateral thinking, unconcerned with logical inconsistencies, and refers to past wrongs or errors which are irrelevant to the argument at hand. Rather than problem solving by meaningfully communicating, these spouses only succeed in frustrating each other further.

Spouses of opposite time gender do not only get frustrated with each other, but also by one or more children of the opposite time gender. This becomes an issue when these children become teenagers and their time gender has fully evolved, and when it begins dawning on the parent that a daughter or son is certainly different from the way the parent is. For example: "Why does this youngster want to drop out and have no desire to get into university?" "Why do we constantly have to sit on her or him? Why this lack of responsibility? I wasn't that way..." Or: "Why can this kid not enjoy life a bit more? Why is she so serious all the time? She ought to take a break from studying once in a while, and have some fun. I had much more fun when I was that age..."

Naturally, these parents often get into conflict about how to raise their teenagers who, outside their home, are constantly exposed to a confusion of fragmented value systems. This affects in particular their alpha children, who are social-context-sensitive and, as a counterbalance, really need structure and consistent control at home. I have already mentioned that alpha parents tend to feel that "as long as the day ends well, all is well," and this is something the alpha teenager readily accepts. The beta parent, on the other hand, constantly looks beyond the horizon, and is therefore more inclined to confront a hostile youngster with consistent corrective measures toward her or his socialization and long-term academic development. All this is less important for beta teenagers, since in their teens they tend not only to identify with their beta parent but, furthermore, are already assuming a future-oriented attitude to begin with.

That one parent is homemaker and the other breadwinner can make a significant difference in this parental conflict because as a rule the homemaker carries more weight. If the homemaker is a beta, a considerably stabilizing influence is exercised on their alpha teenagers, while reinforcing what their beta teenagers are all about to begin with. If the homemaker is an alpha, however, and the "as long as the day ends well, all is well" philosophy dominates, this often is to the detriment of the alpha teenagers, although less so in the case of beta teenagers. In their teens, when time gender characteristics have become pronounced, alpha and beta children must come to grips not only with the parent of the opposite time gender, but also with each other. At this point, alpha and beta siblings tend either to get into conflict with each other, or begin avoiding each other with each going their separate way.

If both spouses are working, as is rather common today, time gender interfacing marriages are not all that different whether the man or woman is alpha or beta. However, the woman being the homemaker and the man the breadwinner may make some difference. An introverted beta-male breadwinner, although usually devoted to his job, tends to seek emotional sustenance in his marriage and family. His wife, being an extroverted alpha, is rather intolerant of her home routines. When social involvements outside her immediate family are lacking, she tends to place additional emotional demands on her beta husband who, himself, is looking for her emotional support. By contrast, an alpha-male breadwinner, being extroverted, tends to seek and find his emotional sustenance outside his marriage, while his introverted beta homemaker is more tolerant of the routines of her home. She therefore places fewer emotional demands on him.

Role reversal with an alpha-female being the provider and a beta-male the homemaker, or a beta-female the breadwinner with an alpha-male looking after the children, has considerable effect on the marriage. Whether male homemaker or female provider, the preferential attention mode of an alpha is the here-and-now in 4-D, which has to provide the main supply of self-esteem. Provided that the untraditional marriage is supported by the social environment and satisfies the dominant alpha's need to control her or his individual niche, the alpha partner sees no problem in role reversal. However, the beta partner (whether male homemaker or female provider) tends to be far less flexible in this regard. Her or his timescape and global self-esteem do not easily allow for a painless role reversal. A beta partner tends to experience role reversal as a situation he or she has been forced into; she or he and resents it while trying to undo it. This, in turn, disturbs the alpha partner. While an alpha-alpha marriage may allow for role reversal and a beta-beta marriage makes this highly unlikely, a time gender interfacing marriage with role reversal is possible but tends to be dysfunctional.

Notwithstanding all the potential challenges in time gender interfacing marriages, the reality remains that alphas and betas have complementary strengths and weaknesses and hence are, in the final analysis, ideally suited for one another. To realize this potential these spouses must abandon the misleading Myth of the Homogeneous Ideal which holds that potentially we all have the strengths of both alphas and betas and the weaknesses of neither. Only then can husband and wife achieve a sophisticated insight into each other's nature, learn to empathize with, and genuinely accept the other and thus adjust their mutual expectations accordingly. If this is achieved, time gender interfacing becomes very satisfying to both, in that both can begin to compensate for their own weaknesses by relying on the strengths of the other, and to apply their strengths more freely. As a result, both are able to genuinely be more themselves and, as such, be more creative and productive.

Concluding summary

This chapter contains a great deal of information. It is therefore helpful to briefly summarize its main points. I must stress once more here that how alphas and betas behave sexually, as intimate partners, or as parents is not a matter of either/or, but reflects statistically significant differences between behavioral trends alphas and betas exhibit.

In respect to partnering, over 80% of betas get into one or more marital-type relationships — there is no difference between beta men and women. In contrast, only 65% of alphas, with over 70% of alpha women but less than 50% of alpha men, enter such relationships. Marriage-minded betas are far more inclined than alphas to prefer legal marriage over a live-in relationship (89% and 63% respectively). The same is also found of men versus women (88% and 69%).

My experience has been that, in picking a partner, people often marry their own hidden conflict. They take a partner whose intra-personal polarization of personality features is opposite to their own, with unresolved dependency needs often playing a major role. Yet despite the fact that alphas and betas have complimentary strengths and weaknesses, and despite Jung's view that extroverts and introverts tend to marry each other, I found that time gender is not relevant in finding a mate. Instead, the distribution of the four time gender combinations in marital type unions appears a matter of chance and availability.

As far as the nature of marriage and the nuclear family is concerned, there is no difference between alphas and betas nor between men and women in remaining faithful to the other. This is not a guarantee that a marriage will endure. Only 30% of alpha women are still in their first marriage compared with only 37% of beta woman. For men, the figures are 40% for alphas and 54% for betas. Since adultery is as infrequent in alphas as in betas, and in females as in males, it does not play a significant role in the breakup of marital unions.

Time gender and sexual gender do not play a role in whether a couple will have natural children or adopt children. Stepchildren, however, are a different matter. Betas are ten times more willing to accept stepchildren than alphas. In fact, only 1% of alpha women and 5% of alpha men had stepchildren, as opposed to 16% of beta women and 22% of beta men.

The four time gender combinations in marital type unions may be grouped into:

1.   identical time gender marriages:

1.1.   *alpha male / alpha female marriages:* all daughters are also alpha, while sons may be alpha or beta (see table 11.1, chapter 11);

1.2.   *beta male / beta female marriages:* all children are beta (see table 11.1, chapter 11);

2.   time gender interfacing marriages:

2.1.   *alpha male / beta female marriages:* all sons are beta like their mothers, all daughters alpha like their fathers (see table 11.1, chapter 11);

2.2.   *beta male / alpha female-marriages:* sons and daughters may be either alpha or beta *(see table 11.1, chapter 11)*.

Each of these time gender combinations have their own strengths and weaknesses, and their own implications for child rearing.

NOTES

1   See Appendix 1 *(The research sample)*.

2   Wherever I speak of "sexual intercourse" I specifically mean "penile-vaginal intercourse," being cognizant of the fact that the term having sex is used in widely divergent ways and may, or may not, include "oral-genital contact" or "penile-anal intercourse" [Sanders and Machover Reinisch (1999)].

3   Michael, Gagnon, Laumann and Kolata (1994), p. 90.

4   U.S. Commission on Adolescent Sexual Health, quoted by Stodghill II (1998), p. 41.

5   Lewin (2002) quoting a report by the U.S. Centers of Disease Control and Prevention.

6   Michael, Gagnon, Laumann and Kolata (1994), pp. 38, 96-101.

7   Michael, Gagnon, Laumann and Kolata (1994), p. 101.

8   Vital statistics of the Province of British Columbia, 118th Annual Report, 1989; Church (1996), p. 20.

9   Church (1996), p. 20; Michael, Gagnon, Laumann, Kolata (1994), p. 100.

10   "Si vis pacem, para bellum".

11   In Chapter 4, I introduced the notion that alphas are extroverts and betas introverts. In Chapter 6, I clarified the differences between Jung's definitions of extroversion and introversion and my own.

12   Jung (1970), p. 65.

13   Jung (1977), p. 517-18.

14   Gray (1994).

15   Michael,Gagnon, Laumann, Kolate (1994), p.101, 105-106; Smith (1991); Billy, Tanfer, Grady, Klepinger (1993).

16   See, for example, Hamilton (1992).

17   Nietzsche, paraphrased, as quoted by Jung (1977), p. 138.

CHAPTER 8

Time Gender And Thinking Styles

Clinical experience with 405 subjects led me to conclude that alphas and betas differ in the way they think. If so, the history of Western scholarly thought which I am familiar with should demonstrate such duality.

Although one's time genderhas nothing to do with the creativity of one's thinking or with the logical quality of one's reasoning, focusing on scholarly thought is helpful in determining time gender differences in thinking because the contrast between the thinking of ordinary alphas and betas is not always discernible. Scholars magnify this duality in pragmatic thinking by moving beyond solving personal problems into unraveling the mysteries of physical and social reality in 4–D, psychological reality in 5–D, autobiographic reality in 6–D and, as logicians and mathematicians, even of abstract reasoning in 7–D. Focusing on this enhanced expression of the time gender duality in scholarly thinking therefore facilitates recognizing its everyday pragmatic version.

Section 1 verifies the existence of the duality in Western thought. Section 2 follows through with a detailed analysis of the thinking of alpha and beta scholars. Section 3 moves the focus from the scholarly back to the ordinary thinking of alphas and betas.

Section 1: A duality in Western thinking

The internationally acknowledged scientist in the domain of time, J. T. Fraser, wrote:

> "Individuals have expressed their personalities in different ways by creating the principles and techniques of the various branches of intuitive and rational knowledge. It should follow that knowledge so created bears the personality marks of its creators, including their views of time."[1]

In the following I frequently draw from Jung's *Psychological Types* which has the history of Western thought as its foundation.[2]

William James' tough-minded and tender-minded philosophers

The American philosopher and psychologist William James (1842-1910) was the first to draw attention to two opposing temperaments which color philosophical thought.[3] He spoke of "tough-minded" and "tender-minded" types which, he said, are responsible for the ongoing clash in the history of philosophy. Their reasons for this is that each has its own bias, making people believe that those of the opposite temperament are out of touch with the true nature of reality.[4]

James described his tough-minded philosophers as empiricists who are lovers of facts or in my terms 4–D oriented, They consider only the observable world in 4–D as real. Their primary concern is to let facts speak for themselves. Only thinking that takes its departure from facts is acceptable. In building theories, concepts should be derived from 4–D and not be induced from 7–D as the starting point. Over time, these tough-minded philosophers may focus on a number of seemingly different areas in 4–D and end up with conclusions which are logically unrelated, if not contradictory; their approach toward 4–D reality is multifocal.[5]

James characterized his tender-minded philosophers as rationalists or intellectualists. They consider the factual, ever-changing world in 4–D as deceptive but hold that beyond it exists an underlying unchanging reality into which one can gain insight through "pure" inductive reasoning in 7–D.[6] In theory building, abstract ideation in 7–D, independent from experiencing 4–D, should play the primary role.[7] Since these tender-minded scholars believe that a single uniformity and coherence underlies the 4–D reality, they start their theories by speculatively inducing into 7–D some theoretical concept about the 4–D reality. Their search for a single theory to account for the 4–D reality makes their overall approach monofocal.[8]

Wilhelm Ostwald's romantic and classic scientists

Early in the 20th century, Wilhelm Ostwald (1853-1932), a German chemist and philosopher, studied the biographies of a number of eminent scientists. He concluded that there were two types: romantic scientists and classic scientists.[9] One readily recognizes major similarities between romantic scientists and James' tough-minded philosophers; and between classic scientists and James' tender-minded philosophers. Ostwald thought, as James did, that his two types are rooted in different temperaments and actually speculated about the nature of these two temperaments. Using a classification as old as Hippocrates (460-377 BCE) he suggested that the romantic scientist reflects the quick reaction time of the sanguine (who is by nature hopeful and cheerful), and that the classic scientist reflects the slower reaction time of the phlegmatic (who may be viewed as cool and calm).[10]

Carl Jung's extroverted and introverted scholars

Jung recognized that philosophers and scientists show a duality in their thinking.[11] He felt that opposing views among scholars are not explained by one or the other using faulty logic, but by basic differences in psychological attitude. His interest went beyond the personality traits of these scholars. He concluded that the tough-minded philosophers of James and the romantic scientists of Ostwald have an extroverted personality whose consciousness is outward- and object-oriented.[12] In developing knowledge, extroverted scholars not only depend on observations of what I would call the physical 4–D reality but also guide their thinking with relevant scientific knowledge and ideas from the social reality in 4–D as transmitted through education. Their extroverted thinking—and I paraphrase Jung—gives a primary role to observations in 4–D, "facts." In building theories, "objective" factors are the decisive ones.[13]

Jung concluded that the personality of James' tender-minded philosophers and of Ostwald's classic scientists is introverted with a consciousness that is inward- and subject-oriented.[14] (In my view this means they are betas.) Their introverted thinking—and I again paraphrase Jung—gives a primary role to abstract ideation in 7–D rather than to observations in 4–D. "Subjective" factors are the decisive ones.[15] Introverted thinking formulates questions and creates theories, leading to new insights. Facts are collected only to support or contradict a theory, rather than being its source.[16] It is important to note in this context that Jung viewed introversion as a preferential orientation of one's consciousness toward the "subjective world of the unconscious," while the time gender model proposes introversion as the result of a preferential orientation of betas toward their timescapein 6–D.

Max Knoll's experimental and theoretical scientists

Because of a growing awareness among scientists that their theories reflect a duality in scientific thought, Max Knoll, a professor in electrical engineering, reviewed the historic evidence for such duality in the 1980s.[17] He concluded that for experimental scientists the 4–D reality comes first and theory formation in 7–Dsecond; for theoretical scientists theory formation in 7–D comes first and proving or disproving it in 4–D second.[18] These conclusions are identical with James's, Ostwald's and Jung's views on how tough-minded, romantic, extroverted scholars and soft-minded, classic, introverted scholars think.

In explaining this duality, Knoll did not focus on extroversion and introversion, as Jung did, but on the role of sensation and intuition (two basic psychological functions which Jung had introduced in addition to thinking and feeling).[19] Jung viewed sensation and intuition as opposite aspects of perception (respectively observational perception of the outside "objective" world, and intuitive perception of the inner "subjective" world). This suggested to Knoll that perception has a built-in duality which accounts for the two types of scientific thinking. Experimental scientists obtain their knowledge primarily through sensation (or observational perception); theoretical scientists obtain their knowledge foremost through intuitive, non-sensory perception of new scientific ideas.[20] Since Jung viewed sensation and intuition as opposite perceptive instruments, Knoll concluded that scientists cannot simultaneously derive their knowledge from sensation and intuition.

There is, however, a problem with defining intuition\as a perceptive instrument which takes its input from an inner subjective world. This position was contradicted by the psychologist Julian Jaynes. He concluded that, when a full-blown idea (such as an atomic model) suddenly emerges in a theoretical scientist, such scientific intuition is the unexpected conscious end product of non-conscious thinking. Although deliberate and conscious thinking is verbal, logical thinking is not always linked to natural language, for logical analysis can also occur in the absence of language, suddenly presenting the person with an unsolicited, spontaneous solution.[21] Jaynes explained that creative thinking goes through several stages. First, a problem is consciously worked over. Next, there is a period of incubation without any conscious concentration upon the problem. Finally, a process of intuitive reasoning occurs without representation in consciousness, yet suddenly leads to the illumination of a discovery which is later justified by logic. A close friend of Einstein told Jaynes that many of Einstein's greatest ideas came to him so suddenly while shaving that he had to be very careful not to cut himself. He also mentioned that a British physicist once said: "We often talk about the three B's, the Bus, the Bath, and the Bed. That is where the great discoveries are made in our science."[22]

Section 2: The thinking styles of alpha and beta scholars

Overview

Experiencing intellectual insights and discoveries can be quite exciting, particularly for scholars who devote their life to unraveling the mysteries of the universe. Such intellectual revelations may gain access to 6–D because they are as emotionally charged as any personal milestone originating in 4–D.

The root of time gender differences between alphas and betas lies in how they store their autobiographic memories. The resulting differences in their 6–D structure should therefore be directly or indirectly responsible for their two contrasting thinking styles.

- *Directly,* because in alphas sequentially occurring but logically unrelated data remain unconnected in time; in betas these data get mapped into their timescape. When in a similar context 6–D contents are used, this dissimilar mapping of personalized data causes the flow of their thoughts to differ.
- *Indirectly,* because the difference in their 6–D structures leads in a similar context to different attention priorities that affect their thinking styles, rendering the thinking of alphas extroverted and the thinking of betas introverted.

Flow and context of thoughts

Since in alpha scholars the mapping of sequentially occurring but logically unrelated data remains without time connections, these 6–D data get mapped in relevant memory islets that are activated in the current contextual thinking paradigm of alpha scholars. If later the same paradigm gets triggered, they readmit these paradigm-specific intellectual 6 D contents to their thinking in 7 D. Because alpha scholars do not put their scientific thoughts in some personalized historic time-perspective, their scientific thinking tends to be situational. Hence, their panoramic view of their area of scientific endeavor tends to become compartmentalized. As a result, they may use the same concept in different contexts, but with different meanings. Jung's thinking style is a good example of this. As one of his followers remarked:

> "Jung often wrote using the abstract language of complex psychology, but he also wrote clinically using *a language that better conveys the flavor of immediate emotional experience*, using such concepts as persona, shadow, anima, animus, and Self.... They are terms to fit clinically useful entities, not theoretical concepts created by fiat [i.e. consensus]. Thus their usefulness is more readily evident than their preciseness..."[23]

The compartmentalized thinking style of alpha scholars is further reflected by the fact that they may embrace contradictory theoretical explanations in different areas of scholarly endeavor. This reflects their natural tolerance for logical inconsistencies between contextual compartments. "The world of science is full of unresolved contradictions," they will say, "That is what the current state of science is all about." Not having the pressure to account for the global entirety of their knowledge with a single unifying explanation permits them to publish early and more frequently than their beta counterparts, often making them more productive in their field and, as a result, well-known at an earlier age.[24]

In beta scholars, personalized intellectual events become part of a sequentially organized timescape in 6–D. This enables them to experience their thinking in a historic context. Darwin, for example, never knew when new concepts would come to him but, in hindsight, could chart their beginnings and growth.[25]

Because betas have access to the emotionally charged intellectual aspects of their timescape, their thinking is global rather than compartmentalized. This results in their intolerance for logical inconsistencies and a search for coherence in their thinking. For example, they are sticklers for consistency in the meaning of concepts, no matter what their context. Their global thinking furthermore makes them realize that their world of science is full of unresolved contradictions. This disturbs their peace of mind and results in a personal challenge to find a theoretical model in 7–D that will unify the disconnected personalized knowledge bits about the 4–D reality. Since this is not a simple matter, they frequently get bogged down for long periods in these attempts to find the unifying model that will create a measure of overall coherence in their frame of reference. In short, beta scholars are system builders who strive in their science toward a monofocal panoramic view. The theoretical physicist Albert Einstein is a classical example of this. He never stopped dreaming of creating a unifying formula which would embrace both the microcosm and macrocosm, although he did not succeed in finding one.[26]

It is in this context interesting to compare how Freud, a beta, and Jung, an alpha, each came to account for the infinite variety of human experience. Freud's monofocal beta thinking led him to account for this with a single example—the Oedipus myth.

Jung's compartmentalized, multifocal thinking, on the other hand, led him to employ an entire body of mythology.

Extroverted versus introverted thinking

The thinking in 7–D of alpha scholars is clearly outward-oriented or extroverted, its conclusions based on input from the observable, perceptual public reality in 4–D. These scientists first observe, then experiment, and then analyze their observations. It does not matter whether this involves the nature of the 4–D reality itself (as in biology, physics, chemistry, physiology, or sociology) or whether the 4–D input conveys information of a psychological, linguistic, logical, mathematical, or musicological nature. Alpha scholars' theories flow with logical necessity from their findings in 4–D. Extroverted scholarly thinking is therefore empirical and deductive in nature. The creativity of alpha scholars lies in their ability to abstract theoretical explanations from factual material.[27]

Since beta scholars unavoidably focus their attention on their timescape, they tend to pursue 4–D information which is related to knowledge they already possess. This leads to selective, in-depth knowledge.

Because beta scholars are inward-oriented or introverted, their scholarly thinking in 7–D takes its dominant cues not from 4–D, but from the emotionally charged scientific experiences in their timescape in 6–D. In developing knowledge they start with what puzzles them about what is already known, and what can be induced from these encountered facts. They use logic intuitively to hypothesize a general theory in 7–D that will fit the 4–D reality as represented by their intellectual 6–D. These scientists turn to 4–D only to prove or to disprove their unifying theory empirically by collecting facts which their theory explains, based on which new facts can be predicted, which in turn can then be experimentally verified.

Instead of turning for guidance to the socially shared world of knowledge in 4–D, betas tend to gravitate toward a private scientific journey in their academic timescape. This often makes betas' scientific language idiosyncratic and difficult to understand, in contrast with the scientific language of their alpha colleagues, who draw extensively on the intellectual tradition and climate of their professional environment.

The significance of the introverted approach in science cannot be overstated. Beta scientists have had a tremendous impact on their field. For example, the English physicist and mathematician Newton (1643-1727), who dominated the scientific revolution of the 17th century, proposed a theory which explains the movements of planets. Darwin (1809-1882) proposed the theory of organic evolution which revolutionized science, philosophy, and theology.[28] And, in the first 15 years of the 20th century, Einstein (1879-1955) advanced a series of theories that proposed entirely new ways of thinking about space, time, and gravitation, long before these theories could be empirically tested.

The introverted thinking of beta scientists tends to render them makers of patterns or theoretical scientists. This stands in contrast with the extroverted thinking of alpha scientists, which makes them accumulators of facts or experimental scientists. One recent scholar divided scientists into "lumpers," who like to draw grand conclusions about the universe based on their study of the big picture, and "splitters," who prefer modest theories teased out from their observations of nature's marvelous details.[29]

Section 3: From scholarly to ordinary thinking

Overview

Young alphas learn to assume that timescape-related words have flexible meanings which can differ from context to context. Young betas, on the other hand, grow accustomed to timescape-related words having a fixed meaning. These tendencies soon generalize to cover the entire language (discussed in Chapter 6). As a result, alpha speak reflects situational language usage, which involves reaching for the right word at the right time. Alpha speak is emotionally more appealing than beta speak, which is more cerebral because it is timescape-oriented and engenders a more consistent usage of word meanings.

The dissimilarity in the ordinary thinking styles of alphas and betas goes well beyond time gender linguistics. This is especially evident in scholarly thinking.

Flow and context of thought

To give an example of the situational context of the every day's thinking of alphas compared with the ordinary thinking of betas which is more globally oriented, an anecdote attributed to Christopher Wren (1632-1723) comes to mind. Wren was an English architect who designed, among many other buildings of note, St. Paul's Cathedral in London. On an inspection tour of the site of St. Paul's, he is said to have asked one workman what he was doing. "Digging a hole" he was told. On encountering another to whom he put the same question, a very different answer explained the same activity: "Building a cathedral."

What clearly exemplifies the compartmentalized day-to-day thinking of alphas is that they behave and think one way in one context, yet quite differently in another. A manager at a corporation, for example, thought differently about relating to the president, an auditor, his secretary, someone of lower rank, or a customer. "You have to think in one situation one way," he said, "and in another situation another way." His view of himself and others was multifocal.

By contrast, the monofocal identity of betas forces them to think and behave with relative consistency—whether in the bosom of their family, at work, or in a religious or political setting. This is not to say that a beta's thinking does not vary with different moods—more optimistic about life and specific goals when feeling good, and more pessimistic in these regards when feeling down. Yet despite their moods or social roles, their basic thinking pattern remains essentially unchanged. This consistency may come across as a rigidity.

A disagreement between a beta-alpha couple who had been together for 20 years serves to further illustrate how the thinking of alphas and betas differ in ordinary life. The argument was about the beta husband having wronged his alpha wife. She naturally assumed that he was to blame for their unhappiness, and he deep down thought that he was totally responsible. She used her alpha speak to her best advantage, and soon shifted from her present hurt to some earlier one, then to an another, and so on. Listening to this, one might gain the impression that their long marriage never had been any good and that her husband always has been wronging her. He, on the other hand, argued in his idiosyncratic beta speak that some of the past experiences she was bringing up had nothing to do with the present situation. As she kept her stream of thought going, he tried to put all this in perspective and exclaimed in utter frustration: "But what about the rest of our marriage over the past 20 years?"

When a good thing happened between the two, the same type of discussion took place, albeit in an emotionally opposite key. To her, everything had always been great, but he, while silently taking responsibility for the good things that had happened, remained cognizant of the not-so-good things in the past for which he also accepted responsibility. In reality, the alpha appeared trapped in emotional opportunism, and the beta in an almost megalomanic sense of responsibility.

Generally, I observed with couples that the alpha may come to view the thinking of the beta as inflexible or, alternatively, think that the beta's approach is too over-inclusive and loses sight of what the alpha thinks is important. The beta, on the other hand, may conclude that an alpha's thinking is too compartmentalized and fails to place matters in their proper perspective.

Extroverted versus introverted thinking

In ordinary life, extroverted alpha thinking and introverted beta thinking follow the same basic patterns as in scholarly thought. When alphas think pragmatically, they tend to reach conclusions based on input from the particular 4–D situation in which they are momentarily involved. Alphas tend not to view matters in their larger context and, despite their adroitness, often confuse appearance with how things really are. This often impresses betas as short-sighted, shallow, one-dimensional, if not highly biased thinking. Or, as Jung put it: the purely empirical accumulation of facts by extroverts paralyzes their thought and smothers their meaning.[30]

One should keep in mind two further features of extroverted thinking. One is that, in guiding their thinking, alphas tend to rely on dominant input from their social reality in 4–D. The other is that the situational self-esteem they derive from a particular context—their nuclear family, peer group, work environment, and so on—significantly biases their conclusions and opinions.

By contrast, when betas think pragmatically, they begin by elaborating on what they know already about the facts they have encountered. In trying to reach agreement between the facts in 4–D and their private reality in 6–D, they may well tilt to forcing facts in the 4–D world to fit assumptions they have already developed in their head. As Jung warned, introverted thinking has a dangerous tendency to adulterate facts or ignore them altogether in order to give fantasy free play.[31] To alphas, this aspect of introverted thinking may appear quite arbitrary, as in the case of the ancient Greek robber Procrustes, who stretched his prisoners on a bed and, depending on whether they were too long or too short, made them fit the bed by either cutting off their limbs or stretching them out. Everyday introverted thinkers are far less inclined to turn to the environment for guidance and are therefore less dependent on any particular social context. Instead, betas' introverted thinking carries the imprint of their timescape, and strives to maintain or improve their global self-esteem. Betas' timescapes certainly makes their introverted thinking rather inflexible.

Since alphas alphacize others and betas betacize others, both extroverted and introverted thinking are biased, focusing selectively on what appears relevant and omitting what is incongruent.

Concluding remarks: Eastern thinking

When I, a Westerner, traced the duality in thinking back through time, I naturally turned to the history of Western thought. This started at the western side of the Eurasian continent in ancient Greece around the fourth century BCE. Only in the late 1980s did I become aware that during the same period, China, at the far-eastern end of the Eurasian continent, went through similar scientific and technological achievements and philosophical insights.[32]

Shortly after I discovered this, a Chinese businesswoman of superior academic background told me she had consulted a Chinese soothsayer. This sage advised her "not to fight Yin and Yang but, rather, to move in harmony with the cyclical process of these two cosmic forces, which by their interaction influence the destinies of creatures and things." The sage was drawing on the Yin and Yang School of ancient Chinese humanistic philosophy.[33] One early commentator in Chinese history noted about the principle of Yin and Yang:

> "As the sun moves on, the moon comes; as the moon moves on, the sun comes. As sun and moon impel each other light is produced. As the cold goes, the heat comes; as the heat goes, the cold comes. As cold and heat impel each other the year is formed. What moves on contracts; what comes expands. What contracts and what expands influence each other, producing what furthers man's activities."[34]

In Chinese thinking, Yin and Yang represent not only a profound duality in the nature of the universe, but also in the nature of people. In this context, Yin and

Yang often refer to the duality in sexual gender, with Yin representing the feminine and Yang the masculine. Yet Yin and Yang may refer also to a personality duality (as I pointed out in Chapter 6) with the Yin person representing "the man of the earth, whose attitude is permeated by the earth under his feet," and the Yang person's chief characteristic being "an attitude conditioned by ideas, often called 'idealistic' or 'spiritual'." In other words, the Yin person represents the alpha, and the Yang the beta. From this followed my assumption that there must be a Yin-Yang duality in the history of Oriental thought which corresponds to the alpha-beta duality in the history of Western thinking.

Focusing on Yang and Yin as an expression of the alpha-beta duality is meaningful not only because of the complementary polarity of these terms, but also because the cooperation between these two poles can produce superior views where previously conflictual positions existed. As Joseph Campbell commented:

> "Yin and Yang interacting produce the order, sense, direction, or way, Tao or Dao, of all things, which is represented geometrically as an ever-turning circle, mixed of black [Yin] and white [Yang]."[35]

Both alpha and beta ways of thinking are necessary for a complete description of the human being. Indeed, the completeness of *any* science depends on the degree to which alphas and betas are allowed to develop their views side by side, demonstrating the complementary nature of their thinking. Thus, both time genders are needed for the formation of modern society which celebrates the bi-polar totality resulting from the union of these opposites.

NOTES

1   Fraser (1966), p. xx.
2   Jung (1977), first published in 1921.
3   Jung (1977), p. 319.
4   James (1907), p. 7 and 12, as quoted by Jung (1977), p. 300 and 301, respectively.
5. Paraphrasing James (1907) , as quoted by Jung (1977), p. 300-301; also Jung (1977), p. 310.
6   James (1907) , quoted by Jung (1977), p. 300-301, as paraphrased by me.
7   Jung (1977) , p.300-301, quoting James; and Jung (1977), p.309, 318.
8   Jung (1977) p. 301, 306, 318.
9   Ostwald (1910/1919), quoted by Jung (1977), p. 322, 324-326, 328-329).
10 Jung (1977) , p.323-324.
11 Jung (1977) , Chapter VIII, p. 300-321; Chapter IX, p. 322-329.
12 Jung (1977) , p. p. 303. 342, 344; Ostwald (1919) quoted by Jung (1977), p. 322.
13 Jung (1977) , p. 373.
14 Jung (1977), p. 309-310, quoting Kant [(1912-22), VIII, p. 400; Ostwald (1919) quoted by Jung (1977), p. 322-323; Jung (1977), p. 325-326, 328-329.
15 Jung (1977), p. 373.
16 Jung (1977), p. 380.
17 Knoll (1983), p. 279.
18 Knoll (1983).
19 Jung (1977) , p. 519, 554.
20 Knoll (1983), p. 270.

21   Gazzaniga (1977).
22   Jaynes (1982), p. 44.
23   Hall (1977), p. 113.
24   Jung (1977), p. 322, 325-326, 328-329.
25   Stone (1982), p. 693.
26   Barnett (1958), p. 110-111.
27   Boernstein (1970), p. 678.
28   Stone (1982), p. 329.
29   Freeman Dyson in *Time* (Winter 1997-1998), p. 123.
30   Jung (1977), p. 381.
31   Jung (1977), p. 381.
32   Fraser, Lawrence and Haber (1986).
33   This philosophy dominated the period of the so-called Hundred Schools, which ended around 221 BCE [Chan (1967)].
34   Quoted from Sivin (1986), p. 151.
35   Campbell (1959), p. 452.

CHAPTER 9

Time Gender And Adolescent Development

Many factors—some nature, others nurture—determine the outcome of the developmental phase called adolescence. This chapter addresses the connection between the social environment and people's time gender.

> "With caring families, good schools, preventive health care, and supportive community institutions, [most adolescents will] grow up healthy and vigorous, reasonably well educated, committed to families and friends, and prepared for the workplace and the responsibilities of democratic citizenship."[1]

The above statement is predicated on a structured social environment in which teenagers and the adults they are involved with (parents, teachers, and other members of the community) share similar expectations about teenage behavior and school attitude. In these circumstances, an omnipresent set of compatible expectations about present- and future-oriented adolescent behavior exercises a powerful positive influence on adolescent development. The presence of shared expectations tends to override the effect time gender might otherwise play.

However, there is a problem. Culturally stable environments have become less and less frequent in contemporary society. There is widespread erosion of neighborhood networks and other traditional social support systems in many communities. Also, both parents often work full time outside the home, and divorce rates are high. As a result, the number of surrogate parents and single-parent families is growing. About half of all young Americans will spend part or all of their childhood and adolescence living with only one parent. Children now spend less time in the company of adults than a few decades ago. Instead, they spend more of their time with their peers in age-segregated, largely unsupervised environments. They spend their time on the street, in front of a computer, or watching television loaded with violent or sexual programming that influences teenagers as much as any commercial. The combination of these conditions threaten adolescents, leading to premature drop-outs, depression, suicide, substance abuse, sexually transmitted diseases (including HIV and AIDS), and gun-related homicides.[2]

Currently, nearly half of American adolescents in families of all economic strata, social backgrounds, and geographic areas are at high or moderate risk in this regard. Studies indicate that one-third of early adolescents (ages 12-15) have contemplated suicide. By the end of middle adolescence (ages 15-17), the total number of teenagers who have used drugs, taken part in antisocial activity, failed at school, or become pregnant) reaches about 25%.[3]

A Canadian sample demonstrated that at age 12, 20% of adolescents showed marked personality dysfunction, with 25% having some personality dysfunction. Although 11% normalized between ages 12 and 15, among late teenagers (ages 17-19) who were still in school, the proportion with personality dysfunction had increased once again to the levels of early adolescence.[4]

Concerning premature, unprotected sex (with the chance of contracting sexually transmitted diseases or having an unwanted pregnancy), my own sample showed that many subjects had already gotten so involved during early adolescence. By age 15, 20% of females and males had experienced their first genital sexual intercourse, and half of females who experienced casual sex had already done so, as had one third of males who experienced casual sex. Of females with one or more abortions (17%) almost 30% had already gone through an abortion at age 15.

There is no general consensus on how healthy, adaptively functioning adolescents differ from those with personality dysfunction.[5] In this context, the question arises as to whether being an alpha teenager or beta teenager influences the degree to which one is either vulnerable or resilient to today's confusing and conflicting value systems which have resulted in the new morbidities of adolescence.

In the following sections I will demonstrate that time gender indeed plays a pivotal role in this regard. Hence, getting to know the time gender of adolescents, and dealing with them in kind, becomes crucially important. It is of fundamental importance that all institutions which contribute to adolescent development (families, the educational system, the health care system, community organizations, and media)[6] come to realize that under unfavorable social circumstances, alpha and beta teenagers tend to respond quite differently. Because they experience reality very differently, they have different social needs. Social institutions must use appropriate approaches in helping alpha and beta teenagers make a successful transition from childhood to adulthood.

To put the role of time gender in adolescence into its proper perspective, I will need to do two things. First, I will review the developments which alpha and beta teenagers share during adolescence. Next, I will shift the focus to how alpha and beta teenagers differ and discuss their vulnerability (or resilience) to high-risk behavior. Corroborating statistical evidence will be given on the topics of alcohol abuse, illicit drug use, run-ins with the law and educational achievement. The chapter concludes by 1) noting that the time gender model can assist parents, teachers, health care workers, and community organizations with the healthy development of teenagers, and 2) recommending teaching this model to youngsters early in their teens.

Developments teenagers share

During early adolescence (ages 12-15), teenagers become capable of sexual reproduction.

But adolescence is also the period in which the human brain weight reaches its full size,[7] which makes adolescence the dawn of the "age of reason"[8] or, as Piaget remarked, the beginning of formal logical operations and therefore the crowning achievement of cognitive development in the human species. In the time gender model, early adolescence represents the emergence of abstract thought within 7–D and the appearance of a paraego XE "paraego:first appearance," the "I" who enables adolescents for the first time to become self-aware, to reflect on their conscious experience.[9] This includes becoming aware of their own reasoning. But as their self-awareness (their conscious personal identity) emerges, adolescents for the first time begin to focus significantly on their bodies and how they appear to others. Understandably, this makes them highly self-conscious.[10]

With regards to how young teenagers experience time, they have already internalized much of 4–D's clock and calendar time into 5–D by the later elementary school years. By early adolescence, they begin to understand that this internalized clock and calendar time as something that is collectively shared.

Although early adolescents sense that one day they may no longer be able to depend on their parents and will have to occupy their own independent niche in society, they still tend to remain rather home-centered. Nevertheless, self-asserting, rebellious behavior may occur. This is particularly true when they are made aware of their dependence on their parents.

During middle adolescence (ages 15-17), bodily changes, including sexual ones, are at an advanced stage. Sexual orientation has, as a rule, crystallized. In addition to their preoccupation with their bodies, mid-adolescents begin to contemplate themselves as persons, judging how their personal identity (current life style, attitudes and beliefs) compares with those of peers and relevant adults.

Hand in hand with this budding self-personification goes a fundamental change in how mid-adolescents experience time.[11] They begin to conceptualize time as having an ever extending past and future. This results eventually, around age 15 or 16, in the abstract concept of universal, infinite time.[12]

Having just become self-aware of their personal identity, mid-adolescents soon try to fit themselves into this new extended view of time. Instead of impersonally referring to *the* future, they begin speaking of *my* future, realizing that, embedded in the distant future of impersonal time lies their own, as yet completely uncharted, personal future. This realization gradually translates into many profound, not easily answerable questions: "What kind of person do I want to become? Whom do I want to be like?" "What are my life goals?" "Will I be able to support myself?" "What sort of education do I need?"

Knowing that one can consciously shape one's future self is easier said than done. Initially, many teenagers *fantasize* about their future, giving it mental representation in 5–D. Imaginary trips into their future often trigger their greatest hopes and deepest fears. For many, never again will life be accompanied by moods of such vividly contrasting emotional colors as in this period. Becoming aware that there exists a personal future triggers a period of emotional destabilization which Erik Erikson labeled the "adolescent identity crisis."[13]

Fantasizing about one's future, however, is not the same as defining and planning for one's future. The real challenge for these teenagers is to *think* their way out of this confrontation with their personal future. As Erikson noted, defining one's future often involves a commitment to some ideology which provides a perspective on one's future. Because their thinking is still mostly of the "black and white" variety and lacks a comprehensive approach, teenagers in the throes of an identity crisis often make rigid, totalistic, intense, even fanatic commitments to their future. Yet just as often they rapidly discard and replace passionately held views. Succeeding in establishing a mature, lasting sense of identity usually occurs well after adolescence.[14]

In dealing with the normal anxieties of their adolescent identity crisis, teenagers often break out of their isolation by making common cause with a best friend, a boy-friend or a girl-friend. Sharing time together provides mutual reassurance and makes one's personal future a shared project.[15] These new peer relationships reflect a shift away from complete dependency on parents toward identification with a peer or peer group. This often translates into holding values that override and are at odds with parental values.[16] Indeed, during mid-adolescence teenagers frequently de-identify with, if not alienate themselves from their parents and their familial values. They often like to emphasize this new sense of belonging by displaying identifying marks of group membership, like nose rings, tattoos, different dress, listening to different music, and so on.

Late adolescence (ages 17-19) more or less coincides with grade 12 in senior high school and the first year thereafter. Although identity formation continues, issues of independence, sexuality, career, and the nature of intimate relationships have, as a rule, been confronted.[17] Any remaining conflicts in these areas tend to be more clearly defined;[18] thus their potential for resolution, with an accompanying stabilization of personality, is greater.[19] Continued parental protection becomes less acceptable. One should begin taking full responsibility for oneself. Failures are no longer readily forgiven and consequences of poor judgment become less reversible. This no longer is a time for promises for the future, but for making final decisions in educational or vocational matters and for making good one's potential to love and to work.

At this time an inner sense of direction and purpose is needed more than anything else. Failing this, circumstances may compel young people to decide what they are going to do with their lives. What often helps at this stage is that one's intellectual perspective has grown more sophisticated, meaning that one can realize that there is more to reality than one's own view of the world.[20] This may in turn make the young adult more accessible to prosocial input.

Some teenagers avoid the upheavals of an identity crisis by deferring consideration of their future "to some point down the road." Since World War II, society has been sanctioning a moratorium on deciding one's future until well beyond adolescence. Young adults supposedly need a few more years to think about what they want to do with their lives. They need "to take a break" from education, "do their own thing" for a little while. Or while making up their mind about their future, they should be allowed to enrich themselves intellectually in pursuing college degrees that are not necessarily relevant to the careers they will choose.[21]

Adolescence and time gender

Erik Erikson thought of the adolescent identity crisis as a step toward developing an inner sense of wholeness in one's personal identity, part of the process of unifying what one wants to become with what one is. He wrote:

> "The young person, in order to experience wholeness, must feel a progressive continuity between that which he has come to be during the long years of childhood and that which he promises to become in the anticipated future; between that which he conceives himself to be and that which he perceives others to see in him and to expect of him."[22]

This implies that everyone ends up with a beta timescape and, thus, with a monofocal, non-partitioned identity. Yet, as self-reflective thinking evolves during adolescence, the compartmentalized identity of alpha teenagers normally emerges and will stay this way throughout life. Similarly, the self-conscious identity of beta teenagers is well on its way to becoming monofocal and will continue to develop along this line.

Erikson opined furthermore that the central feature of the adolescent identity crisis is "being at odds with time itself," which he spoke of as a "diffusion of time perspective."[23] This time perspective, he said, is sometimes experienced as a sense of great urgency and at other times as a sense of loss of experiencing time as a dimension for living.[24] This view implies that, during their identity crisis, adolescents sometimes live anxiously in the future (like betas), yet sometimes purely in the here-and-now (like alphas). But, as I have demonstrated, the time perspectives of alpha teenagers and of beta teenagers are mutually exclusive. Another psychoanalyst, Seton, made this clear by describing two types of adolescents: the one who experiences time as a succession of discontinuous events (alphas) and the other who is able to experience the "imminence of past-present-future"[25] (betas).

Because time gender features become more pronounced with adolescence, one should be able to recognize an adolescent's time gender early in high school. And, just as one should teach early adolescents about the dangers of early, unprotected sex, smoking, drinking and illicit drug use,[26] so one should teach them about time gender. For only then, early in high school, can these young alphas and betas gradually identify their own time gender, and learn that neither its strengths nor its weaknesses are anything to be concerned about. Instead, one should encourage them to use their strengths to their advantage, and motivate them to develop any compensatory mechanisms for their weaknesses.

About alpha teenagers

Alpha teenagers focus habitually on the here-and-now in 4–D. Yet, considering that one's future becomes increasingly important during adolescence, educational and vocational goals should be set and consistently followed through on. In addition, the potential long-term consequences of high-risk behaviors should be considered. The fact that teenage alphas tend not to respond realistically to their future is a definite vulnerability.

What motivates alpha teenagers is the desire to obtain situational self-esteem wherever possible, or to take pleasure in the activity they are currently involved in. Given their appetite for new and varied input, alpha teenagers tend to go for a variety of activities they like, and for which they have some talent, be it intellectual or musical, or a sport, and so on. However, being easily bored and restless, they also may seek out high-risk behaviors. They often search for hedonic excitement, without giving much thought to future consequences.

As a rule, alpha teenagers' extroverted, contextually partitioned personality enables them to fit quite comfortably in any social context with their peers or elders. Their authoritarian-competitive style, reinforced by their flexible alpha speak, renders them increasingly sophisticated in manipulating others to their immediate ends, including their parents. If avoiding confrontation serves them, they may readily behave for the moment in line with whatever is expected from them.

As alpha teenagers become aware of their different identities in various social contexts, each contextual identity may well come to include some relevant past memories or future anticipations. But because their thinking is compartmentalized, these retrospective or prospective memories do not necessarily become time-bound milestones in an overall life story. In any given context, their personal identity is foremost in terms of the present in 4–D. Their compartmentalized thinking usually renders them ignorant about the inconsistency of their behavior across various social contextsi. Even if a friend or sibling whom they trust notices this inconsistency and attempts to make them aware of it, this usually still does not bother them. "Yes, that's the way I am," they may say, testifying to their tolerance for cognitive dissonance between contexts.

In a social niche which provides structure and direction (and is therefore authoritarian, albeit usually in a benevolent way) teenagers have a clearly defined role. Since such a social environment allegedly "knows what is good for you," and expects its teenagers to do their own idiosyncratic, long-term planning only within rather narrow confines, it handles its teenagers with a consistent, benevolent carrot-and-stick approach. "Doing the right thing" means complying with social expectations about here-and-now and future-oriented behavior of adolescents, and results in an ongoing supply of external self-esteem. "Taking the wrong approach" means substantially deviating from social expectations, and leads to sanctions. The social environment, rather than the individual teenager, imposes the confines within which the adolescent should behave.

This habitual carrot-and-stick approach of a structured social environment suits alpha teenagers well. Its authoritarian interpersonal atmosphere feels natural to them, provided adult authority figures are benevolent and trustworthy and supply external self-esteem when deserved. Keeping alpha teenagers focused on a day-by-day basis on "proper" present behavior and on performing their future-oriented educational tasks makes for a comfortable socially structured environment. It compensates for their not having a sustained future oriented sense of direction. Because living in such an environment is attractive, alpha teenagers readily identify with it as their "tribe." This gives them a ready-made group identity with its own social ideology that sets them apart from "outsiders."

In the absence of social structure and direction, adolescents are left to define their own role and values. In these circumstances, alpha teenagers often appear in search of a new identity that satisfies them. Sometimes this leads to a close relationship and identification with a capable beta peer who has rather outspoken values. Such relationship may, indeed, introduce a rather sudden, stable direction and purpose into their behavior, such as a dramatically improved educational performance. In the absence of such a stabilizing influence, alpha teenagers tend to drift into peer groups which not only center around exciting high-risk behaviors, but also, as a rule, celebrate values which are excitingly different from the ones they grew up with. The chance of alpha teenagers ending up in such alienated sub-cultures increases if, prior to adolescence, their childhood was characterized by value conflicts and confusion. Being part of such a group enables alpha teens to experience the group's identity and values as "their own," which means devaluing the identity and values of "outsiders"—parents, teachers, and other peers. It also temporarily satisfies their outgoing nature, their need for excitement, and the reaffirmation of situational self-esteem by others.

When alpha teenagers become intellectually aware of having their own personal future, and begin speaking of "my future," it is quite normal for them not to worry about what lies ahead and to defer real life decisions and long-term commitments for as long as circumstances will allow. After all, they live a day at a time. Their adolescent identity crisis is not anxiety ridden. Yet, like all teenagers, they often enter fantasyland. Sometimes they get involved in what has been referred to as "identity play."[27] They confuse their fantasy about the future with the present by acting out some a future role which appeals to them, although without any actual commitments.[28] For many alphas, this moratorium on making life decisions comes to an end in late adolescence or early adulthood, at which point alphas make long-term commitments to their future, particularly in terms of an occupation or career. This gives them a desired sense of direction and purpose.

Committing a more stable identity to various social contexts (whether educational, career-related, interpersonal or intimate) does not necessarily result in an overall consistency within alphas' partitioned identity. In fact, alphas usually continue to remain unaware of the partitioned nature of their identity. Only a minority develops such awareness, and of those only a few eventually begin to see this as an existential problem: "Who is the *real* me and which values do I really stand for?" Some of these young men and women seek professional help, while for others the problem is alleviated when they join a social institution which provides them with a ready made, institution-derived identity and system of values, such as the army, a religious or political group, a professional organization, or a prestigious firm.

While for many alpha teenagers the moratorium on life decisions comes to an end, in others the moratorium continues in open-ended fashion. These adults usually hide a chronic inability to establish commitments regarding occupation, intimate relationships, or belief systems, and suffer from an ongoing struggle between conflicting identities, which Erikson referred to as "identity diffusion as a life style."[29] Some stay this way well beyond age 30, even if endowed with obvious talent. To watch this may be immensely painful for parents, siblings, or spouses. Yet, to persist in helping them to self-realize may eventually pay off.

About beta teenagers

Beta teenagers experience time in 6–D as an ongoing continuity of past, present, and future. This is why 6–D is their preferred attention mode and why, well before adolescence, their short-term personal future already figures importantly in their motivation.

During adolescence, their pre-livable future continues to extend incrementally from about a season at age 12, to around six months at age 16, to approximately nine months at age 18. This fact becomes increasingly influential in motivating beta teenagers to work toward educational and vocational goals. Instead of becoming bored or restless when faced with an unpleasant challenge, beta teenagers tend to view this as a hurdle to overcome. Reaching their goals is what provides them with the global self-esteem they seek. Hedonistic satisfaction and situational self-esteem remain but secondary considerations.

Their preferred attention mode in 6–D makes these youngsters not only introverted, but also renders their basic personality adjustment progressively less contextually partitioned, more monofocal. Their paraego with its self-reflection, which enters the picture during adolescence, enhances this development. As a result, their personal identity becomes progressively more autonomous from social contexts in 4–D. Since they are introverted, they do not fit comfortably into social contexts which people often expect adolescents to engage in. Rather, they have to try to bring the way they see themselves into harmony with what a given social reality expects of them. This makes them appear shy, or snobbish, or inflexible, and sometimes outright confrontational. Their monofocal introverted personality, plus their often idiosyncratic beta speak, limits their ability to manipulate others to their own ends. Instead, they tend to adopt an egalitarian-cooperative style, without striving to dominate others. As teenagers they are easier for parents to cope with than alpha daughters and sons.

As beta teenagers become increasingly self-aware of their identity, this identity begins to include memories, particularly recent ones, as well as important aspects of their pre-livable future. This development also increases their sensitivity toward behaving inconsistently under different circumstances. In turn, this may lead to internal conflicts with guilt, followed by intense efforts at self-correction. Whether implicitly or explicitly, their central existential problem becomes: "How can I make myself more consistent and coherent?" Of course, they do not take into account that there is an alpha alternative. Instead, they take for granted that everyone's individuality is singular and monofocal. Parents, particularly those who are familiar with the time gender model, can be helpful here by easing the frustration of beta teenagers.

Betas' individuality makes it more likely for them to bond with one or two peers, rather than aligning themselves with the identity and overriding values of an entire peer group. They are inclined to hang onto values they develop during adolescence, but this does not mean that their value system has become fixed. Although somewhat inflexible, they may well amend their values as they grow older, sometimes repeatedly so, even though amending their values invariably causes them a great deal of anguish.

Around age 15-16, beta teenagers begin to realize they have an entirely uncharted personal future which extends far beyond the tip of their anterior pre-livable time cone. Often they will enter fantasy land. Yet since they are future-oriented, the adolescent identity crisis which arises around the question of what to do with their future makes a moratorium on making life decisions less likely than in alpha teenagers. Their introversive thinking gravitates toward autonomous planning for their future. Although they may change theirs plan for the future, their monofocal identity leaves them with fewer options to consider.

For beta teenagers to be part of a structured social environment that provides direction means that they have to align their context-autonomous timescape with surrounding, collective social expectations about adolescents. As a rule, this is not a problem, because their own adolescent values tend to be an extension of the ones they grew up with. However, these introverted teenagers are striving toward a self-conscious, context-free identity. Sometimes this leads to a sense of individuality which no longer fits within the boundaries of behavioral conformity demanded by society. This happens when they become aware of inconsistencies in the value system of their school or family which they previously had accepted. As long as the pressure to conform is not excessive, beta teenagers tend to keep matters inside, rather than act them out and provoke a crisis. If such value conflict occurs in their family, it is helpful to spend less time at home and more with a friend. If the value conflict arises at school, then seeing the "light at the end of the tunnel" by pre-living their immediate goals for the end of the term may do the trick.

A major hurdle beta teenagers can run into late in adolescence is when the future they have built into their timescape deviates from what others expect of them. In this case a confrontation can no longer be avoided. The outcome of the conflict will depend on the one hand on the strength of the betas' inner direction and purpose, and on the other, on the leverage which others bring to bear on them. Such leverage can include blocking the opportunity to realize their plans for their future.

When beta teenagers grow up in a social environment with contradictory, competing value systems that increase the new adolescent morbidities, they respond quite differently than their alpha counterparts. They are less likely to seek variety and excitement when facing seductive, high-risk opportunities and, being future-oriented by nature, they are more preoccupied with consequences, particularly scholastic derailment. Their timescape acts as a compass that provides them with a sense of direction. In developing their self-aware monofocal identity they have become increasingly autonomous, despite the social environment they find themselves in. Their primary purpose remains becoming an increasingly consistent individual. They do not need to search for a new identity, and are less likely to join a peer group with an alienated identity and value system. Under unfavorable social circumstances, alpha teenagers tend to be more vulnerable, and beta teenagers more resilient, to potential problems with health, society, and school.

By late adolescence, most betas have built an inner sense of future direction and purpose into their timescape. Nevertheless, some individuals lack self confidence, which derails this process and makes a moratorium on important life decisions very compelling. However, since their self-awareness is future-oriented, postponing these decisions becomes increasingly uncomfortable. It usually ends by them grasping an opening toward a personal future which happens to come their way, and then rigidly hanging onto it. Unfortunately, this tends to leave young betas with little wiggle room for responding to new, alternative opportunities, and may result in a constricted self-view, which Erik Erikson termed "identity foreclosure."[30]

Adolescence and time gender: statistical data

The baby boom generation, with its flower children of the 1960s, was the first generation in North America to experience the breakdown of traditional channels of socialization. For the first time, the peer group became more important in the socialization process than the parents. Most of the 273 subjects in my research cohort from Greater Vancouver, Canada, belonged to this generation and the next one. Thus, it is worthwhile to look at this cohort to support the assumption that alpha and beta teenagers have different vulnerabilities with regard to high-risk behaviors. Data were available on premature sex, casual sex and abortion during adolescence, as well as illicit drug use, alcohol abuse, behavior resulting in criminal charges, and educational achievement.

Self-reported sexual behavior during adolescence

Chapter 7 showed that, by age 18, 65% of alphas, but only 47% of betas had already had their first sexual (genital) experience (p=0.013). Furthermore, between ages 16 and 20, 65% of the majority of alphas who had experienced casual sex had already been so involved, but only 40% of the small minority of betas with such experience. Regarding unprotected, premature sex, between ages 14-19, 55% of the alpha females with one or more abortions had already gone through an abortion, whereas the only two abortions among beta women in the cohort took place at age 25 and age 41. In other words, alpha teenagers were more likely, and at an earlier age, to have premature, casual, unprotected sex than beta teenagers.

Self-reported alcohol abuse during adolescence

I obtained from 97% of the 273 adult subjects relevant data on alcohol abuse.

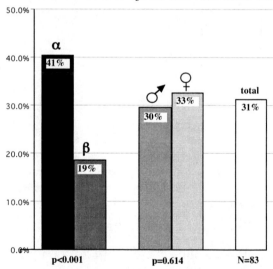

Figure 9.1: Prevalence of self-reported past or present alcohol abuse in 265 adult subjects, broken down by time gender and sexual gender

Figure 9.1 shows that 31% (or 83 subjects) reported past or present alcohol abuse. Forty-one percent of these were alphas and only 19% betas, a difference which was statistically highly significant (p<0.001). There was no statistical difference between men and women (p=0.614) or, for that matter, between alpha females and alpha males (p=0.466), or beta females and beta males (p=0.077). These data clearly indicate the influence of time gender, rather than sexual gender.

Zeroing in on adolescence as a potentially vulnerable period in the 83 adult subjects who reported alcohol abuse, I had data on the age at which this alcohol abuse first occurred in 77 subjects (93%). Figure 9.2 shows the age groups of first alcohol abuse by time gender. It demonstrates that 61% of first alcohol abuse came to pass in the age group 13-18, irrespective of time gender (p=0.340); adolescence was clearly a high-risk period in this regard. However, because the prevalence of alcohol abuse was 41% among alphas, but only 19% among betas (p<0.001), alpha teenagers were at far greater risk of abusing alcohol than beta teenagers.

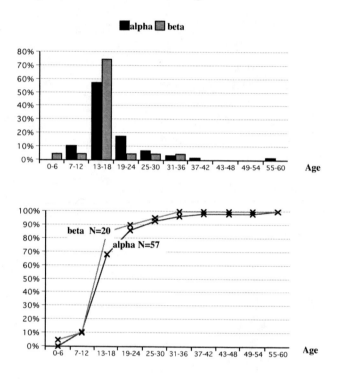

Figure 9.2: Percentage (above) and cumulative percentage (below) of 77 adult subjects who experienced alcohol abuse, broken down by time gender and into age groups in which their alcohol abuse first occurred

Self-reported illicit drug use during adolescence

I obtained in 98% (267) of adult subjects relevant data on past or present illicit drug use (such as marijuana, amphetamine, cocaine, hallucinogens, heroin, sedatives, hypnotics, and anxiolytics).

Figure 9.3 shows that 25% (67) of the adult subjects answered positive in this regard; 32% were alphas and 15% betas, a statistically highly significant difference (p=0.002). There was no significant difference between men and women (p=0.189), although the difference between alpha females (26%) and alpha males (42%) was significant (p=0.049), while the one between beta females (11%) and beta males (26%) (p=0.332) was not.

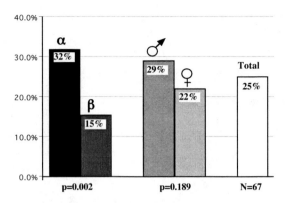

Figure 9.3: Prevalence of self-reported past or present illicit drug use in 267 adult subjects, broken down by time gender and sexual gender

If we focus on adolescence as a potentially vulnerable period, we see that 94% of the 67 respondents (63 subjects) provided information on the age of first occurrence of illicit drug use. Figure 9.4 provides the results, broken down by age groups of first use, and by time gender.

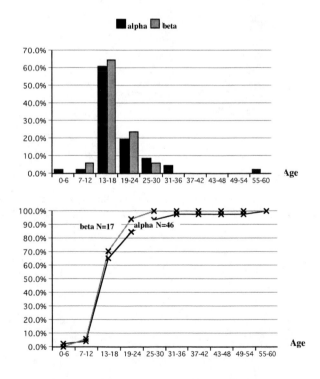

Figure 9.4: Percentage (above) and cumulative percentage (below) of 63 adult subjects with illicit drug use, broken down by time gender and into age groups in which this illicit drug use first occurred

Figure 9.4 shows clearly that the vast majority (62%) of those with a history of illicit drug use had their first experience in the age group 13-18, irrespective of their time

gender (p=0.781). Adolescence was a high-risk period in this respect for all teenagers. Because the overall prevalence of self-reported illicit drug use was 32% among alphas, but only 15% among betas (p=0.002), this supports the prediction that alpha teenagers are at far greater risk of illicit drug use than beta teenagers.

Self-reported legal trouble during adolescence

To study the tendency toward getting into legal trouble during adolescence, I inquired whether there had been, or currently was, any charge under the Juvenile Offenders Act of Canada or the Criminal Code of Canada and, if so, when the first offence occurred. I had data on 98% of 273 subjects. The measure used admittedly has limitations. It does not deal with the seriousness of a charge, nor with whether the case was still before the Court or, if not, what its outcome had been.

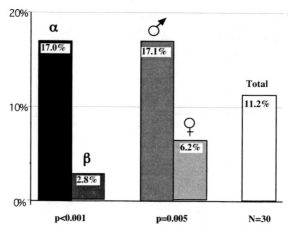

Figure 9.5: Prevalence of self-reported past or present legal trouble in 267 adult subjects, broken down by time gender and sexual gender

Figure 9.5 shows that 11% of adult subjects (30) had experienced, or were experiencing legal trouble. Among this group, alphas were statistically much more likely (17%) to be in trouble with the law than betas (3%) (p<0.001), and men (17%) much more likely than women (6%) (p=0.005). This translated into a prevalence of past or present legal trouble among male alphas of 33%, 8% of female alphas, and only 3% for male betas and 2% for female betas (p<0.001).

Zeroing in on adolescence as a possibly vulnerable period for self-reported legal trouble, I had in all positive respondents data on the age at which their run-in with the law first occurred.

Figure 9.6 presents the percentage and cumulative percentage of these 30 adult subjects, broken down by time gender into age groups in which contact with the law first took place. It shows that 47% of these 30 subjects been in trouble in the age group 13-18, namely 52% of the 14 alphas, yet none of three betas. Although this difference is not necessarily significant (Fisher Exact test p=0.228), the overall time gender difference between alphas (17%) and betas (3%) (p<0.001) suggests that alpha teenagers are far more likely to have trouble with the law than beta teenagers.

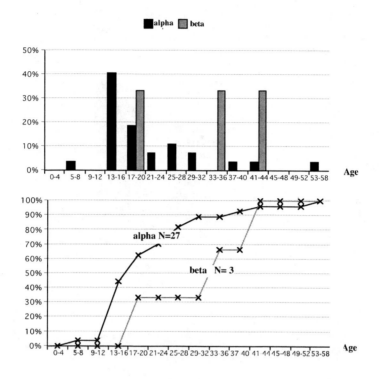

Figure 9.6: Percentage (above) and cumulative percentage (below) of 30 adult subjects with past or present legal trouble, broken down by time gender and into age groups in which their legal trouble first occurred

Educational achievement during adolescence

My theory correctly predicted that the likelihood of alcohol abuse, illicit drug use and legal trouble would be significantly greater in alpha teenagers. Therefore, the likelihood of academic success should be significantly higher in young betas.

To put my sample of 98.5% of my subjects (269 out of 273) into some realistic perspective in this context, I began by comparing its distribution of three basic educational levels (before grade 9, between grade 9-13, after high school) with that of the 1986 Census data of the general population of Greater Vancouver, BC, Canada. Figure 9.7 shows that the distribution of these educational levels among my subjects was very similar to that of the general population to which they belonged.

The fact that all my subjects sought counseling suggests a certain psychological sophistication, which cannot be taken for granted in the general population and could reflect a somewhat better education in my group of subjects. To test this I took a closer look at the two higher educational levels (grade 9-13 and college/university) in figure 9.7. I found that in my cohort the proportion of high school drop-outs was lower than in the general population, and among those with an education beyond high school, the proportion with a university degree was higher. My cohort probably under-represents high school drop-outs, and perhaps over-represents those with a university degree.

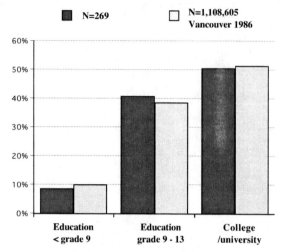

Figure 9.7: Comparing 269 subjects with the population of Greater Vancouver (Census 1986), broken down by education below grade 9, grade 9-13, and beyond high school

In this context, let us review the role of time genderin terms of educational level. Figure 9.8 represents a detailed distribution of educational levels among 269 subjects, broken down by time gender (above) and sexual gender (below).

The upper part of figure 9.8 shows that 5% of alpha and beta teenagers dropped out in grades 7-8 of high school. However, between grades 9 and 11, 16% of the alphas, but only 9% of the betas dropped out. Over 30% of alpha teenagers ended up with only a high school education, far more than the roughly 20% of beta teenagers. This contrast becomes understandable when one realizes that only 16% of alphas ended up with a university degree, compared with nearly 40% of the betas. These differences were statistically highly significant (p=0.002), unlike female-male differences (as shown in the lower part of figure 9.8) (p=0.344).

Corroborating the significant difference in the distribution of educational levels among alphas and betas and the insignificant difference between the sexes, figure 9.9 reflects the average of the total years of education, broken down by time gender and sexual gender. For alphas the average years in education is 12.6, for betas 14.4. This difference is statistically highly significant (p<0.001), unlike the one between females and males (p=0.419), or the one between alpha females and alpha males (p=0.120) or between beta females and beta males (p=0.101).

In sum, my statistical data on educational achievement support the hypothesis that the likelihood of more education is significantly higher in betas than in alphas.

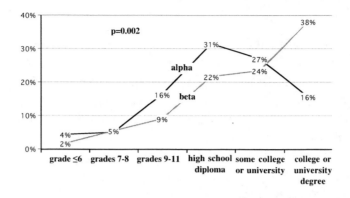

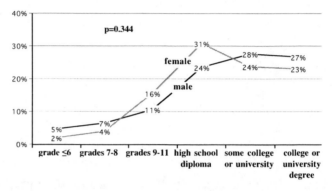

Figure 9.8: Distribution of educational levels among 269 subjects, broken down by time gender (above) and sexual gender (below)

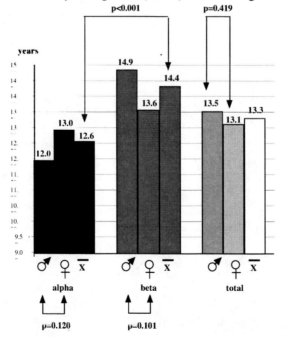

Figure 9.9: Mean of total years of academic education (high school grades+college/university years), broken down by time gender and sexual gender (N=267)

Concluding remarks

Culturally stable environments contribute to a healthy adolescent development and facilitate education. The reason is that a relatively omnipresent set of compatible social expectations about present- and future-oriented adolescent behavior exercises a powerful positive influence. A culturally stable environment tends to neutralize the effects time gender may have on adolescent development. In contemporary society, such favorable social circumstances are becoming less frequent. This has resulted in the new morbidities of adolescence: teenage depression and suicide, substance use (alcohol, tobacco, and drugs), gun-related accidents and homicides, premature sexuality with abortion and sexually transmitted diseases, all of which contribute to dropping out of school. Under these circumstances alpha teenagers tend to be more vulnerable, and beta teenagers more resilient, to derailment in their health and social adjustment.

If society is to improve the chances for healthy adolescent development, it is mandatory that all institutions which contribute to adolescent development (families, the educational system, the health care system, community organizations, and media) come to realize that there are two types of teenagers: alpha teenagers and beta teenagers, each experiencing reality very differently and, as a result, having different needs, and often requiring different approaches in their transition from childhood to adulthood. If these institutions, particularly parents, become familiar with the time gender model, learn the time gender of their teenagers, and, familiarize them with the implications of the time gender model, society can expect much healthier adolescent development.

NOTES

1   Hamburg (1997), p. 7.
2   Hamburg (1997), p. 7-8.
3   Hamburg (1997), p. 7.
4   Stein, Golombek, Marton and Kornblum (1991).
5   Stein, Golombek, Marton and Kornblum (1991), p. 16, 19.
6   Hamburg (1997), p. 7-8.
7   Kerwin et al. (1973), p. 128-129.
8   Muuss (1975).
9   Beard (1972), p. 122.
10   Chamberlain (1980), p.38.
11   Wessman and Gorman (1977), p. 32.
12   Fraisse (1966), quoted by Wessman and Gorman (1977), p. 32.
13   Erikson (1959), p. 142.
14   Erikson (1964), p. 96, 142, 181-182.
15   Green (1975), p. 7-8.
16   Chamberlain (1980), p. 39; Wessman and Gorman (1977), p. 30.
17   Bettelheim (1971); Arnstein (1979).
18   Stein, Golombek, Marton and Kornblum (1991), p. 19.
19   Blotkey and Looney (1980); Stein, Golombek, Marton and Kornblum (1991), p. 16.
20   Chamberlain (1980), p. 40.

21   Erikson (1959), p. 111.
22   Erikson (1968), p. 87.
23   Erikson (1959); Rappoport, Enrich and Wilson (1982), p. 57-58.
24   Erikson (1959), p. 126; Rappoport and Enrich (1985), p. 2-3.
25   Seton (1974) in Rappoport, Enrich and Wilson (1982), p. 62; Golombek, Marton, Stein and Korenblum (1986); Stein, Golombek, Marton, and Korenblum (1991).
26   Hamburg (1997), p. 8.
27   Stein and Vidich (1960), p.24.
28   Rappoport, Enrich, and Wilson (1982), p. 59.
29   Compare Rappoport , Enrich and Wilson (1982), p. 56-57.
30   Stein and Vidich (1960), p.19-20.

CHAPTER 10

Time Gender And Occupation

Factors that determine one's career choice include education, personality traits, special talents, acquired personal preferences, and opportunities. Despite the reigning democratic principle that proclaims equal opportunities for all, actual options are determined by a multiplicity of factors, such as socio-economic status, sexual gender, ethnicity, and disability. The available job market is another consideration, in that necessity may force one into a certain occupation.

Choosing a particular vocational stream is not at issue here. Rather, we are concerned as to how time gender modulates one's career choice. People also often gravitate toward a job that provides a natural fit for the strengths and weaknesses of their time gender. Also, being alpha or beta puts a stamp on how people define their job.

Chapter 8 discussed how time gender influences one's thinking in general and how this applies to philosophers and scientists. Naturally, these different thinking styles affect anybody's job definition. In this chapter, I will restrict myself to examples from my counseling experience to demonstrate the relationship between time gender and occupation.

Section 1: About occupations

Novelists

Anyone familiar with the plots of successful novels, movies, plays and soap operas, knows of the excitement that generated by the polarity between the main characters. One may be good, the other evil; one generous, the other selfish; one smart, the other foolish; one elicits the audience's sympathy, the other is repellent to the audience. No matter what their sexual gender or time gender, readers can read their own lives into the characters and plots because these are, in some way, invariably true to life. Once familiar with the time gender model, it is not difficult for readers to recognize alphas and betas among the main characters. Successful writers apparently have an intuitive grasp of the creative or destructive impact of time gender interfacing.

Take one of the most successful movies in history, *Doctor Zhivago* (1965), based on a novel of the same name by the Russian author Boris Pasternak (1890-1960).[1] The novel plays against the background of a painful period in modern Russian history (from the early 20th century, through World War I, ending in the Russian Revolution, civil war and the Stalinist period). Its main characters include the poet-physician Dr. Zhivago, a beta; the beautiful young woman Lara, an alpha; a despicable, philandering lawyer Komarovsky, an alpha; and an ardent revolutionary student, Pasha Antipov, a beta, who during the civil war transforms into the brutal executioner Strelnikov. The movie clearly illustrates therefore, that both alphas and betas can be "good guys" or "bad guys." Although alphas and betas may reach their moral positions along different pathways, neither road automatically determines their morality.

The movie explicitly highlights a human duality which cuts across sexual gender. While Lara is in her late teens, Komarovsky, the lover of her mother, seduces Lara. And when Lara becomes engaged to Pasha Antipov (a beta), Komarovsky ravages Lara. When she berates him, contrasting him with her devoted Pasha Antipov, Komarovsky responds, "There are two kinds of men, and two kinds of women." Komarovsky thus puts himself and Lara in one category and Lara's fiancée, whom he describes as endowed with great moral purity, in the other (this is well before Antipov turns into a brutal executioner).

Eventually, a tragic love affair between Doctor Zhivago and Lara becomes the focus of the movie. Their love affair takes place during Russia's civil war, which followed the October Revolution. In the middle of the harsh Russian winter, the two are hiding in a lonely house in the country. At one point, Zhivago is writing a poem, called "Lara." When she enters the room and looks over his shoulder, reading what he is jotting down, she exclaims that his description of her is all wrong. Whereupon Zhivago turns around and, facing her lovingly, says something like: "Yes, yes, this is exactly the person you are!" Zhivago sees Lara through his own eyes, thus betacizing her, but Lara resists this perception.

Good novelists must be astute observers of others, otherwise they could not hatch true-to-life characters and plots. They must be aware of the fact that, hidden beyond the female-male duality, there exists another human polarity, leaving one with two kinds of men and two kinds of women. It is my contention that, although unaware of the exact workings of the time gender model, many writers have intuitively grasped this human duality.

Beyond being good observers, authors need a lot of creativity. It is exactly in applying creative imagination to a mix of alphas and betas that the authors' alphacizing or betacizing biases shine through. This happens when authors describe events outside their own experience, and have to solely depend on their imagination. As a result, alpha authors may have a beta character transiently behave as an alpha; and beta authors may briefly endow an alpha character with a timescape. In his novel, *Dr. Zhivago*, Pasternak sometimes has Lara, an alpha, behave beta-like. Someone sensitized to the alpha-beta duality can usually discern such contradictions and recognize the time gender of the author.

There is yet another way authors alphacize or betacize. Some authors appear to assume that the human duality reflects two poles of a continuum so that an alpha can be transformed into a beta, or the other way around. However, alpha and beta characters cannot change their time gender, no matter how the plot molds their personalities. The challenge for alpha and beta authors alike is to try to keep their characters as true to their time gender as possible.

Actors

Russian teacher and director Stanislavski suggested that actors, in their approach to a scene, must credibly assume and act out someone else's identity.[2] Because alphas have a multifocal, contextually partitioned identity, they can, in a given situation, act out the sub-identity which fits that script. This makes them natural actors. The Irish dramatist, George Bernard Shaw (1956-1950), said that he had to become an actor and create for himself a fantastic combination of different identities in his personality. Only then could he fit in the various parts he had to play as author, journalist, orator, politician, committee man, and man of the world.[3]

Two other alpha men of fame come to mind, who ended up in public life, but were much concerned with professional acting in the beginning of their career. I am referring to Karol Joseph Wojtyla (1920-2005), who eventually became Pope John Paul II of the Roman Catholic Church,[4] and to Ronald Reagan (1911-2004), who became the 40th President of the United States of America.[5]

The natural ability to energize various identities is a blessing for professional actors who are alphas. They can set up a sub-personality within themselves which corresponds to whatever character they are playing; they are unencumbered by a constantly interfering, dominant, monofocal identity. They simply become the character they are playing. As a professor of English and creative writing, married to an actor, wrote:

> "Living with an actor is like living with someone who keeps getting kidnapped. And longs to be kidnapped...I began to understand that a job is more than just a job to an actor. It is more than the money or fame. It is the chance for transformation. As a writer, I rely on words to create a voice, an identity. But an actor goes a step further—he or she literally embodies the voice, the created self."[6]

This professor was obviously married to an alpha actor. By contrast, professional beta actors are inclined to pursue roles which reflect a type of character in line with their own singular, monofocal identities. They cannot portray a character alien to their own identities. An example is the Welsh stage and motion-picture actor Richard Burton (1925-1984), known for his portrayals of highly intelligent and articulate men who are world-weary, cynical, or self-destructive.[7]

Salespeople

Salesmanship refers to the adeptness of selling products or services, particularly when a potential buyer is unsure of exactly which product or service he or she actually needs. Successful salesmanship involves a strong motivation to sell, coupled with a finely honed skill of persuasion (a highly specific, yet multi-factorial social skill).[8] This skill includes being a good communicator and being comfortable in dealing with people but, above all, an ability to earn others' trust.

Since alphas are extroverted and therefore more socially perceptive, skilled and comfortable in dealing with people than their introverted beta counterparts, salesmanship comes more naturally to alphas. Alpha salespeople are interpersonal tacticians who use their flexible, situational alpha speak to reach for the right word at the right time. They are able to establish an atmosphere of familiarity and quickly form attachments with their clients, even though they tend to seek a variety of clients as opposed to forming long-term relationships with specific customers. They win people's confidence by selling themselves, rather than trying to make the customer want the product. Since they are not product-bound, their salesmanship ability consists in being good at selling various things to different buyers. Given their competitive-authoritarian interpersonal style, they experience selling and buying as a game which they want to win. This is more important than any monetary gain itself. Making a sale provides them not only with the momentary thrill of success and its accompanying situational self-esteem, but also with the ongoing external praise that goes with being a top salesperson.

Betas are salespeople are quiet different. As introverts, betas tend not to be comfortable in dealing with people. However, in their role as salespeople they acquire through training and experience the social perceptiveness, comfort, self-confidence, and appropriate language needed to sell the products or services they have to offer. Rather than quickly forming attachments and creating an atmosphere of familiarity as alpha salespeople do, their attitude tends to be more emotionally detached. Their social skills are rather specialized at a professional level and do not necessarily generalize to other products or services. To instill in their clients confidence in their credibility, beta salespeople must have not only full confidence in their ability to handle their particular sales situation, but also in the quality of what they are selling. Beta salespeople are product-bound. Because of their timescape they are prepared to professionally deal with a client over a longer period of time. Hence they are concerned with whether their product or service is appropriate and reliable. Because of their inclination toward an egalitarian-cooperative interpersonal style, they tend to treat their customers as they wish to be treated themselves. In the end, their global self-esteem derives from their reputation as successful but ethical salespeople, rather than from successfully closing an individual deal.

Management style

Economists, sociologists, and others often classify business executives as either entrepreneurs or managerial types. Although these definitions may vary, I will use these terms to clarify how time gender impacts on the managerial style of leaders of large organizations.

The best entrepreneurs are usually business executives of the alpha time gender. They are not preoccupied with constraints and maintaining a smoothly running organization as is, but prefer creating a new organization, or reorganizing an existing one. Good at improvisation, these business men and women are constantly on the look-out for new opportunities, and prefer being immersed in the ongoing wheeling and dealings of new business ventures and the excitement of risk taking that goes with it. They are after acquiring wealth through short-term speculative coups and deals, rather than through long-term consolidation and slow painstaking labor guided by forecasting. For many of these business executives, the opportunity to make one's mark on the external world, with its accompanying ongoing situational self-esteem, often means as much, if not more than the possibility of profit.[9]

By contrast, the best executives of the managerial type belong to the beta time gender. They see their function first and foremost as running an existing business. They usually prefer a stable and smoothly operating organization over one that constantly involves new business ventures and intermittent risk-taking. Usually, these business leaders are more guided by forecasting than by improvisation, and therefore tend to be motivated to achieve ordered, long-term growth in line with the possibilities and constraints of the business. They are not interested in producing fast growth based on improvising short-term speculative coups and deals.

The fact that the best entrepreneurial executive tends to be an alpha and the best managerial one a beta may lead to some misinterpretation. Not all alpha executives are entrepreneurial innovators. Many seem preoccupied with just keeping their own position secure or profitable, even at the expense of the organization. And far from all managerial beta executives are at the bureaucratic pole of the continuum. Many of them turn out to be innovators by achieving an organizational breakthrough. However, how an entrepreneurial alpha and a managerial beta approach organizational innovation is determined by their time gender. The alpha entrepreneur tends to bring about innovation rather suddenly, often through a succession of tactical dare-devil improvisations. By contrast, the beta managerial type tends to plot a strategy first, and then executes it over a longer period.

Apart from a chief executive's time gender there is a second important factor in achieving a successful business operation. This has to do with policies that take into account the strengths and limitations of individual staff members. Implicitly this includes the strengths and weaknesses which alphas or betas bring to their particular jobs. Peters and Waterman found that top-performing companies consider it essential to take their employees' individual strengths and weaknesses into account in order to achieve quality and productivity. In labor relations these companies avoid "we-they" attitudes, and they do not view capital investment as the principal factor in improving efficiency. For example, IBM's Thomas J. Watson Jr., said that respect for the individual is the most important company philosophy. Observing this philosophy requires a major chunk of management time.[10]

Explicit awareness of the time gender model will facilitate much smoother management-employee relations. I remember an industrialist who concluded that his long-term financial planner was an alpha and his sales manager a beta. Having them switch positions resulted in an increased efficiency in both departments with the managers becoming more comfortable in their work.

The story of the two bankers

The story of two vice-presidents at the same bank, one an alpha, the other a beta, illustrates that, although alphas do not spontaneously manage their future in a sustained fashion, they may be more efficient in completing a long-term than their beta counterparts. They story began one day when the president called the two vice-presidents in and told them that he wanted them both to complete a review of their divisions' efficiency within six months.

The alpha vice-president had learned the hard way from past experience that she had a problem executing long-term goals. She had learned to successfully complete any long-term task by transforming it into a daily challenge to be met. Following the meeting with the president she went to her office, took her agenda and blocked out the last two weeks prior to her deadline. She estimated she would need one week to write her report and prepare a summary and wanted an additional week just in case she needed more time. Over the following two days, she consulted with her senior staff members. Based on her discussion with them she was able to organize her task into sections with the number of hours maximally needed to complete each section. She then calculated that until the two weeks prior to the president's deadline, she needed to work two hours on the report for three days a week. Having blocked out the needed hours on the appropriate days in her calendar, she then made clear to her secretary that she was not to be disturbed at these times, except for emergencies, or if the president wished to see her. This permitted her to be her flexible and pleasant self the rest of the time and deal with whatever crossed her desk. In sum, her approach consisted of first dividing the required work up into discrete, wholly programmed pieces and then putting the pieces back together in a truly optimal fashion.[11]

The beta vice-president felt good about having six months to complete his task. He did an outline and began working on it whenever he was not absorbed by one of the crises that go with the job of a vice-president. Initially, he would handle these crises quite competently, feeling confident that there was still a lot of time left to deal with his assigned task. However, as the weeks went by and he began looking more closely at the time left to him, he gradually grew more and more tense, and began feeling that these emergencies were interfering with what he really had to do. Eventually, by the time two weeks were left to the deadline, he blocked everything else out, locked himself in, and completed the task only at the very last moment. In this context it is worth mentioning that one particular study of how effective managers use their time found that they don't regularly block out large chunks of time for planning, organizing, motivating, and controlling.[12]

The story of the two vice-presidents demonstrates that, although alphas do not spontaneously manage their future in a sustained fashion, they can learn to do so, while betas who spontaneously attend to future goals can become distracted by a variety of competing influences.

Law students and lawyers

When alpha students enter law school (time gender plays no role) and find they do not like it, they tend to drop out. Even if they like being in law school, they often quit when they find that they have to work very hard to keep up. By contrast, once beta students have entered law school, they tend to stick it out whether they like it or not, regardless of the workload. The upshot of this is that alpha lawyers tend to like their job, and be intellectually more gifted than beta lawyers.

This is not to say that there are no brilliant beta lawyers who love their work. Since among betas there are fewer dropouts, the total number of beta lawyers is larger than the total number of alpha lawyers, which should leave the number of brilliant alpha and beta lawyers about the same. There are also alpha lawyers who are not particularly brilliant and who do not like their job. One lawyer exemplified this:

> "I lived with my mother on whom I was completely financially dependent. She was very controlling. She literally dragged me through high school; otherwise I might have dropped out. We lived in a small town close to a university with a law school. She had set her mind on me becoming a lawyer, whether I liked it or not, and I didn't. So, first she pushed me through my BA. Everyday she would see to it that I got up in time to attend my lectures and that I did my home work. The same happened in law school. So here I am, and I still don't like what I am doing."

I made similar observations about students and graduates of other professions.

One issue, however, specifically relates to criminal defense attorneys and prosecutors (Crown attorneys in Canadian criminal courts). Criminal defense lawyers must be able to comfortably separate their own personal value system from that of the accused. It is their professional duty to give their client the best possible defense. Alpha criminal defense lawyers find this much easier to handle emotionally than betas because their value system is flexibly multifocal and situationally partitioned. Beta criminal defense lawyers have a rather inflexible monofocal value system which frequently leads to a conflict between their own values and those of their client. Hence, they tend to drop out as criminal defense lawyers. The role of prosecutor as major reinforcer of the law of the land suits them much better. Alpha lawyers can pick either role.

Medical doctors and nurses

A busy medical emergency unit is full of professional excitement and variety. Doctors and nurses working in such an environment must be able to emotionally walk away from one emergency after another. Usually they do not get involved with any follow-through. Either a patient is admitted and other members of the hospital staff take over or, when a patient is discharged home, a general physician will do the follow-up. The natural ability to walk away from disasters which alpha physicians and nurses have, and their need for variety of input, makes them a natural fit for this type of work. Betas, on the other hand, are more inclined to want to see each case through. They become dissatisfied with pure emergency work and burn out much earlier than their alpha counterparts. These outcomes have nothing to do with the professional attitude of doctors and nurses, but depend directly on their time gender.

Another example is provided by surgeons and nurses in the operating room. Surgery is often a one-time affair from which surgeon and nurse walk away, moving onto the next case, with grateful patients providing an ongoing supply of situational self-esteem. Alphas adapt much more readily to this scenario than betas, particularly because a patient occasionally dies on the operating table. In these circumstances, alpha surgeons tend to have a more "professional attitude" than beta surgeons, in that they can literally and figuratively walk away from these tragedies, saying to themselves: "You win some, you lose some." Beta surgeons, on the other hand, may for some time suffer from self recrimination, something others may consider as "too much personal involvement." This is not to say that over time beta surgeons cannot develop a certain emotional blocking in this regard: a more "professional attitude." However, some types of surgery are more suited to beta surgeons such as re-constructive surgery that involves multiple operations on the same patient over a long period.

As physicians, betas are better suited to a medical practice in which they are exposed to a narrowly defined group of patients over a long period, as in a family practice, or internal medicine (such as gastro-enterology, nephrology, respiratory medicine, or oncology). Their global self-esteem makes them invest more of themselves in each patient. Alpha physicians who have to deal with the same problem in the same patient over a period of time tend to get bored and become impersonal with "the case." Alpha general practitioners soon refer the long-term patient to some appropriate specialist. Among these specialist physicians, alphas tend to concentrate on the diagnostic, and betas on the therapeutic side of their specialty, the diagnostic approach leading to a far greater number of short contacts and the therapeutic approach involving long-term contacts with a smaller number of patients.

Finally, I will say a few words about the potential role of time gender in my own specialty, psychiatry. Young alphas may be unwittingly attracted into psychiatry in part because psychiatry supposedly provides them with the necessary insights to gain not only control over themselves, but also over others. Such work will, they intuit, provide them with ongoing situational self-esteem. Later, in their work as psychiatrists, they tend to crave variety, resulting in short-term commitments, with emphasis on providing short-term therapy or diagnostic services, as in forensic psychiatry.

By contrast, young betas may be attracted to psychiatry because of an unwitting belief that their acquired knowledge will provide them with therapeutic manipulation to control their own future, and especially the future of others. This will upgrade their global self-esteem. Later, in their work as psychiatrists, they tend to concentrate on a therapeutic, narrow, in-depth focus with long-term commitments, and therefore a practice with fewer patients.

I am talking here about tendencies. There are long-term alpha therapists such as Jung. And there are excellent beta diagnosticians.

Section 2: About politicians

Since no one escapes the control of politicians, the discussion about politicians will be more detailed than the preceding ones.

The time gender model cannot explain why someone goes into politics or why some politicians achieve greatness. But it is safe to say that politicians have a need to dominate others, with a special appetite for public power and an ambition for senior status, if not leadership. In this respect, the time gender model can explain that public power means different things to alpha and beta politicians. Since alphas are preoccupied with controlling their personal life in the here-and-now in 4–D, it follows that alpha politicians try to gain public power in order to play a dominant role in controlling their current political arena. And since betas are preoccupied with controlling their personal future in 6–D, beta politicians try to gain public power to manipulate the political arena to translate their present convictions into a future reality.

To become a successful politician, one must excel at selling political ideas and be an actor who can take on the role of protector of these ideas. To translate projected ideas into reality, one also must have the managerial skills of an innovator. With regard to each of these variables, the time gender of a politician makes a considerable difference.

In the context of selling political ideas, the situational and compartmentalized thinking of alpha politicians tends to adjusts itself to changing political circumstances. As a result, as political salesmen, alphas are not product-bound; they are not rigidly tied to a political framework or party loyalty, but more focused on acquiring and maintaining power. Gaining political influence is not so much a matter of demonstrating a deep, persistent belief in particular political ideas, but in the ability to sell themselves. These extroverted politicians have a natural ability to project a public image commensurate with their current political ideas and office. They diligently apply their social skills, perceptiveness and flexible, situational alpha speak not only in their personal lives, but also with their political audiences and other politicians. Often, they are charismatic orators.

Since the thinking of beta politicians is timescape-oriented, it is more consistent and coherent over time than that of their alpha politicians. As political salesmen, betas are product-bound. They are tied to the political framework of their party and are also more loyal. To these introverted politicians, gaining political influence does not mean selling themselves, but rather convincing others of their personal belief in the veracity of their political ideas. They establish themselves on the public stage as people with firm and enduring convictions. Although they have to be able to wheel and deal tactically, in the end political conviction rather than the pursuit of power dominates their strategic decisions. They do not think or speak in terms of broad conceptual ideas or rousing generalities that are easily understood by political colleagues and the public, but tend to be more logical and cerebral, rather than charismatic. Often, their social skills and perceptiveness do not extend beyond their political colleagues to people in general. There are, of course, exceptions to this rule. Bill Clinton, for example, learned to speak to and feel comfortable with a wide variety of audiences despite being a beta. I based this insight on his biography,[13] particularly because, notwithstanding a very dysfunctional childhood and adolescence, he functioned very well as an adult. Given their introverted attitude, however, beta politicians are generally speaking rather shy in their private, non-professional relationships.

Given their generally authoritarian attitude, alpha politicians tend to pay more attention to the power others hold than to listen to, let alone solicit input from their colleagues. Since their self-esteem is situational they do not like criticism from others and prefer positive praise. In the absence of the checks and balances of a democratic system, alpha leaders are more likely than beta leaders to surround themselves with sycophants and often end up functioning in isolation from the general public. All this renders their decision-making largely autonomous.

The interpersonal egalitarian inclination of betas, their gut instinct to respect individuality, and their penchant toward inclusive thinking, usually make beta politicians good listeners and tolerant of criticism. When in leadership, these tendencies certainly lend themselves toward consensus building and participant decision-making.

As managers of their public office or party, alpha politicians tend to be political entrepreneurs and innovators who are guided by populist visions and who bring about political change through tactical improvisation. Usually, they are not particularly interested in maintaining a smoothly run political apparatus, unlike beta politicians, who usually are very good at this. As political innovators, beta politicians have goals which are anchored in a firm, broad-based belief system which derives from their party's thinking. They tend to plot their strategy first, and then execute their objectives over a longer period.

Short of electoral defeat, alpha politicians tend to hang onto positions of power for power's sake for as long as circumstances permit. Frequently, they retire not because they realize that their time has run out and that they are becoming an impediment to their party, but because they are forced to quit. If not defeated in an election, beta politicians in positions of power usually leave office because of inner motives rather than external pressure. They quit because they have concluded that their future role in serving their party is no longer feasible or desirable.

For several reasons, there are more alpha politicians in democratic governments. First, salesmanship and acting ability come more naturally to alphas than to betas. Secondly, alphas, unlike betas, readily adopt an ideology which appears to have current political potential. Perhaps another reason is that getting involved in an election for public office not only places one in the political spotlight, but also involves considerable risk-taking, opportunism, and wheeling and dealing. Finally, getting elected provides security only for the elected term, rather than securing a career with a stable future. Some betas get involved in politics because of the strength of their political convictions, others because of family tradition, yet others simply because they can afford, both mentally and financially, to suffer a defeat or two.

I want to highlight the time gender duality among politicians by contrasting two 20th century world leaders: the alpha politician, Winston Churchill (1874-1965),[14] prime minister of the United Kingdom, and the beta politician, Lyndon Johnson (1908-1973),[15] the 36th President of the United States. The personalities and behavior of these two leaders clearly demonstrate strong time gender differences.

Several biographies have dissected in great detail the characters of these two sometimes glorified, sometimes maligned politicians. Churchill's and Johnson's time gender difference cannot account for the fact that both were born leaders who could be ruthless in achieving their goals; that both loved dealing with new challenges; and that both had occasional temper outbursts, drank more than their share, loved the good life, and were interested in enriching themselves. Their difference in time gender will, however, speak for itself.

Churchill, the alpha politician

Churchill's greatness as a politician does not lie so much in his career in general but in his success as wartime prime minister of Great Britain from 1940-1945. This was in no small part due to his charismatic and persuasive personality. Producing the right words at the right moment, his public alpha speak, was a superb ability of his. Alexander Scott, Churchill's parliamentary private secretary at the War Office, already saw in 1905 the charismatic leader in Churchill who at the time was only thirty:

> "He does the inevitable act which no one had thought of before; he
> thinks the original thought which is so simple and obvious once it has

been uttered; he coins the happy phrase which expresses what all men have longed to say, and which thereafter comes so aptly to every man's tongue."[16]

Churchill demonstrated his topnotch extroverted social skills not only in everyday life by successfully manipulating people to his best advantage, but he also had the gift of the populist touch in the public arena:

> "When the prime minister toured the scorched and shattered remains of Bristol after a particularly hellish air raid in April 1941, a woman who had lost everything and was awash with raging tears, on seeing the jowly face and cigar, stopped crying and waved her hanky, shouting herself hoarse, "Hooray, hooray!"[17]

Churchill's down-to-earth language made it the language of the people.[18] According to Clement Attlee, the Labour Party leader in Churchill's War Cabinet, Churchill turned out to be the only leader who could take on Adolf Hitler's manic logorrhea and wipe the floor with it.[19]

Arguably, Churchill would never have been prime minister but for World War II,[20] for he had long been kept from his party's leadership due to others' suspicion about his loyalty. He constantly appeared to put his own ideas above party allegiance.[21] He represented an autonomous brand of politician who, in order to maintain political influence and power, felt no compunction about changing his ideas and his party. By his own words, Churchill was not bound or loyal to a particular ideology. In his early twenties, he wrote with a startling frankness to his mother about what he called his one "mental flaw":

> "I do not care so much for the principles I advocate as for the impression which my words produce & the reputation they give me...I think a keen sense...of burning wrong or injustice would make me sincere, but I very rarely detect genuine emotion in myself."[22]

His political career bears this out. In 1900, within three years of beginning his political career as a Conservative, Churchill sensed that the political mood of the country was swinging toward the Liberals. Consequently he began speaking of himself as an English Liberal[23] and, in 1904 (age 29), joined the Liberal Opposition benches and became a major player in persuading the public of the merits of Liberalism and discrediting Conservatism.[24]

He could not have described his position better when he admitted to one of his Conservative friends that his switch from Conservative to Liberal was open to criticism not because on account of his motives. He had had to make a choice between fighting and remaining on the sidelines and he wanted to fight with everything that was in him, although staying on the sidelines would have been more socially correct.[25]

Churchill's desertion of the Tories was followed by a meteoric rise in the Liberal Government: from Colonial Under-secretary, to the Board of Trade, to Home Secretary, and finally to the Admiralty (1911-1915).[26] In the Admiralty Churchill strongly advocated a British naval attack on the Turkish Dardanelles. However, the attack had such a disastrous outcome that he lost his job.

Having unsuccessfully pleaded with the Prime Minister for whatever role in the war, and with nobody paying much attention to him in Parliament, he abruptly left for France to join the army on the Western front late in 1915. But his commitment to the Army never outstripped his political ambitions. His soldiering only lasted for just under six months,[27] as he kept up his political machinations. In May 1916 he returned to London and after much political manipulation,[28] the Liberal prime minister, Lloyd George, made Churchill Minister of Munitions over strong Conservative protest.[29] In the fall of 1922, when Churchill was in charge of the Colonial Office and the Turks wanted to reoccupy the Dardanelles neutral zone, Churchill urged a firm stand against them. A political debacle ensued which brought down the shaky coalition government and cost Churchill his Parliamentary seat.

When the weakened Liberals formed a coalition government with the Labour Party, Churchill saw his chance to return to Parliament by moving back to the Tories. He asked the Conservative leader Baldwin to let him act as leader of 50 Liberal MP's who were willing to cooperate with the Tories. The Conservatives fixed him up with a safe constituency. In May 1924, Churchill stated that there was no longer any place in British politics for the Liberal party. He was elected to the House of Commons with Conservatives in the majority, was offered the post of Chancellor of the Exchequer, and rejoined the Conservative party.[30]

When in 1929 the Conservative government fell and the Labour Party formed a minority government with Baldwin accepting the role of Leader of the Opposition, Churchill resigned from Baldwin's shadow cabinet. By this time, every party had come to distrust Churchill's independent brand of politics, his lack of party loyalty, his dislike for the necessary compromises of practical politics, and his preference for associating with influential people. By 1935, Churchill began giving public voice to his view that Hitler's Germany was a growing menace that should be taken seriously.

In May 1937, when Neville Chamberlain became conservative Prime Minister, he ignored Churchill's warnings, although the accuracy of Churchill's information on Germany's aggressive plans was repeatedly confirmed by events. However, in March 1939, when Churchill finally pressed for a truly national coalition, the sentiment in the country began to change. People started to recognize him as the nation's spokesman against Hitler, and began to agitate for his return to office. Chamberlain continued to ignore him until September 3, 1939, when Britain declared war on Germany. Only then did Chamberlain appoint the 65-year-old Churchill to his old post in charge of the Admiralty. When on May 10, 1940, the German invasion of the Low Countries came on top of the German seizure of Norway in April 1940, Chamberlain resigned. Churchill, at age 66, became prime minister of a coalition government.

Churchill's period of supreme power and political splendor began. Now he was the prime minister of an all-party government. His sole focus was the defeat of Hitler's Germany. He gave the British people the collective will and confidence to fight. When Clement Attlee, the Labour Party leader in the War Cabinet, commented about this period of war, he said that Churchill was "a supremely fortunate mortal" but "the most warming thing about him was that he never ceased to say so."[31]

When party politics began to revive in 1944 in the face of victory, the 70 year old Churchill wanted to continue his position as prime minister of an all-party cabinet at least until Japan was defeated. But, by May 1945, all parties wanted an early election. Churchill therefore had to run as Conservative prime minister. By identifying wholly with the Conservative cause and flamboyantly indulging in prophecies of disastrous results of a Labour victory, he became his own worst enemy. Although personally re-elected, his party was left with a minority of seats. Rather than resign as leader of the Conservative party, Churchill would not abandon political power, and accepted the role of opposition leader although he never felt fully comfortable with it. Rather than being preoccupied with domestic policy, he focused more on the Soviet threat and the unification of Europe.

In February 1950, the 75-year old Churchill had once again the opportunity to seek a personal mandate. This time, he abstained from the extravagances of the 1945 campaign. Although the general election shook Labour, it left them in office. It would take Churchill "one more heave" to defeat Labour. This happened in October 1951 when his Conservatives gained a narrow majority, and when Churchill, almost 77 years old, became prime minister for the second time. In June 1953, the 78-year-old Churchill was partly paralyzed by a stroke, but he continued to hang onto office until age 80 when his powers were too visibly failing. Rather than accepting a peerage, he remained, however, a member of the House of Commons and in 1959, at age 84, was re-elected. In January 1965, at the age of 90, he died at this London home.

Roy Jenkins, one of Churchill's biographers,[32] succeeded better than many biographers before him in recognizing in Churchill the political animal. Churchill's impatient appetite for power and strenuous exertions to secure it were often hidden beneath the grand opera of his speechifying. He was smoke, certainly, but he was also mirrors.[33] Thus Jenkins brought into sharp focus what I call the alpha politician in Churchill—the man who, in order to maintain political influence and power, never felt any compunction about changing both his ideas and his party.

Being an alpha politician, Churchill was autonomous in his decision-making and was not a good listener to the input from others.[34] Given his situational self-esteem, he was rather sensitive to criticism from others. For example, when Churchill asked his brother to give his "candid" opinion about a maiden political speech Churchill had given in 1897,[35] Churchill stated that he only wanted to hear something positive "because hostile criticism is of no value."[36]

Churchill's overall political alpha thinking was, as would be expected, situational and compartmentalized, if not sometimes downright impulsive. Jenkins pointed out that for more than once in his career in government, Churchill was the author of policies he later attacked as shortsighted. Thrice he was the impassioned advocate of reduced arms expenditures: as Tory, as Liberal Secretary of War in 1919, and as Tory again. And thrice he was gung-ho for rearmament: in the naval arms race immediately before the First World War, in the 1930s, and during the Cold War.[37] Paul Addison pointed to Churchill's tendency to favor trigger-happy solutions for difficult problems — calling out the troops in 1911 and 1926 to deal with industrial strikes, for example.[38] And Robert Rhodes James rightly remarked that Churchill's career was not only full of impulsive blunders as the Dardanelles affair in 1915, but also was characterized by a quixotic devotion to deservedly doomed causes. These include his restoration of the gold standard while at the Exchequer, a disastrous measure that led to deflation, unemployment, and the miners' strike that led to the general strike of 1926. As well, in 1936, he grossly misread the political and public mood when he opposed prime minister Baldwin by publicly championing King Edward VIII in the King's abdication crisis.[39]

However, as even his most severe critics have conceded, all of Churchill's shortcomings could be forgiven in light of his supreme accomplishment of giving Britain the collective will to fight at the time no one else would or could.

Johnson, the beta politician

Lyndon Johnson, who became President of the United States after the assassination of John F. Kennedy in November 1963, made his place in the history of his country by achieving within the first two years of his presidency (1964-1965) what no other President had achieved. He brought into law the so-called *Great Society Legislation* which covered an agenda that had been with the Democratic Party since Roosevelt. The most extensive civil-rights legislation since Reconstruction, it included the introduction of Medicare, educational legislation for children and college students, environmental laws for clear air and clean water, and consumer protection laws.[40]

Sadly, the name of President Johnson is also connected with the Vietnam War, during which he had to deal with a confusing and divisive foreign policy he had inherited from his predecessors. This was unlike Churchill in World War II, who was dealing with the sheer survival of his nation. Nor was Johnson a charismatic politician like Churchill who, by the very strength of his personality and use of oratorical skill, could make national policy understood by the general public. Johnson did not have a knack for talking to the general public. Yet he went a long distance in his attempt to get the North Vietnamese to conclude a peace that was acceptable to him. It was a tragedy that he failed to realize that the way he applied power to achieve results in the US Congress did not work nationally or internationally.[41]

During his 37-year public career, first as a Congressman, then as a Senator, next as a Vice-President and finally as President, Johnson was a political salesman who was, in contrast to Churchill, very much product-bound. As he himself stated in 1968, in his last and famous State of the Union message:

> "Throughout my entire public career I have followed the personal philosophy that I am a free man, an American, a public servant, and a member of my party, in that order always and only."[42]

Johnson's strong belief in and adherence to the principle of loyalty, as well as many of his political beliefs, well preceded his political career. His biographer, Rulon, pointed out that Johnson developed his set of values in the late twenties, when he served as an editor of the school newspaper at Southwest Texas State College. Among these values were the importance he attached to education, the worth of teachers to society and his emphasis on the provision of an education for poor and underprivileged youth in rural areas. Until his dying day, Johnson believed that schooling would open doors for those on the lower end of the socioeconomic ladder. Another recurrent theme was Johnson's loyalty, in this case to his school and its faculty, and the state, which had made his education possible. For him a staff member's greatest sin was not to be dedicated to the policy or program at hand.[43]

In 1937, Johnson ran successfully for a seat in the US House of Representatives. For 12 years he represented his congressional district of Texas. In 1948 he became a Senator and remained so for 12 years, becoming Democratic whip in 1951 and then, from 1955 to 1961, Senate majority leader. He was unwavering in his service to those in superior positions, such as the Republican President Eisenhower and the Democratic House Speaker Rayburn.[44]

Johnson did not think or speak in terms of broad conceptual ideas that could be easily understood by his political colleagues and the public. He felt that speaking in rousing generalities or in terms of broad principles was divisive and would narrow his area for political maneuver. Instead, he became a master in handling very specific political issues. During his enormously effective time as Senate Majority Leader, he avoided divisive generalities and showed himself to be a consensus builder, a good listener to the input from his colleagues, and a man who was able to bring together colleagues from both sides of the isle to support specific measures.[45] His skilled leadership was largely responsible for the passage of the civil-rights bills of 1957 and 1960 — the first in the 20th century.

In 1960, Kennedy picked Johnson as his running mate. As Vice-president, his life with the Kennedys was unhappy and full of tension. Some tension was of his own making due to his insecurities as a person, but they were played upon by the "mystique of

Camelot." Even so, his relationship with President Kennedy was free of friction, stress, competition, and politicking.[46]

As a typical beta, Johnson always kept an eye on his future, particularly as to whether his political role would continue to be meaningful so that he could maintain his global self-esteem. It is hard to believe that on the night of Kennedy's assassination, November 22, 1963, Johnson had planned to tell President Kennedy that he didn't wanted to run for Vice-president again in 1964,[47] because he had no choice but to do exactly what the President wanted him to do. He could not set his own goals and therefore felt that his time in Washington was over.[48]

From accounts of what happened the very night when Johnson returned to Washington as President by two men who worked for him during his presidency, Horace Busby and Jack Valenti, there can be little doubt about his deep commitment to his political party, his penchant toward inclusive thinking, and his genius. He told Busby that when he came to Washington as President that night, on his desk were the same things that were on his desk as a freshman in Congress in 1937: civil rights, federal aid to education, Medicare and federal assistance for hospitalization. He felt totally committed to overcoming all that stood in the way of realizing these issues by the end of his term.[49] Valenti recalled that on the first night of Johnson's presidency, his senior staff remained until early the next day as Johnson mapped out his vision of the Great Society. In five hours Johnson wove into a tapestry his political agenda for governing America. Johnson impressed Valenti with his all-embracing mind—he had an ability to think six moves ahead in the political chess game while everybody else was still preoccupied with the first move.[50]

Far from being autonomous in his decision making, Johnson paid considerable attention to the opinions of others. Judge Abe Fortas, who worked with Johnson, said that he had never before worked with someone who insisted on hearing different viewpoints. Fortas found that, while there was very little dialogue and give and take with Johnson, he was a good listener. Johnson felt particularly ill at ease when during his cabinet meetings everybody in attendance expressed the same view. In these instances, he would ask friends outside the government, especially lawyers, to take the other side. Basically, Johnson liked to hear different points of view and in the end make up his own mind.[51] This did not make for decision-making by committee, of course, but it certainly enabled participant decision-making.

Johnson's brilliant politicking lay in working the two ends of Pennsylvania Avenue, but his introverted social skill was limited when dealing with individual strangers. For example, when he first became President, he was loath to ask White House telephone operators to dial a number for him, but rather dialed his own.[52]

Despite his discomfort with strangers, Johnson did have a feeling for people, and where the country ought to go, and what the relationship with the people through their government ought to be.[53] But he was often out of touch with what the American public thought and felt. For example, although he lived and worked in the mid-sixties, he had no idea what the Beatles or Bob Dylan meant to the younger generation.[54] His thoughts were on another plane. And he had a deep sense of self worth which overrode any concern with his popular public persona. He felt that "they either took him like he was or they should find themselves another boy." Although he was President, he never listened to an image maker or a public relations counsel.[55]

Since his persuasive skill was more logical or cerebral than charismatic, Johnson was not good at speaking to wider audiences, as is true of many beta politicians. One of his main speech writers, Harry C. McPherson Jr, said that Johnson did not have much "plebiscitary sense," and that one of Johnson's main weaknesses as President was his inability to make a speech. He even couldn't read a speech well. He was just an amateur compared with Reagan (an alpha), sounding "like a Methodist Bishop at a meeting of the Board of Bishops."[56]

Johnson, the beta politician, was not only a strategically oriented innovator, but also a superb manager with a relentless energy that pervaded his entire life. As long as there was work to be done he wouldn't sleep nor let others sleep. When in 1925 he was Head of the National Youth Administration he ran it as a twenty-four-hour-a-day enterprise. The same thing happened when he became a Congressman: he had his staff work in two shifts to make his office a twenty-four-hour-a-day operation. One could call his office early in the morning and if Johnson himself wouldn't respond someone else would. And when he was President his staff was not allowed to leave until they had returned every phone call by a member of Congress.[57]

Johnson was not interested in power for power's sakes but he had a very clear idea of how to use personal power to realize what one believes in.[58] He used power to serve his global self-esteem as determined by the future. What was very special about Johnson was his ability to create a power base where nobody else could see this as a future possibility. Busby recounted that time and again, from college to Senate, Johnson would enter a situation without a power base and then build the base that gave him the power he needed. He was possessed by what he felt had to be accomplished.[59]

As a beta politician, Johnson could abandon power when it no longer served his global self-esteem:

> "On March 31, 1968, after three of the most turbulent years in U.S. political history, Johnson startled television viewers with a national address that included three announcements: that he had just ordered major reductions in the bombing of North Vietnam; that he was requesting peace talks; and that he would neither seek nor accept his party's re-nomination to the presidency."[60]

Later, Johnson told Jack Valenti some of the reasons behind his decision not to run again. He said that the presidency was no longer any fun, but had become a heavy burden "filled with hollows and dark demons." Although he felt that he could have beaten Nixon, he thought he would have done so only with the slightest majority. As a result, he would have had to preside over a divided, polarized nation full of poison and bitterness. This he considered an impossible task. He thought that, rather than tainting the presidency, some new face should take over and heal some of the wounds. He had concluded that he could no longer lead.[61]

Johnson sought not to pick a successor, and he eventually made himself available to both major parties' nominees, Hubert Humphrey and Richard Nixon. Thus, the 36th president of the United States ceased to be a politician and made the full transition to statesman.[62]

In sum, it could be said that Churchill, the alpha politician, won the war but lost the peace; and that Johnson, the beta politician, won the peace but lost the war.

NOTES

1   The screenplay of the motion picture *Dr. Zhivago* was written by Robert Oxton Bolt (1924-1995). It was directed by Sir David Lean (1908-1991) and produced by Metro-Goldwyn-Mayer. The screenplay deviates in some significant aspects from Pasternak's novel [Pasternak (1958)].

2   Stanislavski (1980), quoted by Rowan (1990), p. 150.

3   Shaw (1952) quoted by Erikson (1960), p. 44, as paraphrased by me.

4   For Pope John Paul II's biographical details see, for example, Weigel (1999).

5   For Ronald Reagan's biographical details see Edwards (1987), Cannon (1991), and Vaughn (1994).

6   Muske (2000), p.116.

7   Ferris (1981), Junor (1985), and Bragg (1989).

8   See, for example, Pratkanis and Aronson (1992).

9   Compare, for example, Person (1986), p. 260-261; Peters & Waterman (1982), pp. 3-8

10   Peters & Waterman (1982), p. 8, 14-15.

11   Frederick Taylor as mentioned by Peters & Waterman (1982), p.5.

12   Henry Mintzberg of Canada's McGill University, quoted from Peters & Waterman (1982), p.7.

13   Maraniss (1995

14   My opinion that Churchill was an alpha is based on Gilbert (1991).

15   My opinion that Johnson was a beta is based on Thompson (1986), Rulon (1981), and Caro (1982).

16   Alexander MacCallum Scott quoted by Gilbert (1991), p. 172.

17   Schama (2002), p. 15, quoting Orwell [Orwell and Angus (1968)].

18   Schama (2002), p. 16, quoting Orwell and Angus (1968).

19   Clement Attlee, the Labour Party leader who served in his War Cabinet, quoted by Schama (2002), p. 16.

20   Schama (2002), p.16.

21   Paraphrased from Schama (2002), p. 16.

22   Churchill wrote this letter to his mother from Bangalore (India) in May 1898; quoted from Gilbert (1911), p. 88.

23   Gilbert (1991), p. 158.

24   Gilbert (1991), p. 167.

25   Quoted from Gilbert (1991), p. 170.

26   Gilbert (1991), p. 174, 194-195.

27   Gilbert (1991), p. 339, 350-351, 353, 353, 359, 360.

28   Gilbert (1991), p. 365-367, 369, 372-373.

29   Gilbert (1991), p. 374.

30   Gilbert (1991), p. 460-468.

31   Schama (2002), p. 15, quoting Attlee (1965), p. 35.

32   Jenkins (2001).

33   Schama (2002), p. 15.

34   Gilbert (1991), p. 350-353.

35   Gilbert (1991), p. 71.

36   Gilbert (1991), p. 78.

37   Schama (2002), p. 17, quoting Jenkins (2001).

38   Schama (2002), p. 15, quoting Addison (1992).

39   Schama (2002), p. 15, quoting James (1970).

40   McPherson (1986), p. 53-54.

41   Fortas (1986), p. 10 - 12.

42   Quoted from Rulon (1981), p. 286.

43   Rulon (1981), p. 37.

44   Fortas (1986), p. 6-7

45   I paraphrased here Justice Abe Fortas (1986), p. 9, 14.

46   Fortas (1986), p. 6-7

47   Busby (1986), p. 253.

48   Busby (1986), p.253, 266-267.

49   Busby (1986), p,. 257.

50   Valenti (1986), p. 22, 24.

51   Fortas (1986), p. 10.

52   Busby (1986), p. 253-254.

53   McPherson (1986), p.48.

54   McPherson (1986), p. 47-48.

55   Busby (1986), p. 258.

56   McPherson (1986), p. 47-48.

57   Valenti (1986), p. 23, 25-26.

58   McPherson (1986), p. 48.

59   Busby (1986), p. 268-269.

60   Encyclopedia Britannica, Inc. (1994-1999).

61   Valenti (1986), p. 30.

62   Rulon (1981), p.290.

CHAPTER 11

Time Gender, Nature And Nurture

In explaining how people's personalities work, theories tend to stress either the influence of the genetic constitution (nature) or of the environment (nurture) while paying little attention to the ongoing interaction between the two. This is unrealistic.

> "...Nature and nurture stand in reciprocity, not opposition. All children inherit, along with their parents' genes, their parents, their peers, and the places they inhabit...[Development] unfolds in an ecological and social setting that, like its genes, is species-typical for the organism."[1]

The reciprocal relationship between nature and nurture engenders behavioral differences both within and across cultures, as is evident by the wide variations in human behavior. Similarly, nature and nurture also have a strong influence on the expressions of people's time gender.

Yet the renowned, developmental cognitive psychologist Jean Piaget claimed that children develop through the same stages of cognitive development in the same order in spite of vast differences in their cultural milieu, educational training, and personal experiences, which was born out by comparing, for example, North Slope Eskimos of Alaska, Mexicans, Costa Ricans and Koreans, Rwandese, French-speaking Canadians, Iranians, Norwegians, and Hungarians.[2] This makes it hard to deny that a child's basic cognitive development has a genetic underpinning. Similarly, it is hard to conceptualize how the two distinct ways in which elementary school children begin to encode their autobiographic memories (which lead to their time gender differentiation) can be anything but genetic in nature. Although environmental : actors influence how children behave and experience reality, the alphas among them still develop a preferential attention mode in the here-and-now of 4–D, whereas the young betas still will generate a preferential attention to their timescapein 6–D. These two different ways of experiencing reality introduce, in turn, dissimilarities in mood regulation, self-esteem, motivation, self-talk, identity, social behaviors, thinking, and attitude toward education and occupation.

The conventional view among psychiatrists, psychologists and sociologists is, however, that time perspective is the learned product of environmental influences, including the particular orientation toward past, present and future in one's family, social class, or culture. This view holds that people may sometimes live in the past, and at other times in the present or future. For example, a soldier confronted with immediate danger focuses on the present, a student on the future, and a person faced with terminal illness on the past. When it is time for hedonistic enjoyments, one naturally suspends planning and goal seeking. This conventional view assumes that one is not stuck with a dominant time orientation. If it does not serve us well, one adjusts one's time perspective.[3]

Although explanations based on learned or acquired behavior contradict the fact that time gender differentiation begins only around age 6-7, the nurture or environmental explanation of time perspective (or time gender) need to be confronted because it is so widely shared. Therefore, the first section of this chapter examines some popular environmental factors often advanced as having a formative influence on our personality and which are used to account for different time perspectives. It examines the role of family size and birth rank, of being an immigrant, and, perhaps most importantly, of growing up in a broken home, or with parental substance abuse, sexual abuse, or physical abuse. Finally, we will look at the possible impact of being born under a specific Zodiac sign.

The second section of this chapter focuses on the role of genetics or nature in accounting for time gender. This requires explaining the methodology used in assigning time gender. Then follows a discussion of my present view on the genetics of time gender (the duality in autobiographic memory) follows, which replaces my previous view as expressed in the e-book version of this work.[4] My present view considers time gender to be an expression of a gene (or possibly more genes) on the X-chromosome, with the X-linked alpha-genotype being dominant and the X-linked beta-genotype recessive. The discussion indicates that methods are underway to localize several human mental functions in the genome, notably on the X-chromosome. Localizing time gender has therefore become possible.

Section 1: Confronting nurture explanations of time gender

The family of origin

In 1908 the Austrian founder of the school of Individual Psychology, Alfred Adler (1870-1937), introduced the assumption that the size of one's family and birth-order position have a formative influence on one's personality, both normal and abnormal. He suggested that parents, as well as siblings tend to treat the oldest, middle and youngest child differently, and that these children behave accordingly. I found that a parent's own birth rank often influences how he or she treats offspring in a similar birth rank. Although alpha and beta children and teenagers will respond to how they are treated, the point needs to be made that the size of family of origin and birth-order position are not associated with generating the time gender duality.

I had relevant information for 268 out of 273 subjects (98.2%). The number of children per family was, on the average, 3.4 children from the same parents.

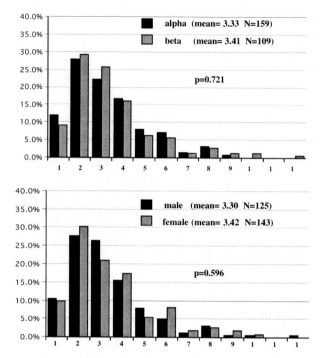

Figure 11.1: Size of family of origin by number of children (in percentages),
broken down by time gender (above) and sexual gender (below) (N=268)

Figure 11.1 shows that the size of the family of origin in alphas (with an average
of 3.30 children) and in betas (with an average of 3.41 children) is only a matter of
chance (p=0.721), just as it is in men (with an average of 3.30 children) and in women
(with an average of 3.42 children) (p=0.596). Growing up in a large or small family
has therefore nothing to do with being alpha or beta.

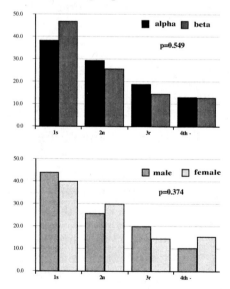

Figure 11.2: Birth rank, broken down by time gender (above) and sexual gender (below) (N=268)

Concerning the birth-order position, figure 11.2 shows that 42% of the subjects were first-born (the oldest or only child), 28% second born, 17% third born and 13% fourth or later born. Neither alphas nor betas showed a significant association with any birth-order position (p=0.549), and neither did females and males (p=0.374).

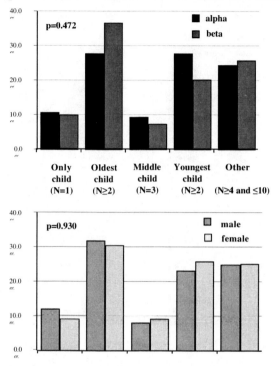

Figure 11.3: Sibling position in family of origin (in percentages)
broken down by time gender (above) and sexual gender (below) (N=268)

Then there is the question addressed in figure 11.3, namely whether the alphas or betas were more likely to be an only child (31%), or in a family of more than one child the oldest (31%) or youngest (25%), or being the middle child in a family of three (9%) (25% accounted for all the left-over positions). Whether alphas or betas belonged to any of these groups turned out to be just a matter of chance (p=0.472). The same applied to men and women (p=0.930). In sum, neither family size, nor birth rank, nor being the only, oldest, middle or youngest child was associated with being alpha or beta.

Figure 11.3 addresses the question whether alphas or betas were more likely to be an only child (31%) or, in a family of more than one child, the oldest (31%) or youngest (25%) or, being the middle child in a family of three (9%).[5] The figure shows that it was just a matter of chance whether alphas or betas belonged to any of these groups (p=0.472), just as being female or male was (p=0.930).

The immigration factor

Immigration may affect personality development.[6] Mobility and acculturation demand adjustment to a new socio-cultural environment which often are challenging due to language barriers or cultural alienation. To exclude the role of these factors in creating the time gender duality, I looked at the time gender distribution among Canadian-born subjects, as opposed to Canadian immigrants.

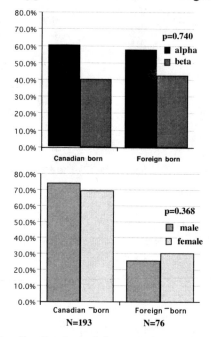

Figure 11.4: Comparing the distribution of time gender (above) and sexual gender (below) among Canadian-born and foreign-born subjects (N=269)[7]

Figure11.4[8] shows that 72% of my cohort were Canadian-born and 28% foreign-born. The difference in time gender distributions of these two group was a matter of chance (p=0.740), as was the difference in sex distributions (p=0.368).

Similar results pertained when comparing among foreign-born subjects those born in the USA, the UK, the rest of Europe, and the rest of the world. Neither their time gender distribution (p=0.846)[9] nor sex distribution (p=0.983)[9] differed statistically. In addition, in the Canadian-born group, the alpha-beta distributions among those born in Vancouver, in the rest of British Columbia, in Quebec, and in the rest of Canada were also only a matter of chance (p=0.425),[10] as were their sex distributions (p=0.896).[11] Acculturation or mobility certainly cannot be responsible for the time gender duality.

These results testify to a remarkable stability of the Vancouver sample of 405 subjects in terms of its time gender distribution (about 60% alphas and 40% betas), and sex distribution (53% females and 47% males), when comparing this sample with various sub-groups (according to where subjects originated) which renders similar results. This lends some credence to the assumption that the time gender distribution of the Vancouver sample may not be just a local phenomenon, but has significance for Canada as a whole and beyond.

Dysfunctional childhood

It is hard to avoid speculation about the role of childhood maltreatment in becoming an alpha or beta because the prevalence of dysfunctional childhood is rather high in the general population.[12] In addition, some influential streams of thought in Freudian psycho-analysis acknowledge a duality in how people experience time, although not viewing them as two normal genetic options.

The first stream of thought attributes the cause of this blocking to poor nurturing early in life—poor mothering in particular.[13] Poor nurturing results in a "primitive" personality structure characterized by a sense of timelessness—an absence of a sense of continuity or duration (the alpha mode)—as opposed to a more "advanced" personality structure that displays a sense of duration and continuity (the beta mode).[14]

The second stream of Freudian thought considers one's functioning-in-time as starting with a timeless here-and-now experience (the alpha mode). Normally, this mode shifts during adolescence to a second stage of "psycho-temporal adaptation," when experiencing duration and continuity begins, which enables one to acquire a sense of one's own history (the beta mode).[15] Harmful life events, such as child abuse, may cause some to get stuck in the first mode. Hence the duality in time experience.

I considered dysfunctional childhood in terms of growing up in a broken home, with parental substance abuse, with sexual abuse, with physical abuse, or with several of these factors[16] and looked at the prevalence of these factors in my cohort.[17]

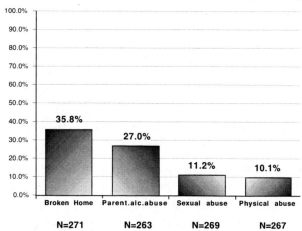

Figure 11.5: Prevalence of four dysfunctional childhood factors[18]

Figure 11.5 shows that these dysfunctional experiences were absent in the vast majority of subjects, so that a dysfunctional childhood cannot account for the time gender duality. In any case, the majority of maltreated children grow up to be well-functioning adults.[19] A further reason as to why maltreatment in childhood cannot account for the time gender duality is that this maltreatment may occur not only *before* time gender differentiation begins around age six,[20] but also, and more frequently, *after* the differences between alphas and betas already have begun to show.

While subjects were not responsible for the broken home in their background, or parental alcohol abuse, their childhood personalities could have played a minor role (less possibly a major role) in and, particularly, physical abuse. Could these tendencies have affected the time gender distribution and sexual gender distribution in subjects with these problems in their background?

Although the number of subjects with sexual abuse in childhood was only 30 out of 269, comparing the time gender distribution and the sexual gender distribution of these 30 subjects with those in the overall sample of 405 subjects resulted in statistically significant differences between the four conjoint genders in the prevalence of sexual abuse (p=0.028); the vulnerability to sexual abuse being greatest among alpha females, followed by alpha males, then beta females, and least among beta males.

The number of physical abuse victims was also only 27 out of 267. Even so, the difference in time gender distribution and sexual gender distribution between these 27 subjects and the overall sample of 405 subjects was insignificant. Time gender and sex did not appear to have played a role in causing this problem.

In sum, I concluded that dysfunctional childhood experiences do not play a role in *creating* the time gender duality.

Astrology

Astrology is a belief system that can be traced back to the beginning of civilization in Sumeria around 3,200 BCE. Its contemporary form dates back to the ancient Greek astronomer and mathematician Claudius Ptolemy whose principles of cosmic influence still lie at the heart of modern astrological practice.[21] Astrology holds that the snapshot of the position of the sun, moon and major planets, as seen from one's place on Earth at the moment of birth, determines one's personality and bodily constitution. It also defines one's future, which is further fixed by the day-to-day positions of the "planets" (which in astrological tradition also embrace the sun and moon).

Daily horoscopes in most newspapers and on the Internet testify to the fact that Western astrology retains millions of adherents. During his presidency of the United States, Ronald Reagan and his wife Nancy were devoted believers in astrology. They were in good company, for Carl Jung stressed "the curious psychological qualities of the Zodiac," and called astrology "a complete projected theory of human character."[22] Since some clients in my practice also initially assumed that the Zodiac sign under which one is born may play an important role in determining whether one becomes an alpha or beta, it made sense to attempt to disprove the role of astrology.

The Zodiac is the circular belt of twelve star constellations, each taking up 30° in the 360° imaginary circle through which the sun appears to move around the earth every 24 hours. Ptolemy named and listed each of these 12 star constellations as follows: Aries, Taurus, Gemini, Cancer , Leo, Virgo, Libra, Scorpio, Sagittarius, Capricorn, Aquarius and Pisces.[23] In addition to its daily move through the circle of 12 constellations, the sun also appears to move on a month-by-month basis counter-clockwise from one sign of the Zodiac to the next and thus, on an annual basis, through the entire Zodiac belt.

Since astrology holds that the personality and the destiny of each person depends on the sign of the Zodiac under which that person was born, it assumes that there are 12 basic Zodiacal personalities,[24] each bearing the name of the constellation for which it was originally named two millennia ago.[25]

Figure 11.6 shows that astrology also holds that each Zodiac sign should be considered not only in its own right, but also in contrast with its opposite, and whether it is feminine-receptive or masculine-direct in nature. Furthermore, each sign is a unique combination of one of four elements: fire (enthusiastic), earth (practical, stable), air (intellectual, communicative), or water (emotional, intuitive). And of one of three qualities: cardinal (enterprising, outgoing), fixed (resistant to change), or mutable (adaptable).[26]

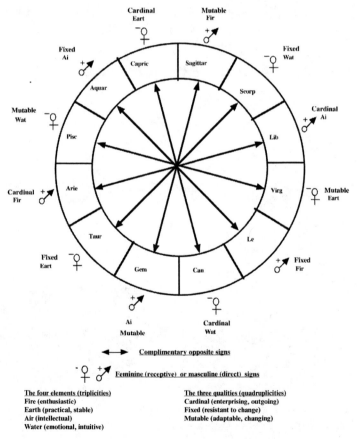

Figure 11.6: The Zodiac signs, feminine or masculine, with their opposites,
divided into 4 elements and 3 qualities

However, popular Western astrology has fallen prey to emphasizing that one's Zodiacal birth sign is sufficient to describe not only one's character, but also to predict one's life events.[27] An equally serious flaw is the wide spread confusion about how the twelve Zodiac signs fit precisely into our annual calendar. This confusion occurs because the sun's annual movement through the twelve signs of the Zodiac does not correspond with the calendar in a fixed manner. The beginning and ending of each sign shifts somewhat from year to year, especially in leap years. This means that subjects born between the 18th and 24th of any month (that is, seven days out of each month) may be uncertain about which Zodiac sign they were born under. Even so, many astrologers feel free to schedule the beginning and ending of each Zodiac sign as they see fit. On the same day one may be a Virgo in one newspaper and a Libra in another, for example. Even a recent publication by three physicians used a schedule of fixed dating in comparing the birth dates of 171 Nobel laureates in medicine and physiology with those of 375 scientists and scientific trainees at a Canadian medical research institute. They claimed a significant statistical association between Zodiac signs (in particular Gemini and Leo) and the likelihood of having received the Nobel Prize in Medicine and Physiology (p=0.042).[28] Since such a schedule of fixed dating might involve an error rate of up to almost 25%, researchers should only allocate Zodiac signs to subjects who were born between the first and the 17th, and between the 25th and the last day of any month.

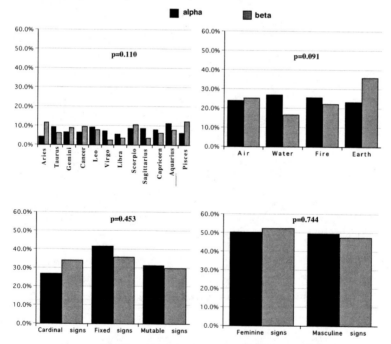

Figure 11.7: The time gender distribution among the twelve signs of the Zodiac and their derivatives

With this in mind, I now can deal with the question whether being alpha or beta has anything to do with the Zodiac sign under which one is born and its several aspects.

Restricting my subjects to those born between the 1st and 17th, or the 25th and last of any given month led to 92% of the 273 subjects having an assigned Zodiac sign, including its elements (Air, Water, Fire or Earth), its quality (Cardinal, Fixed, Mutable), and its grouping (feminine-negative and masculine-positive, broken down by time gender.

Since one's sex is not related to one's Zodiac sign or its derivatives, I anticipated that men and women would be equally distributed among these astrological categories. This hypothesis indeed turned out to be the case not only for the 12 Zodiac signs ($p=0.856$), but also for the four elements ($p=0.717$), the three qualities ($p=0.747$), and the grouping into feminine and masculine signs ($p=0.547$). Since, in my view, time gender is determined genetically, I furthermore predicted that the distribution of alphas and betas among the Zodiac signs and their derivatives would not be statistically significantly different either. Figure 11.7 demonstrates that this, too, was borne out for the twelve Zodiac signs ($p=0.110$), the four elements ($p=0.091$), the three qualities ($p=0.453$), and the feminine and masculine groupings ($p=7.444$).

People have always wanted to believe in stars; they still do. It invests our lives with cosmic importance. Even so, one need not look at the stars and planets in trying to account for time gender.

Section 2: About nature and time gender

About time gendering

Genetic research in the domain of time gender depends entirely on how one assigns people their time gender. For the time being, this "golden standard" must depend on carefully executed time gendering by qualified experts.

The two different ways of storing autobiographic memories find secondary expression in certain behavioral and experiential personality aspects, as outlined in previous chapters. Hence there is a returning inclination to think of the time gender duality as two distinct sets of quantifiable personality traits, particularly because these secondary traits (as described in several of this book's chapters) are not of the black-and-white variety, but may vary in strength in individual alphas and betas. Such traits may be uninhibited and unmistakable, or moderated, if not covered up altogether by a variety of other genetic or environmental factors. To quantify these secondary personality traits, many psychologists and psychiatrists in research would favor the use of the "NEO-PI-R Self-report Inventory," which represents the most prominent contemporary model of normal personality, namely the "Five-Factor-Model."[29] It assesses five allegedly independent, mutually exclusive personality domains or traits, namely neuroticism (N), extroversion (E), openness to experience (O) , agreeableness (A), and conscientiousness (C).[30] But even if such research would come up with scoring patterns that have reproducible high correlations with one or the other time gender, these scores could only indicate the *probability* of being an alpha or a beta. Even so, such research has to be based on cohorts of subjects who had been individually time-gendered by experts.

Eventually, far more efficient in diagnosing one's time gender will be genetic screening, although here, too, research will have to start with cohorts of subjects who had been individually time-gendered by experts. Either approach requires that my method of time gendering has to be reviewed.

I used both a *direct* and an *indirect* method. The *direct method* of time gendering was applied to all 405 subjects of my four-year research cohort and was based on personally assessing the type of autobiographic memory storage a subject displayed during chronologic life history taking.[31] Eventually, however, the presence of clusters of secondary personality traits in alphas and betas as described in this book, became a co-determining factor in time gendering. This raises the question whether these clusters of secondary personality traits eventually biased my judgment as to how a subject stores autobiographicmemories. Or, the other way around, whether my judgment about the type of autobiographic memory storage was generating a bias toward preferentially focusing on one of the clusters of personality features. Such biases might create a systematic error in assigning time gender to a subject.

In Chapter 1, I pointed out that I had divided my cohort of 405 subjects into an "early" group of 273 subjects from whom I collected data during the 1987-1989 period, and a "late" group of 132 subjects from whom I collected data during the 1989-1991 period. The female-male distribution appeared stable over the four years of data collecting ($p=0.514$) and indeed similar to that of the general population of Greater Vancouver, BC. Hence, the overall sample of 405 subjects approximated a general population sample. It is in this context remarkable that the alpha-beta ratio in the early group as compared with the late group also was stable ($p=0.545$). This leaves little room for a biased interpretation of observations (intra-observer variation). In addition, I noted in Chapter 1 that the results of my research described in the chapters of this book, amass into a consistent, coherent body of facts, and that the coherence of these data, which took four years to accomplish, suggests that my direct method of assessing time gender in 405 people must have been both precise and consistent; and that the method therefore appears to represent a definite golden standard for the assessment of time gender.

For purposes of future research, an important question is whether one can educate others to use this method of time gendering. Having taught the method to one professional counselor and having been in a position to supervise her work for several years, I am satisfied that it can be done. Naturally, in future research projects it will be desirable for two adequately trained professionals to perform a time genderevaluation of each involved subject. In case of disagreement, a third one should be consulted, with the final time gender assignment to be made by consensus after discussion.[32]

Indirect time gendering is based on third-party information — that is, information obtained from a subject's repeated descriptions about the personality of a significant other (such as a marital partner, parent, sibling or child). However, when using the indirect method one is looking through a subject's eyes at the significant other, the obtained information may be colored by a particular bias of the reporting subject. Certain subjects may be projecting their own time gender on their marital partner (alphacizing or betacizing the partner), for example. Science rightly advises that one should approach such data with some reservation, speaking of indirectly obtained information as "soft," rather than "hard" data.

When I time-gendered the marital partners of 100 subjects to study the choice of marital partners, I had the advantage of having 48 partners in conjoint counseling, so that I was able to use the direct method in both. But I had to apply the indirect method of time gendering in 52 marital partners of subjects.[33] In retrospect, I have in this case *some* confidence in the indirect method because the time gender distribution of the 100 subjects whose partner's time gender had to be assessed (51.0% alphas, 49.0% betas) did statistically not change significantly when adding the 100 time-gendered partners (52 of whom had been assessed indirectly) (48.0% alphas, 52.0% betas; p=0.624).

In the unabridged e-book version of this work[384] I used the indirect method also to time gender parents and siblings of research subjects to see whether there was any preliminary support for the suggestion that alpha-alpha marriages produce only alpha children; beta-beta marriages only beta children; and that half of the children from marriages between an alpha and beta are alphas, the other half betas. This tentative suggestion could not indicate the exact genetic mechanics of such time gender transmission, nor did it explain why the ratio of alphas to betas in my 405 subjects was about 50%-50% among men, but around 70%-30% among women.

While I remain totally committed to the genetic basis of the time gender duality, a recently published research on the DNA sequence of the human X-chromosome[35] led me to accept an alternative version of time gender transmission. This alternative version does not only account for the difference in alpha-beta ratios among the men and women of my research cohort but, in addition, it offers exact details as to how the time gender transmission from parents to children is achieved. There is, however, a price to pay for this more promising explanation: it clearly demonstrated the unreliability of the indirect method which I had used in assigning a time gender to some parents and siblings of my research subjects.

A hypothesis aboutf the genetic transmission of time gender

In 2005, geneticist Mark Ross from Hinxton, England, and his team of international scientists published the complete DNA sequence of the human X-chromosome of which women have two copies (XX) in all cells of the body (one X inherited from the father and one X from the mother), and men only one (XY) (the X inherited from the mother, the Y from the father). Despite the fact that females have two X-chromosomes, males and females have in large part the same dosage of gene products, since women inactivate one of the two Xs early in their development (their body cells randomly choose either the maternal or paternal X to be the active X-chromosome).[36]

That the 1890 US Census noticed that more boys than girls were mentally disabled,[37] reflects a preponderance of genes for brain function on the X-chromosome, for a woman uses only one of her two X-chromosomes in each cell, so that, only some of her cells will suffer, while men with only one X express invariably any defective brain gene from that X-chromosome.[38]

Ross' team confirmed that an unusually large number of almost 1,100 genes of the X-chromosome code for proteins important to brain function (there are 14x more genes on the X-chromosome than on the tiny, male Y chromosome). Because women have two X-chromosomes and men only one, the X-chromosome in men gets a chance to shine (if it expresses a desired mental ability), or fail miserably (if it expresses a genetic defect that causes mental impairment).[389] Since successful males have the potential to sire children with multiple partners, mutations on the X-chromosome that are advantageous to both sexes can spread rapidly through a population.[40]

"..there is...some indirect evidence that genes on the X-chromosomes are involved in higher cognitive functions. One hint comes from a study of 4,000 sets of British identical twins. Each female male twin inherits two X-chromosomes, one from her mother and one from her father, but each individual twin randomly inactivates one of her two X-chromosomes. So identical twin sisters can express different X-chromosome genes. In contrast, male identical twins inherit only one X-chromosome, from their mothers, and so must activate the same X-linked genes. In the British study, researchers led by Ian Craig of King's College London found that in some traits linked to intelligence, such as verbal skills and good social behaviour, male twins were more alike than female twins."[41]

As a result of all these developments, the DNA sequence of the "feminine" X-chromosome has become a prime hunting ground for geneticists interested in the evolution of the cognitive and cultural sophistication that defines the human species.[42]

All this naturally re-focused my attention on the genetic transmission of time gender. Since the characteristic pattern of X-linked inheritance (which, apparently, not only involves many genes involved in higher mental functions, but also diseases such as hemophilia) is that it affects males, but that there is no male-to-male transmission. Thus, if the gene or genes that are the underpinning of time gender are located on the X-chromosome, then in men whose single X-chromosome comes from their mother, it always must be their mother who determines their time gender, never their father. In women are located on the X-chromosome,, however, who receive an X from their father and an X from their mother, either one could determine their time gender.

Time gender analysis of my 405 subjects showed that 47.89% of the 190 males were

THE GENDER BEYOND SEX: TWO DISTINCT WAYS OF LIVING IN TIME   213

alphas and 52.11% (99) betas. In other words, men showed an almost equal alpha-beta ratio, so that among the two X-chromosomes of women (the mothers of men) the distribution of alpha-causing genes and beta-causing genes should also be about equal. Yet the actual time gender distribution among the 215 women of my cohort did not show an almost equal proportion of alphas and betas, but 70.70% alphas and 29.30% betas. This can only mean that, if one of the two X-chromosomes a female has carries the alpha-causing gene and the other X-chromosome the beta-causing gene, then the alpha-causing gene must be dominant and the beta-causing gene recessive. In that case, the woman will be alpha. This, in turn, may indicate that perhaps about 1/3 of the women in my sample carried an alpha-gene on both X-chromosomes (AA, resulting in the alpha time gender), about 1/3 an alpha-causing gene on one X-chromosome and a beta-gene on the other (Ab, resulting in the alpha time gender), and about 1/3 carried a beta-gene on both X-chromosomes (bb, resulting in the beta time gender). This explanation of the genetic time gender transmission sufficiently allows for the alpha-beta ratio among the men and women of my 405 subjects (given the fact that the alpha-beta ratio among men is not *exactly* 50%-50%, and that the distribution of time gender genotypes among women (AA, Ab, and bb) does not need to be *exactly* 1/3–1/3–1/3).[43]

Table 11.1 demonstrates how the possibility of a dominant alpha gene or a recessive beta gene on an X-chromosome influences the time gender of children in each of the four possible time gender combinations in marriage.

marriage - type		---husband--- TG	X-TG	-----wife------- TG	XX-TG	-----sons------- TG	X-TG	--daughters- TG	XX-TG
alpha male x	alpha female	alpha	A	alpha	AA	alpha	A	alpha	AA
				alpha	Ab	beta	b	alpha	Ab
alpha male x	beta female	alpha	A	beta	bb	beta	b	alpha	Ab
beta male x	alpha female	beta	b	alpha	AA	alpha	A	alpha	Ab
				alpha	Ab	beta	b	beta	bb
beta male x	beta female	beta	b	beta	bb	beta	b	beta	bb

TG	time gender phenotype	alpha or beta	
X-TG	time gender genotype	for male X:	A or b
XX-TG	time gender genotype	for female XX:	AA or Ab or bb

Table 11.1:
The potential time gender of children in the four time gender combinations in marriages

In alpha-alpha marriages, sons may of either time gender, while all daughters will be alpha; in beta-beta marriages all children will be beta; in marriages between an alpha husband and beta wife, all sons will be beta, while all daughters will be alpha; and in marriages betweem a beta husband and alpha wife, all children may be of either time gender.

In the original e-book version of my work I produced in its Chapter 11 data which are in conflict with table 11.1, for they indicated, for example, that two sons from an alpha-beta marriage were alphas and that five daughters from an alpha-beta marriage were betas.[44] The only explanation I have for this is that the method of obtaining these and similar data — the indirect method of time gendering parents and siblings of subjects in my research cohort — was unreliable.

Concluding remarks

Can the time gender gene or genes be located in the human genome? Erika Check, Washington's biomedical correspondent of the journal *Nature* wrote:

> "In London, Craig's team plans to identify twins who score high or low on certain 'people skills,' such as sharing their toys and volunteering help to others. The researchers will then use gene chips to scan the twins' DNA, looking for particular genetic variations that correlate with these traits. Once they find a region of DNA on the X-chromosome to link up to a particular trait, the group will look at the detailed sequence of individual chromosomes to try to pin down the exact gene involved."[45]

This indicates that, once a group of twins is properly time-gendered by experts, we are but a step away from identifying the detailed DNA sequence of the gene or genes responsible for the human duality in autobiography knowledge memory that is the underpinning of the two time genders.

Complementary to this molecular genetic approach, a research technique, called positron emission tomography (PET), may also be able to verify the biological nature of time gender. This technique creates images of the brain which allow for a degree of precision in measuring localized brain activity that was altogether unimaginable a few years ago. These scans have demonstrated, for example, that different brain loci are in action during different types of working memory tasks.[46] By using this technique in time-gendered subjects, we will be able, perhaps, to demonstrate what differences exist in the autobiographic memory of alphas and betas.

NOTES

1   Eisenberg (1995), p. 1563, 1568.
2   Green (1989), p. 188.
3   Gonzalez & Zimbardo (1985) paraphrased.
4   Pos (2004).
5   25% accounted for all the left-over positions.
6   Leacock (1957).
7   I had relevant information in 99% of my 273 subjects.
8   The mean time gender distribution was 58% alphas and 42% betas.
9   The mean sex distribution was 58% females and 42% males.
10   The mean time gender distribution was 60% alphas and 40% betas.
11   The mean sex distribution was 52% females and 48% males.
12   Rutterand Maughgan (1997).
13   Balint and Winnicott [Meissner (1985), p. 394].

14   Kernberg (1985).

15   Erikson pioneered this thinking (Chapter 9); Seton (1974), Finagrette (1977), and Masler (1973), as quoted by Rappoport, Enrich and Wilson (1982), p. 60-62.

16   All four dysfunctional factors were equally likely to occur in combination with one or more others except that a history of physical abuse was more likely to be part of a multiple factor picture than a history of a broken home.

17   Concerning the presence or absence of a broken home I had data in 99% of 273 subjects, on parental alcohol abuse in 96%, on sexual abuse in 99%, and on physical abuse in 98%. 'Broken home' was defined as the breakup of the parental marriage and childhood bereavement due to the death of one or both parents, prior to a child leaving home or reaching age 18, whatever came first. 'Parental alcohol abuse' was either by the father, mother, both, a stepfather or a stepparent and a parent. 'Sexual abuse' was defined as having been subjected to exhibitionism, fondling, masturbation, oral sex, or genital intercourse. The sexual abuser actually turned out to be either the father, mother, brother, cousin, grandparent, stepfather, or non-family, including a foster father and a priest. No sexual abuse by a sister was found. The physical abuse was either by the father, mother, stepfather, stepmother, brother, or by a non-family person. No physical abuse by a sister was found.

18   The prevalence of these four dysfunctional factors in childhood is expressed as a percentage of those on which relevant information was available.

19   Rutter, et al. (1975); Farber & Egeland (1987); Werner (1989); Rutter,(1990); Paris(1998); Widom (1989).

20   See Chapter 2.

21   Parker & Parker (1990), p.16.

22   Jung (1968b), p. 245, 343.

23   Parker & Parker (1990), p. 68.

24   Innis (1970), p. 13-15; Parker & Parker (1990), p.106-129; Goldschneider & Elffers (1994), p. 20-79; Jones (1970), p. 60-71].

25   However, there is a problem. The circular belt of 12 star constellations moves very slowly clockwise in the skies at the rate of about 30 degrees every 2,000 years. As a result, the name of each of the 12 Zodiacal personalities, which was assigned according to the particular position of the constellations two millennia ago, no longer coincides with the present position of these constellations, but now refers to the constellation west of the one from which it took its name. Today, for example, Aries is found in the astronomical constellation Pisces. This discrepancy has led to a broad schism in astrology. On the one hand, contemporary astrology practiced in India takes account of the gradual movement of the stellar constellations and observes planetary positions against the background of the actual stellar constellations. Contemporary Western astrology, on the other hand, considers this an esoteric practice [Parker & Parker (1990), p.42], and disregards the precession of the Zodiacal belt altogether. Instead, it assigns the position of the traditional Zodiac signs in relation to the first day of spring, the Astrological New Year. As a result, the 12 Zodiac signs of Western astrology should not be confused with the moving stellar constellations from which they derived their name.

26   The figure was drawn up based on information according to Parker & Parker (1990), p. 85.

27   Goldschneider & Elffers (1994).

28   Pollex, Hegele and Ban (2001).

29   Costa and McCrae (1992).

30   Costa and McCrae (1995 and 1998

31   See *Appendix 2: The chronologic biographic interview.*

32   DeLisi et al. (2002), p. 804.

33   See Chapter 7 under: *Choosing a partner (3): the role of time gender.*

34   Pos (2004).

35   Ross et al (2005); Carrel & Willard (2005)

36   Ross et al. (2005). Early in female development, cells randomly choose either the maternal or paternal X to be the active X-chromosome. This means that females, but not males, are mosaics of two cell populations with respect to X-linked gene expression (i.e. their specific protein production). Yet only 75% of the genes in an *inactivated* X chromosome are actually subject to inactivation; 15% escaping inactivation to some degree (a majority showing robust expression, a minority only partial expression, but all expressing higher levels of making proteins in females than in males) and 10% sometimes being inactivated, but not at other times. This means that on the inactivated X-chromosome in women up to

15% - 25% (200-300 genes, a hugh number) remain active [Carrel & Willard (2005), p. 400, 403].

37   Johnson (1997).

38   Check (2005), p. 266.

39   Check (2005), p. 267.

40   Check (2005), p. 267.

41   Check (2005), p. 266-267 quoting Loat et al. (2004).

42   Check (2005), p. 266.

43   What is actually needed in my research cohort of 405 persons is that the proportions of A and b genes on the activated X-chromosomes of women (ready for transmission to sons) approximate 49.89% A's and 52.11% b's, and that the proportion of women with the genotypes AA or Ab (representing the alpha phenotype) approximates 70.70% and the proportion of women with the genotype bb 29.30%.

44   Pos (2004), table 11.1. This means that table 11.2 in the e-book edition must also be wrong. At the time I fortunately pointed out that these were only preliminary and tentative data and that, hopefully, future research would replicate or amend these preliminary findings with hard and more extensive data. The recent findings by geneticist Ross and his team [Ross et al (2005)] certainly made such amendment possible.

45   Check (2005), p. 267.

46   Jonides et al. (1993).

CHAPTER 12

The Evolution Of The Modern Mind

In the study of the evolution of the human species, available information concerns itself almost exclusively with anatomical structures. Psychological functioning has received comparatively little scholarly attention.[1] In an attempt to address this neglect, this chapter focuses on our psychological evolution. This chapter is therefore neither intended to support the time gender model nor to argue against the validity of the alpha-beta duality. In this sense, the chapter has its own validity or lack thereof, independent of the time gender model.

In fact, this chapter does not solely focus on the evolution of the alpha-beta duality in 6–D, but also traces the psychological evolution of other aspects and conscious dimensions of the theoretical model I described in Chapter 3. Based on this theoretical, developmental model, I discuss the evolution of aspects and conscious dimensions in the following sequence:

1. the reality of 4–D as modern humans experience it;

2. our long-term memory recall (including dream recall) and the world of imagination in 5–D together with the development of spoken language;

3. the internalization of 4–D (particularly of the spoken language) into the privacy and silence of 5–D, together with the emergence of our autobiographic memory (alphacization) in 6-D due to a dominant genetic mutation on the X-chromosome;

4. the genetically recessive mutation in this autobiographic memory in some people (betacization) with the appearance of the time gender duality in 6–D;

5. the shift from pre-logical thinking to concrete, operational logical thinking with an awareness of concrete cause-and-effect relationships (as witnessed by the agricultural revolution);

6. our abstract thinking with the appearance of the paraego in 7–D (as documented by scientific rather than technological thinking); and finally,

7. the chapter concludes with a discussion of the evolution of our silent self-talk.

Because the evolution of 5–D occurred rather early in our development, we have to go back in time to the origin of modern human beings. Molecular biologists suggest that about 100 million years ago, placental mammals began diversifying into today's

18 living orders,[2] which includes the one of primates ("Chiefs"). The evolution from lower primates (lemurs, lorises, aye-ayes, and tarsiers) to higher primates (monkeys, apes, and humans) is of particular interest.[3]

Around 23 million years ago, apes originated in Africa, which was a continent that had been drifting around in the southern Indian Ocean for 87 million years. When around 15 million years ago, Africa bumped into the Eurasian landmass, these apes began to disperse around the forests of the world,[4] which covered most of the continents. However, following a significant climate change that led to extensive deserts in northern Africa, the Middle East, and India, apes were no longer able to migrate between Africa and Asia. As a result, African apes became restricted to that continent's equatorial zone, where they became larger and evolved into the gorilla, the chimpanzee, and the hominid line of great apes. Climatic changes periodically wreaked havoc on Africa's forests. These changes drove the hominid line of great apes, which were in search of food, into the grassland savannahs that had replaced the tropical forests.[5]

Unfortunately, there is a fossil gap between 10 and six or seven million years ago that creates "a yawning void" in the evolution line of humans.[6] Scientists presently assume that the split between African apes (chimpanzees and gorillas) and the hominid or pre-human lines occurred six to four million years ago.[7] Researchers define the hominid or pre-human apes as different based on the fact that their pelvis had rotated so that they had evolved into upright-standing apes who had begun walking on two legs, leaving their hands free to manipulate things.

The Savannah theory has been particularly popular in accounting for hominid bipedalism.[8] It claims that in the savannahs, natural selection favored apes who could stand up and walk upright because they could see over the tall savanna grass, allowing them to spot their pray and escape their predators. They also had their hands free to manipulate things and could walk long distances holding food or children.[9]

Some fossil findings contradict this theory, however. For one, bipedal prehuman apes did not solely live on the savannah but also in the forests. More importantly, the preoccupation with bipedalism does not explain a package of adaptations which modern humans share with aquatic mammals (whales, dolphins, seals, manatees, and sea otters) but not with our closest relative, the chimpanzee.[10] These adaptations include loss of hair, the presence of subcutaneous fat, tears and the ability to cry, face-to-face copulation, the un-apelike human fondness for swimming, and the diving reflex in babies. The aquatic ape theory explains the existence of these adaptations by suggesting that there was a period of aquatic adaptation of certain great apes, followed by their return to land.[11] The turned pelvis which enabled their bipedalism is explained as the result of swimming and the frequent upright position in the water as seen in other aquatic mammals, such as sea otters, dugongs and manatees.[12] A geological plausible locality where aquatic evolutionary processes leading to bipedalism could have occurred has been postulated near the Afar region where human evolution occurred.[13]

No matter which theory is closest to the truth, fossil finds dated between four and two-and-a-half million years ago suggest that humans evolved from one of several bipedal lines of the Southern Ape or Australopithecus which overlapped in time.[14] Instead of reflecting a simple transition from the Southern Ape to the modern human, there were many false starts and dead ends. We know little about the exact origin of our own genus Homo.[15]

Homo habilis and Homo erectus

Modern humans evolved from their hominid ancestors during the ice age that began about 3 million years ago. By 2.5 million years ago, glaciers were beginning to expand repeatedly across the continents while sea levels were dropping, and these glacial period alternated with warming interglacial episodes and rising sea levels. New fossil finds and advances in dating techniques over the last decades have greatly added to our knowledge of the history of this period in human evolution.

One line of Southern Apes of Africa developed traits linking them both with the earlier Australopithecus and later members of the genus Homo. They became the first primates to produce primitive tools and are hence considered the first species of the genus Homo. They are given the name "Handy Man" or "Homo habilis." For some 500,000 years (between two and one-and-a-half million years ago), they lived as contemporaries of other descendant lines of the Southern Ape, which later became extinct.[16]

In many ways Homo habilis still looked like a Southern Ape, being still small in stature (on the average 1.52 m. and weighing under 45 kg)[17] but with a somewhat larger brain, (about half the size of our brain). Even so, they were still ambidextrous like great apes, throwing stones with either hand. They had not yet evolved lateralization of their brain, with accompanying right- or left-handedness, as has modern man.[18]

Homo habilis appear to have been the first forest-living great apes who lived in stable, small, close-knit troops, usually less than 50, or sometimes less than 30 individuals. Hence they were in regular, close contact, which helped enhance their communication skills. Yet, conscious voluntary verbal communication was still far beyond their horizon although their social closeness and learning facilitated iconic gestures and emotive vocalizations. Handy Man's brain still lacked important prerequisites for language development: it had not yet lateralized and still was without conscious long-term memory recall, which allows for a well-developed 5–D.

Their social also closeness enhanced their tool-making skills. Once an individual had acquired stable tool-making habits through opportunistic trial-and-error, these habits could be transmitted through social learning.[19] However, modern humans would be able to produce these simple tools with little practice. The symbolizing and designing abilities of these early humans were therefore not much beyond that of chimpanzees or gorillas. Their tool making did not yet reflect the presence of a stable 5–D and imagination.

Bones from different animals at the same location as Handy man's fossils suggest that Homo habilis carried food back to a home base for sharing. It is not clear when this shift from the feed-as-you-go of the great apes, to the common human pattern of gathering food for collective consumption occurred. It is well to keep in mind that bipedalism, manufacturing tools, transporting food, and food sharing are not exclusively human traits. Each trait can be found also in other great apes. However, Homo habilis developed all of these together, and to a much higher level of importance in sustaining them.[20]

Around 1.8 million years ago, one line of Homo habilis yielded a taller (average five feet six inches), stronger, smarter variety of human species, Homo erectus or Upright Human. They had a rather human-like body but were still primitive above the neck, with a flattened forehead and prominent brow ridges, as in gorillas or chimpanzees, and with massive teeth and rounded jaws without a chin. No longer mainly vegetarian as Homo habilis, they had become increasingly carnivorous and active hunters.[21] Their time span covers the period from about 1.8 million to perhaps 100,000 years ago. during which period their brain size increased. This time span constitutes the main formative period of some typical human faculties. For example, the majority of tools used by Homo erectus found in northern China (Beijing man) were chipped by right handers.[22] This indicates that the uniquely human lateralization of brain functioning (the functional specialization of each brain half) was underway and with it the rewiring of the brain that eventually would allow for language.

The early Homo erectus were found in Kenya about 1.8 million years ago,[23] while the first evidence of the use of fire at their campsites is about 1.4 million years old. Fire remained associated with them where ever they went.[24] In Africa, Homo erectus were contemporaries of Homo habilis for about 300,000 years, but since they were carnivores who needed immense home ranges, they eventually overran Homo habilis. Indeed, many African Homo erectus were ultimately forced out of their homeland by their own and migrated to Europe and Asia. For almost a million years African, European and Asian Homo Erectus developed apart from each other. Among the latter, Java Man in Indonesia is older than Beijing Man in northern China who, despite his cannibalism, is generally considered somewhat less primitive.[25]

For one million years, Homo erectus in East Asia did not change substantially and continued to employ crude stone choppers and chopping tools.[26] But about 450,000 years ago, the western group (the European Homo erectus) produced a superior implement: a sharper, thinner, lighter, symmetrical, almond-like flint hand ax. This represented the so-called Acheulian tradition and lasted until about 100,000 years ago,[27] well after the European Homo erectus had disappeared.

There is no scientific consensus as to when Homo erectus was replaced by early forms of Homo sapiens Neanderthaliensis. Part of the problem is that during the 1.5 million years of their stay on the planet, western Homo erectus evolved considerably, so that it is not always clear whether to classify fossils as late Homo erectus or early Homo sapiens.

Our Neanderthal cousins

The Neanderthals entered Europe 250,000 years ago. They lasted until 30,000 years ago by which time modern humans, called Cro-magnon, had replaced them.[28] The Neanderthals were short and stocky, more powerfully built than modern humans, had massive skulls with sloping foreheads and protruding faces, projecting noses, and rather heavy bony ridges over their brows, but lacked a chin. Their brain had a volume of 1,300-1,425 cc, [29] compared to the human brain volume of 1,400-1,500 cc.[30]

However, Neanderthals fall outside the range of genetic variation found in the modern human. They are a separate species.[31] Nevertheless, this extinct branch of the human evolutionary tree is of great interest as Neanderthals show clear transitions from subhuman features to uniquely human features: the first burials and grave offerings; early language development; and a new inventiveness that made them both excellent toolmakers[32] and first-rate hunters who could kill animals by driving them over a cliff. This is not, however, evidence of planning, but rather of trial-and-error learning transferred by social learning. Many animals (wolves and lions, for example) demonstrate hunting patterns of comparable complexity.

By 100,000 years ago, Neanderthals had replaced the Acheulian tradition (created by the European Homo erectus) with their own Mousterian culture, which was characterized by an impressive inventory of tools. They were the first to produce hafted hand-axes with a design of increased complexity and also scrapers and saw-like blades to work wood, bone, and horn into tools and weapons. But their tools, and thus their technology, stayed more or less the same over 65,000 years.[33] Their inventiveness was therefore minimal, meaning that the Mousterian culture represents a prolonged sluggish cultural advance.

Having found 100,000 year-old Neanderthal grave sites and "offerings," some scientists assume that Neanderthals were modern-humans-in-the-making. These scientists maintain that the "careful disposal of their dead" shows that Neanderthals already had a special regard for the dead, and therefore a uniquely human self-awareness and a self-conscious death anxiety that modern adults experience in anticipating their own death.[34] Another speculation is that they were already troubled by a metaphysical intuition of a possible continued existence after death,[35] and even, perhaps, that they had some vague notion of eternity.[36] Some experts have gone as far as assuming that, for Neanderthals, the future must have stretched not merely far into the known, but into the unknown as well; and that the human capacity for dealing with time does not seem to have increased markedly since Neanderthals walked the earth.[37]

In my terminology, for this last hypothesis to be true would have required that Neanderthals had already evolved an autobiographic 6–D; that some of them were betas; and furthermore that they could already think abstractly and possessed 7–D.[38] Any idea of death, soul, life after death, or eternity depends on a well developed language with stable abstract concepts, and this the Neanderthals did not yet possess. Marija Gimbutas, a renowned archaeologist, wisely remarked:[39]

> "A serious and continuous obstacle in the study of ancient societies is the indolent assumption that they must have resembled our own. Bachofen warned [already] in 1859 that 'the scholar must be able to renounce the ideas of his own time and transfer himself to the midpoint of a completely different world of thought,' but the existence of 'a different world' is the hardest thing to admit."

There is concrete evidence negating the idea that Neanderthal burials indicate a vision of life after death. Since there lived a few million Neanderthals across the globe at any given time,[40] those who believe that Neanderthals envisioned an after life would expect more than the dozen or so graves found to date. There is reasonable doubt that Neanderthals habitually buried *all* their dead, only select ones. Furthermore, in western Europe, only one out of four co-existing Neanderthal cultures appears to have been associated with graves in the first place.[41] Indeed, graves and burials were not only rather selective among Neanderthals, but even among modern man, for in Europe personal graves did not become common until 10,000-8,000 BCE.[42]

The emergence of 5–D and language

Why did Neanderthals, through burials, protect the bodies of only a select few against scavenging animals? And why were grave offerings made at only some sites? My answers rest on two assumptions. The first assumption has to do with the fact that all levels of mammals dream (from the oldest existing mammalian, the opossum, to the highest level of primates, humans). The physiological earmarks of dreaming (rapid eye movements, flattening of muscle tone and a waking type of electroencephalogram) indicate this.[43] Since mammals other than humans do not experience occasional dream-recall -upon-awakening, the Neanderthals were the first who could recall some of their night dreams. They must therefore have evolved 5–D. the uniquely human mental platform for conscious long-term memory recall, which also enabled the uniquely human feature of imagination, of which their Mousterian tools were the first expression and the appearance of which support the advent of their 5–D. To hold select burials the Neanderthals must in addition have acquired sufficient language to communicate these dream contents to one another. As one expert wrote,

> "...as hominids became enchanted and troubled by memories of dream images, a need for symbols to define and order meaning emerged. Such symbols then could be used to communicate not only remembrances of

dreams but to share memories of what was seen or done during the day with others after returning to camp."[44]

This quantum leap in the evolution of the modern mind—evolving conscious recall of long-term memories in 5–D, together with a nascent ability to convey this private information to others—apparently reflects a recent development in human evolution. The theory that individual development is a repetition of the development of the species may be of help in this context.[45] Although babies dream from the moment they are born,[46] conscious memory recall (independent of what is happening in 4–D) does not become operant until around 18 months, when memories of past experiences begin to be displayed in an infant's emerging 5–D. Conscious recall also enables the recall of night dreams, but it is not until around age three or four that children become able to verbalize occasionally remembered dreams, such as a nightmare.[47]

How might dream recall, communicated in semi-speak, have led to select burials? Just as the 4–D and 5–D of modern preschoolers are still intertwined, so that these youngsters do not yet experience 4–D as "reality" and 5–D as "in the mind," so there would have been no difference to the Neanderthals between their dream world and their waking reality. One's place in the hierarchy of the Neanderthal tribe might have determined whether or not one had a right to a burial. These hierarchies were, as outlined in Chapter 4, typically mammalian, based on competitive dominance-submission fights, which probably involved occasional hand-to-hand battles.[48] As a result, Neanderthals behaved in line with their tribal power structure. While most members who died may have been given some type of farewell, a select few were given a grave. A burial took place because, I assume, someone communicated in semi-speak that this dominant member had made a dream appearance. Hence the troop used a burial to protect this member against scavengers and gave him some flint flakes, food, flowers and, occasionally, one or more companions in the world of dreams.[49]

Like Neanderthals, modern infants begin language development hand in hand with an evolving 5–D, but they are, within the context of modern civilization, swamped by pressures for verbal language over the following years. In exchanging private experiences in 5–D among each other, Neanderthals were trailblazing verbal language some 100,000 years ago. It would take them many millennia to shift from a mammalian auditory and gestural communication system solely based on emotions, to a new auditory-verbal language that communicated far more than purely emotional states. In addition, their phonological speech apparatus—their larynx—had not reached its full potential and may have had only 10% of the speaking ability of modern man.[50] Moreover, the Neanderthal brain, although already lateralized, was not yet wired to permit fully evolved language.[51] Finally, just as burials in western Europe apparently did not occur in all contemporaneous Neanderthal cultures, so the evolution of their 5–D and language may well have been out of step with each other across their world.[52] Under these circumstances, it is unlikely that any of their emerging languages reached the so-called "steady state," which all known languages, including languages of extremely isolated, simple cultures, have reached.[53]

Just as prior to age six or seven, modern preschoolers cannot yet think or fantasize silently in 5–D, so Neanderthals did their emerging verbal thinking aloud in 4–D, rather than silently in their head. Spoken monologue must have accompanied their actions in 4–D, like a running commentary on what they were doing. In this sense their talking often must have been thinking aloud rather than communicating. Neanderthals must also have displayed their fantasies visibly in 4–D, including loud, imaginary discussions with others (self-talk), particularly with those in a higher position whom they had to fear and obey.

Neanderthals did not yet practice cults or possess art

In some Neanderthal caves, bear skulls have been found, some of these with little stones arranged around them, others set on slabs, and yet others with long bear bones beneath the snout, or with long bones pushed through the orbits of their eyes.[54] Some archaeologists state that these displays were a kind of "magic" practiced to guarantee a successful hunt, as is true of contemporary hunters of the northern Arctic. And, as European and Asian Neanderthals occasionally massacred and ate their own kind,[55] some have compared this behavior with primitive cannibalistic cults in modern times.[56]

However, any cult, no matter how primitive, holds 1) a belief in hidden forces that dominate the life of one's group, and 2) a belief that magic can control these hidden forces. The presence of these qualifications presupposes a full-grown linguistic capacity which any primitive, contemporary, cult-practicing tribe possesses. Contemporary tribes, no matter how primitive, are some 40,000-120,000 years ahead of Neanderthals in terms of cultural and neurological evolution..

In short, the linguistic and cognitive development of the Neanderthals argues against the existence of Neanderthal cults. The fact that some Neanderthal behaviors appear ritualistic, similar to the practices in some contemporary primitive cultures, does not give them the same meaning as the corresponding rituals in these cultures. On the other hand, we should not be unwilling to compare Neanderthal cannibalism with the behavior of some primates that occasionally eat their young.

Along somewhat different lines, it has been suggested that Neanderthals were the first to establish some tradition in art.[57] The fact that their new inventiveness, based on their 5–D, featured the first engraved squiggles[58] does not indicate a first step toward art. For, in my view, these early squiggles were no more than the early, playful expression of a visual pattern, much the same as a modern child begins to produce twenty different basic scribbles—proto-drawings, patterns and devices—after acquiring 5–D around the age of 18 months. The use of a visual pattern by itself is no indication of art. [59]

The African Cro-magnon

Although Neanderthals dominated Europe and the Middle East from 130,000 to 35,000 years ago, the ancestors of modern humans (Homo sapiens sapiens) had split already from the ancestors of the Neanderthals 500,000 years ago, as suggested by recent mitochondrial DNA studies.[60] Concerning fossil evidence, the oldest skulls of what is currently thought of as the intermediate between archaic African forebears of modern humans and the anatomically modern Cro-magnon of 45,000 years ago, were found in Ethiopia and are 160,000 years old.[61] These skulls lack the features of classic Neanderthals and have instead almost entirely human characteristics.

This archaeological evidence, supported by estimates obtained by genetic analysis, suggests that modern humans evolved in Africa probably 150,000 years ago, when the only people in Europe and Asia were Neanderthals.[62] Modern humans subsequently spread outwards from Africa (the "Out of Africa" theory).[63]

The first migration of early Homo sapiens out of Africa into the Middle East occurred 100,000 years ago, as climate changes had made the Middle East an extension of tropical north-eastern Africa. The population of modern humans in what is now modern Israel used Mousterian tools very similar to those of their Neanderthal contemporaries. With the acceleration of the last ice age around 80,000 years ago, these modern humans abruptly disappeared. In some cases, they were supplanted by Neanderthals.[64]

Meanwhile, the savannahs of eastern Africa had gradually turned into steppe and desert, except in a narrow coastal zone, where the early humans congregated. By following the coast of eastern Africa over thousands of kilometers to southern Africa, they migrated relatively rapidly.[65]

In spite of possessing all anatomical elements of modern people (including a speech apparatus capable of producing the full range of modern vocalizations),[66] the pace of innovation of these modern Cro-magnon was not much faster than that of their Neanderthal cousins in Eurasia—at least until about 60,000 years ago.[67] Then, between 60,000-50,000 years ago,[68] the African Cro-magnon overtook their Neanderthal contemporaries in a sudden cultural quantum leap. Their tools began to differentiate wildly from century to century, and region to region, innovations that exceeded all those of the preceding million years.[69] Evidence of this first occurred in Africa, followed by Asia, and finally Europe. The people who stayed in Africa and the ones who left were technologically, culturally and artistically at the same level.[70]

Several scientists have concluded that the best explanation of this cultural quantum leap was a crucial genetic development in the way brains were wired that enabled the full exploitation of language.[71]

Some scientists think that in modern children a comparable development occurs around age two, when youngsters begin to create and understand complex sentences that convey much more information than single nouns and verbs alone.[72] This development can be explained, they say, by a genetically determined increase in working memory that allows the youngster to understand the meaning of a complex sentence rather than only a single labeling word.[73]

The internalization of language: silent thinking in 5–D

My explanation of the sudden cultural advance of the Cro-magnon differs in important aspects. I assume

1) that, prior to the Cro-magnon's cultural quantum leap, their language had already evolved into a stable Adamic proto-language which allowed them to communicate their private experiences in a completely verbal manner (something contemporary Neanderthals never achieved), although the Cro-magnon still thought aloud in 4–D;[74] and

2) that the genetic mutation that occurred around 60,000-50,000 years ago resulted in a significant increase in the span of their working memory which enabled them to internalize not only their 4–D reality in general, but their already well-advanced speech in particular so that they began to think and fantasize silently in 5–D.

This language internalization would have taken many centuries, just as early in middle childhood a modern child does not shift abruptly from thinking aloud in 4–D to thinking silently in 5–D. Thinking aloud can still account for 20-60% of remarks in a child under 10 years of age.[75] Thus the foundation was laid for silent thinking, silent fantasy and imagination, and silent self-talk.

In this context, one should once again keep in mind that a modern child, who is internalizing 4–D into 5–D, is under pressure by the surrounding culture in shifting its intuitive, illogical ("pre-logical" or "pre-operational") thought processes that do not use even simple rules of logic, to the thinking of the elementary schooler who begins to apply such rules in its thinking ("concrete operational" or "concrete, logical" thinking). This is in contrast with the internalized, silent thinking of the Cro-magnon that, without the outside cultural pressure on its 5–D thinking which the modern child experiences, remained intuitive and illogical ("pre-logical") in nature. It was not until the beginning of the agricultural revolution, around 12,000 years ago, that simple cause-effect relations became evident for the first time.

One must guard here against uncritically drawing analogies between the pre-logical reasoning in contemporary, albeit primitive cultures, and the pre-logical reasoning of the Cro-magnon. In contemporary primitive cultures, many significant matters are "explained" and dealt with through cult magic. However, the Cro-magnon were much more like modern preschoolers who, left to their own pre-logical thinking, do not yet seek to "make sense of, or "explain" the world around them, let alone try to do so through supernatural spirits. Preschoolers do not have cult-like beliefs. Neither did the Cro-magnon.

Cro-magnon burials and mythology

Since the Cro-magnon had sufficiently internalized their 4–D world and language into 5–D, they could intuitively separate their public 4–D reality from their private 5–D with its silent thinking, imagination, and fantasy. Still, with their pre-logical mind they continued to believe in the reality of dreams, a belief they had shared with the Neanderthals. The public world in 4–D and the remembered world of dreams in 5–D were equally real to them. Their dead continued to be real in their dreams, and they reinforced this perception by speaking about the dead and holding conscious memories of them. Thus, the Cro-magnon were preoccupied with appropriately burying at least some of their tribe, even more so than the Neanderthals before them. Cro-magnon burial sites, in contrast to Neanderthal graves, have revealed a relative wealth and variety of goods.[76]

Concerning the origin of mythology, it has been suggested that in a preliterate society, orally transmitted genealogical information may stretch, perhaps reliably, for about 150 years. Any event older than this tends to be relegated to the nebulousness of "a long time ago," and certain members of the tribe become mythological characters. These deceased members are, in the mind of their tribe, still living and part of the tribe. They need occasional attention, even though they are no longer connected with any known generation.[77] It is perhaps through the transmission of such information that the Cro-Magnon created an ancestral proto-mythology which, as they spread across the Earth, became in due course fashioned to fit local circumstances. This may well be how mythologies of so many widely different cultures across the globe came to share many similar themes.[78]

The Cro-magnon take-over of the Earth

Endowed with their intellectual advantages, language and silent, pre-logical verbal thinking, the nomadic hunting-gathering Cro-magnon spread from Africa to all over the Earth. In summarizing Cro-magnon migrations across the Earth, I have followed the major lines of Spencer Wells' *The Journey of Man: A Genetic Odyssey,* an approach based on changes in Y-chromosome sequences in the DNA of men and, to a lesser extent, mitochondrial DNA sequence changes in women.[79]

As previously noted, some 80,000 years ago, as forests began to shrink and were replaced by savannah and steppe grasslands, modern human populations began congregating in coastal areas of East Africa. Immediately after the earliest archaeological evidence for the sudden quantum leap of the African Cro-magnon, the exodus out of Africa of modern humans began, starting in Northeast Africa (Ethiopia and Sudan).[80]

Between 60,000-50,000 years ago, a very early migration of coastal dwellers appears to have proceeded along the coast of South Asia, ultimately reaching Southeast Asia (where they became "the southern Chinese") and Australia.[81] The resources along the sandy highway of coastal Eritrea were pretty much the same as those in coastal Arabia, western India, Southeast Asia or Australia. Circumnavigating the continents and having to cross only short stretches of open water, most likely in rather simple boats — probably a few logs lashed together — allowed relatively rapid migration. Furthermore, this coastal route was infinitely preferable to anything further inland.[82]

Between 50,000-45,000 years ago, the northern hemisphere warmed slightly for a few thousand years. This brought the eastern Sahara in retreat, and opened a gateway for the hunters and gatherers who had stayed in the interior of Africa to move into northeastern Africa and the Middle East. This time they came, unlike their predecessors, with an inventory of modern tools, advanced technology and a complex culture. By 40,000 years ago, the Cro-Magnon in Southwest Asia had replaced the Neanderthals completely.

However, these Middle Eastern Cro-magnon were locked into their new home when the Sahara became its driest between 40,000-20,000 years ago. A small number moved into the Balkans — the first modern humans in Europe — but they did not leave a lasting trace. Some 40,000 years ago, Middle Eastern Cro-magnon began instead migrating eastward, apparently attracted by the continuous steppe highway with its large grazing mammals (not unlike the African savannah) that stretched from the Gulf of Aqaba to northern Iran, and beyond into central Asia and Mongolia. There, these steppe hunters faced the great mountain ranges of southern Asia. Until 20,000 years ago, a significant decrease in precipitation led to deserts in Iran and prevented these Eurasian Cro-magnon from mingling with their Middle Eastern brethren.

These Eurasian Cro-magnon split into two groups: one moving to the north of the mountain ranges toward central Asia around 35,000 years ago; the other moving south of the mountain ranges into Pakistan and the Indian subcontinent some 30,000 years ago. The northern Cro-magnon, who were trapped in Central Asia, had to adapt to the harsh lifestyle of the icy open steppe and tundra. They had to develop portable shelters, clothing to protect them against the intense cold, and far more efficient tools, like small stone points, which were fitted onto wooden shafts like arrow heads. Having adapted to these harsh conditions, the Cro-magnon of Central Asia moved further east around 35,000 years ago and entered northern China (where they became the "Northern Chinese"), and then Korea and Japan.

Between 35,000-30,000 years ago, the central Asian Cro-magnon moved also westward into the milder climate of Europe. The steppe zone in Central Asia extended westward well into present-day Germany, where reindeer were common. The Cro-magnon coexisted with the Neanderthals in Europe for several thousand years. However, concerning remains dating after 30,000 ago, only Cro-magnon remains have been found. The semi-speaking Neanderthals who thought aloud were probably not slaughtered by the Cro-magnon, for there is very little evidence of butchery on Neanderthal skeletons and the Cro-magnon appear to have been rather peaceful people. The Neanderthals may simply have been crowded out by the far more intelligent and efficient Cro-magnon.

Finally, by 20,000 years ago, Cro-magnon from Central Asia took hold in Northeastern Siberia and the Asian Arctic. When the ice age intensified and sea levels dropped, a land bridge between Siberia and Alaska was created. Some Siberian Cro-magnon moved across. Initially, these first American Cro-magnon could not cross the continuous sheet of ice that covered eastern Alaska and northern Canada. This ice sheet did not begin retreating until after 15,000 years ago. Perhaps 10,000 years ago, the first trickle of Cro-Magnon made it to the vast grasslands on the plains of North America. In just 1,000 years they traveled to the tip of South America.

In sum, by 10,000 years ago, in a space of just under 40,000 years, the Cro-magnon had colonized every environment in which humans live today.

As the Cro-magnon settled into different habitats around the world, their original, Adamic proto-language turned into various different proto-languages,[83] which eventually led to the Babylonian language confusion that has plagued humankind ever since. And, as these Cro-magnon spread across the globe, they also adjusted their proto-mythology to fit local circumstances.

Language and mythology are, however, not the only human features that adjust to variations in geographical nature, climate and food supply. Our genome, too, has always responded to changes in our ecological niche. In other words, some genetic refinements and purifications occurred among Cro-magnon the world over. Indians in the Andes mountains of South America have larger chests with larger lungs and a larger supply of blood then those living at sea level where there is more oxygen in the air. The short fingers of Eskimos may have lessened the danger of frostbite. The dark skin of the Negroid race may have developed to protect them against the tropical sun.[84] And so on. Regional differences in bodily appearance as we know them today are therefore only of relatively recent origin and have not compromised our inter relatedness as the planet's one and only population that descended from the Cro-magnon.

The Cro-Magnon's European civilizations

Between 34,000 and 9,000 BCE, the Cro-magnon civilizations in Europe stretched from the Atlantic Ocean to the Urals, and from the Baltic to the Mediterranean. They were characterized by magnificent stone tools, the first appearance of bone tools and mural and portable art, the earliest use of body ornaments, the intensive use of red ochre in habitation sites and burials; and the curing of animal skin. They also had needles, which they used to make proper garments.

Each of the Cro-magnon civilizations is named after the place in France where the archeological evidence corresponding to each civilization was first found. As a result, scientists have classified these civilizations according to their tool-making industry,[85] rather than the prehistoric art for which they are famous and which, as I will discuss shortly, points to an emerging time gender duality. Without going into detail about their characteristic tools of stone, bone, and ivory, and the variety of body ornaments which characterize these civilizations, I simply will enumerate their time frame.

33,000-26,000 BCE: The Aurignacian civilization

27,000-19,000 BCE: The Gravettian civilization

20,000-16,000 BCE: The Solutrean civilization

16,000-10,000 BCE: The Magdalenian civilization

10,000-8,000 BCE: The Azilian civilization.

The appearance of art

The first dating of mural art at the entrance of caves, which the Cro-magnon inhabited, or hidden in deep subterraneous caves, suggested to leading specialists that the 30,000 years of subsequent Cro-magnon civilizations showed a linear development of increasing sophistication, just as their tool industry did.[86]

According to this view, around 30,000 years ago, the Aurignacian civilization made the first prehistoric art, which was line drawings of isolated animals, small in size, and simple in contour. Next, the Gravettian elaborated this prehistoric art further with engravings, paintings and sculptures. Then, the Solutrean produced monumental sculpture and bas-relief friezes. Finally, the Magdalenian civilizations represented the high point of Paleolithic art with, for instance, the 17,000-year-old extraordinarily dazzling paintings in the Cave of Lascaux—the "Sistine Ceiling of the Paleolithic"—or the 13,000-year-old exquisite wall paintings in the Altamira Cave in northern Spain.[87]

In 1994, the discovery of the Chauvet Cave in southeast France,[88] with its highly sophisticated wall paintings that are some 31,000 years old, made it necessary to revise the original assumption that cave art evolved in an entirely linear fashion. Clearly, there were in certain regions already some great artists among Aurignacians, who coexisted with the last Neanderthals, and who already possessed the same artistic capabilities as the Magdalenians some 30,000 years later. They used sophisticated techniques for wall art, including various ways of rendering perspective, the use of shading, and reproducing movement. The drawings in the Chauvet cave present exquisitely rendered likenesses that use the cavern's natural contours to heighten a sense of perspective. "Our view of the beginnings of artistic creation and even of the psyche of these first modern humans has been changed by this," said Jean Clottes,[89] Scientific Advisor on Prehistoric Art to the French ministry of Culture.

The discovery of the Chauvet Cave makes it clear that the artistic and psychological development of the Cro-magnon was far from the same everywhere at the same time. This view is supported further by comparing the 31,000-year-old Chauvet Cave paintings with the 18,500-year-old paintings in the Cosquer Cave on the Mediterranean coast of France. The technique in the Cosquer Cave was sure but cursory, and showed an apparent lack of sophistication; the Cosquer Cave art is less visually striking that that of the Chauvet Cave.[90]

The emergence of the time gender duality in 6–D

The Cro-magnon's wall paintings and engravings in Europe present two basic categories that coexisted in the same periods. Jean Clottes and Jean Courtin, the authors of *The Cave Beneath the Sea: Paleolithic Images at Cosquer,* wrote in 1994:

> "In European Paleolithic art, there are two categories of sites: those in daylight—cave entrances or shelters—and deep caves, where darkness is total. The former most often served as habitats so that all members of the group—men, women, and children—lived in the immediate vicinity of engraved, sculpted, and/or painted walls. Little by little, debris mounted, matter accumulated from erosion, and layers of sediment were laid down, until the decorated walls were covered...On the other hand, Paleolithic people did not usually make more than very short trips into the farthest galleries [some galleries are hidden 1.2 km away from the entrance, inaccessible to the tribe on a daily basis, if at all.]. They left their drawings there, where they have been preserved (willful destruction such as that of the hands in the Cosquer caves remains a very rare event). Thus, we are observing two different ways of thinking...(These) two ways of thinking have...coexisted in the same period."[91]

The wall art at the entrance of caves or shelters where the Cro-magnon lived, enabled tribe members to relate emotionally to the animal icons, on a day-to-day basis, in a here–and–now fashion, for as long as the tribe lived there. When the tribe moved, fresh icons were created at the entrance of the new habitat. Thus, entrance wall art at different habitats continued to fulfill the (admittedly undefined) need of these Cro-magnon to have animal icons in their sight on a daily basis. Entrance wall art therefore suggests a mental attitude of most if not all members of tribes who lived in the here-and-now of 4–D and were alphas.

This mental attitude is in sharp contrast with the mental attitude of the Cro-magnon who created their murals in the total darkness of deep caves. Indeed, even today with all the aids of modern technology, many of these murals cannot be made accessible to the ordinary visitor. In creating their murals, the artists often had to face a macabre ordeal. They had to overcome the terror of the unknown and risk losing their way in the darkness of a subterranean labyrinth full of blind passages, and sudden, dangerous drops which their primitive animal-fat lamps could only feebly illuminate. Then they had to work in these cold, slippery, dark caves, using only the dim light their lamps provided.[92]

To overcome all these difficult obstacles, Cro-magnon artists must have had some strong, pre-logical belief that it was somehow essential for their tribe to go beyond creating icons at the entrance of the caves they inhabited and, instead, create vibrant frescoes of the animals they honored, hidden on sub-terranean walls. Surely, these Cro-magnon must have envisioned and emotionally related to their creations and the trials and tribulations involved ahead of time. And, long after their task had been finished, they must have continued to be emotionally sustained by these out-of-sight murals. In other words, both prior to, and after creating their frescoes, these Michelangelos of the ice age must have related to them in their head, that is, in their time in 6–D.

Whatever meaning these Cro-magnon attributed to their hidden murals, the members of the tribe had to be able to communicate with each other about the importance of the envisioned dangerous mission in the caves. Those who gathered and hunted in the light had to excuse those who painted and sculpted in the dark from the daily search for food. The proto-languages of these artists and their tribes must have been sufficiently sophisticated to convincingly describe to each other the importance of what the artist or artists intended to do, or had achieved. Furthermore, in order for these invisible murals to realize their (to us undefined) meaning on an enduring basis, a sufficient number of tribe members had to be able to sustain emotionally charged visions of these hidden murals (before and after they had been created), if they were to maintain their emotional connection with these hard-to-reach wall paintings and sculptures. This kind of a connection would have been possible only if a majority of tribal members possessed a timescape in 6–D.

Thus, I conclude that the duality in the siting of wall art in different, albeit contemporaneous cultures of Cro-magnon reflects the earliest indication of an emerging time gender duality. Although future or past images in 6–D were for the early beta Cro-magnon as real as 4–D perceptions, their silent thinking in 5–D was still pre-logical, despite their timescape.

The question "why?" (in the sense of asking to describe the goal of something) or the idea that something was a "cause" and something else an "effect" and, hence, that they could "plan" something did not yet occur to them.

It makes sense from the technical point of view to assume that, originally, the development of techniques to create wall art at the entrance of Cro-magnon habitats must have preceded the application of these techniques in the darkness of subterranean caves. This makes sense also from the evolutionary point of view. First, there were only alphas (with their cave art at the entrance of caves or shelters) whose particular autobiographic memory is an expression of a dominant gene on the X-chromosome. Then, at some point in human evolution, this dominant alpha gene mutated into a recessive beta gene in some of their women (leading to the genotype

Ab). This recessive beta-mutation translated into male betas (with the genotype b) who apparently were favorable for the survival of all tribe members. Since these male betas sired children with multiple partners, the beta mutation on the X-chromosome spread rapidly through the Cro-magnon tribes. As a result, female betas (with the genotype bb) began to appear, further advancing the spread of the recessive beta gene.

The original beta mutation within the Cro-magnon population first spread within a certain tribe, and then from that tribe to another and another. This would have taken many generations. While some tribes remained alphacized, in others alphas and betas were living together, and some tribes eventually became betacized. In these latter tribes the incremental spread of the beta mutation catalyzed a vitally important change in their nature. Eventually, the mental attitude of Cro-magnon who created murals in the total darkness of deep caves made its appearance.

About the Cro-magnon experience of time and their autobiographic memory

Studying the appearance of the time gender duality among the Cro-magnon, one wonders as to how they experienced what we refer to as "time." The answer is that they probably had evolved a concrete way of "timing" or organizing their day according to a succession of discrete moments that corresponded to the position of the sun. During the night, stellar movements may have served the same purpose. Their rhythm of living would have been elastic in the extreme and, except when motivated by hunger or necessity, their activities were probably dictated by external circumstances or by whim. The life cycle of individuals may well have been divided into a number of maturation stages (baby, walking child, sexual differentiation, adult, old one) rather than in terms of years.[93]

Since the time gender duality is based on a duality in autobiographic memory, it follows that the alpha-type of autobiographic memory in 6–D must have been introduced into the Cro-magnon prior to the appearance of betas, probably while or shortly after the Cro-magnon began to internalize 4-D into 5-D so that 6-D could develop. These proto-alpha Cro-magnon would have remembered important personal events through personalized milestones. They may have told stories to the effect of "this happened when it was snowing," "this happened when we were on that hunting camp site," "this happened when there was a famine," "this happened when I was so big," and so on. [94] But when the beta mutation appeared, the pre-logical timescape of the first proto-beta Cro-magnon made their past and future emotionally more meaningful and real, so that they could continue relating emotionally to something that was no longer in their present (as with the murals in the underground caves) or to some future event they anticipated (as with descending underground to create murals). In addition, the new ability of Cro-magnon betas to intuitively sequence significant life events that were unrelated must, in due course, have led from individual story telling to the Cro-magnon proto-mythology.

About the meaning of Cro-magnon art

The role of the time gender duality in determining the location of wall art by one or more artists, and the acceptance by a given tribe of its siting at the entrance of the tribe's habitat, or in the darkness of a subterraneous cave, does not say much about what this mural art actually meant to the Cro-magnon. Interpreting such art without reference to the cultural context that inspired it (which and is now forever lost) is an undertaking full of pitfalls. One can only rely on the scientific analysis of these works of art and on more or less logical theories derived from direct knowledge in this area.[95]

The wall art in deep caves was clearly not painted or carved for its aesthetic effect, for this cave art was not accessible to admiration. Also, cave paintings and engravings were frequently superimposed, so that earlier work was obliterated or defaced; or they overlapped in ways that spoiled the decorative effect.[96]

One clue to the meaning of Cro-magnon wall art is that the pre-logical Cro-magnon were not yet preoccupied with themselves and the human form, for in Paleolithic wall art human figures are very uncommon and, if present, poorly drawn.[97] Instead, animals (not necessarily hunted ones)[98] are the predominant subject matter of wall art, whether in the bright daylight at shelter entrances, or in the dark bowels of the earth. Animals were of fundamental importance to the Cro-magnon. The pre-logical Cro-magnon assumed, like preschoolers, that animals and humans were similar and could talk to each other. (anthropomorphism) (compare the Bible's snake in the Garden of Eden who seduced Eve into doing the wrong thing, or the role of the wolf in the fairy tale of Red Riding hood; or think about how young children often talk to their stuffed animals).

In the context of animal art, another aspect of pre-logical thinking may have come into play. Animal icons did not simply represent painted or carved animals, but were experienced and treated as the creatures themselves; they *were* the animals. There was no sense of logical contradiction between what was apparent, and what was real.[99] Even modern adults, when overcome with emotion, may experience the portrait of a loved one as that very person and actually kiss it. People also cross themselves before or pray to religious statues or icons, which is yet another aspect of modern pre-logical thinking, namely one involving magical wish-fulfillment. It is the belief that persistently wishing for something in 5–D alone can cause it to happen in 4–D.

The blurring of the line between imagination and reality would explain why the Cro-magnon engraved, carved or painted the animals that were important to them. Experiencing animal icons as the true apparition of the animals made it possible to talk to, if not plead with these animals, just as a Catholic may use an icon of a saint. Since the Cro-magnon believed in magical wish-fulfillment, their art indicates perhaps that they introduced prayer to animals long before the humans who followed them introduced praying to spirits and gods.[100]

This explanation only makes sense when one assumes that the animal icons the Cro-magnon prayed to when they first began making art had to be visible to every member of the tribe. They had to be painted or carved on the walls and roofs of their shallow rock shelters or entrances of caves. Only later did some tribes become preoccupied with making these animal icons independent from their temporary habitats and hiding them instead out of sight in underground caves.

It is frequently assumed that these underground caves were sanctuaries, used perhaps for puberty rites or for magic to increase the number of animals they were hunting.[101] But, as previously discussed, the pre-logical Cro-magnon nomads were not yet preoccupied with invisible spirits of a supernatural world. They had not yet imagined spirits that influenced important events and that needed to be controlled through magic. They did not yet engage in cults. Alpha-dominated tribes were accustomed to pray to icons at the entrance of their temporary habitats. Praying to invisible icons in subterranean caves while the tribes were in the neighborhood, but also after these nomadic tribes had moved on, simply suggests that beta-dominated tribes had emerged.

Were the cave artists men or women?

The tools which the Cro-magnon produced were mostly used in the hunt and slaughter of animals, or in self-defense. Since the men hunted and the women gathered and tended their young, it makes sense to assume that the men who used these tools also produced them. In other words, the tool industry reflected a necessary and widely shared skill among the hunters.

In southern France, the Cro-magnon probably lived in small hunting bands that each required a territory with a radius of 30-40 kilometers.[102] Wall paintings and carvings of animals represented a skill which only a few members possessed, or which was lacking altogether in some tribes. Perhaps a special group of artists served several tribes with their artistic skills, which might have varied from the crude and primitive to outstanding mastery of graphic and sculpturing techniques.

Various authorities take it for granted that the Cro-magnon artists of the great murals in the subterranean caves must have been also hunters—that is men—[103] rather than women. It may be doubtful that a definite conclusion can ever be reached as to whether the cave artists were men or women. Yet the question is worth raising,[104] since I assume that the underground cave art was created by betas. My view that the beta gene on the X-chromosome is a recessive mutation of the alpha gene, and that the beta mutation therefore began among gathering women with the first beta phenotypes being hunting men, does not solve the issue. But two simple points favor the hypothesis that these artists were women. The first is that gathering women, rather than hunting men, likely collected the pigments for the four basic colors which cave artists used (black, white, red and yellow),[105] mixed these colors in animal fats or blood to produce a paste-like paint, and then painted the surface of carvings with them. The second point is that women not only gathered food, but also looked after their young. In some deep caves with brilliant wall art, footprints of women and children, sometimes three to six years of age, have been preserved along with those of men.[106] It would not be unreasonable to assume that, if women were painting in the deep caves, they took their young with them. Men may have been there simply to assist them. Or, perhaps the women were the painters, and the men, who were routinely trained at tool-making, were the engravers and sculptors.

In dealing with the debate over the sexual gender of the artists, one should further take into account the special position of women among the Cro-magnon. Given the pre-logical thinking of the Cro-magnon, they did not yet have insight into the causal relationship between sexual intercourse and pregnancy and birth. Hence, Cro-magnon women, who through pregnancy and childbirth re-supplied the tribe with new members, were held in mystical adoration, not unlike the Holy Virgin. In line with this thinking, Cro-magnon all over Europe and as far as Siberia carried with them little female statuettes, made of bone, ivory or stone, most of them faceless, curvaceous depictions of the female body with the maternal attributes grossly exaggerated.[107] That there are no traces of a father figure in Paleolithic art[108] supports the idea that the Cro-magnon did not yet connect sexual intercourse with pregnancy.

While most experts think that these female statuettes represent images of a mother-goddess whom the Cro-magnon revered,[109] in my view the Cro-magnon's pre-logical thinking did not yet allow for a goddess or gods. The Cro-magnon used these statuettes of pregnant women more or less in the same way as they used their wall art of animals, namely to help them to concentrate on making come true what they wished for most: the pregnancy of their females.

The mystery of the female as giver of new life and as the restorer of life through the healing power of some of the plants they gathered, gave women a prodigious power among the Cro-magnon. This makes female artists more likely candidates for having created wall art to facilitate the Cro-magnon's prayers.

The agricultural revolution

Between 13,000 and 8,300 BCE, glaciers began to retreat northbound, leaving lakes with an abundance of fish and fowl in their trail, while steppe and tundra began giving way to forests. The melting of the polar caps also caused flooding of coastal plains that previously had been fertile grazing grounds for large animal herds. The end of the Ice Age brought many other changes to the Earth's ecological systems. The nomadic hunters and gatherers of the planet, perhaps 5-10 million in number,[110] had to adapt.

To catch animals that were out of easy reach, people invented new hunting and fishing techniques: spears and bows and arrows for land animals, harpoons for seals, ingenious traps for wildfowl, and nets for fish. But this was not just a period of increasing practical ingenuity. It was also a gradual but fundamental transition from the era of the nomadic hunter-gatherer to the agricultural revolution. The ability to domesticate wild plants and animals meant that people gained control over their own food supply for the first time in their existence. For thousands of years, people had witnessed wild plants growing from seed and seen wild herds of animals. Yet, the idea of agriculture had never occurred to them. How did these people turn into tillers of the earth and husbanders of animals?

The emergence of agriculture and animal domestication was not simply a matter of shifting from a nomadic to a settled existence. Farming did not necessarily lead to a sedentary life,[111] nor did a sedentary life necessarily lead to farming.[112] Towns, such as Jericho, had already come into existence at the juncture of trade routes well before the agricultural revolution.

Agriculture requires deliberate planting of seed stock in prepared seedbeds that leads to the separation of these plants from wild populations. The deliberately planned isolation and domestication of herds of animals in order to control their reproduction leads to their dependence on humans.[113] The pre-logical adult thinking that dominated the hunting-gathering civilizations of the Cro-magnon could never have achieved this shift. For one of the prerequisites of agriculture is the ability to have practical cause-and-effect insights, particularly into serendipity, which becomes possible only after a shift from pre-logical to concrete, logical thinking. This shift in thinking was likely due to yet another genetic mutation of a gene on the X-chromosome (remember in this context, for example, that the 1890 US Census found that more boys than girls were mentally disabled,[114] which reflects a preponderance of genes for brain function on the X-chromosome).[115] In early betas, the gradual shift from pre-logical to concrete, logical thinking would have gone hand in hand with a slowly increasing depth of their timescape (as is the case in contemporary beta children during the elementary school years), which would have enabled planning deliberately for a progressively more distant future, while consistently keeping working toward these plans.

The agricultural revolution became the most visible expression of this shift from pre-logical to concrete, logical thinking. Yet, although this shift made the agricultural revolution possible, it was by itself not enough to initiate the revolution. Other factors had to be involved. The transition from hunting-gathering to the domestication of wild plants and animals did not begin in one region and then spread from there. It started independently in seven areas across the globe during different periods, involving different people and different types of plants and animals. First it began around 10,000 years ago in the Near East, coming to full fruition about 2,000 years later. Next, agriculture appeared in the Central Highlands of Mexico around 9,000 years ago, and then surfaced in the Far East, first some 8,500 years ago in the Yangtze River Corridor in South China, and then, a thousand years later, around the Yellow River in North China. The domestication of plants and animals emerged in the South Central Andes, Peru and Bolivia, about 7,000 years ago, and 2,500 years later in what is today the Eastern United States. Finally, around 4,000 years ago, it developed in Sub-Saharan Africa.[116]

Despite of all these differences, the transition from hunting and gathering to the domestication of seed plants and animals appear to have involved a similar motivation. All these people wanted to increase both the economic contribution, as well as the reliability of one or more wild species they depended on for survival. This way, they could reduce risk and uncertainty. This shared motivation led to a sequence of similar steps. First, hunter-gathering communities had to discover an aquatic zone with lakes, marshes, or rivers rich in animal resources, and with moist, fertile soil and high quality wild species that ensured reasonably reliable high-yield harvests. These attributes encouraged permanent settlement with considerable reliance on local plant and animal resources. In due course, there had to be a shift from pre-logical to concrete, logical thinking that would enable insight in cause-and-effect relations. For only then would such an environment become for the betas among gathering women a natural laboratory for the deliberate planning and experimentation involved in the domestication of plants and animals. Once agricultural techniques had been mastered, hunting-gathering activities would no longer be essential for a community's survival, meaning that hunting-gathering became progressively more supportive, if not disappearing altogether.[117]

The shift from pre-logical to concrete, logical thinking that created insights into causal relations was in my view not only the prerequisite for the agricultural revolution. It also permitted people to become aware of the relationship between sexual intercourse and pregnancy. As a result, men began to feel equal to women, because they too supplied the tribe with new life, and there ensued a battle for dominance between the sexes, which is still going on today. Agricultural civilizations initially created optimum conditions for the continuation of the privileged status of women. This was because agriculture was developed by women. Early in agricultural times, women remained at the apex of their influence in farming, arts and crafts, and social and religious functions.[118]

The disappearance of animals in Cro-magnon cave art

I previously introduced the assumption that Cro-magnon cave art and portable art were the medium through which the Cro-magnon expressed their pre-logical prayerful anthropomorphism and magical wish-fulfillment. It is reasonable to assume that, as their thinking moved toward concrete, logical levels, their animal paintings and portable art would no longer serve a purpose and, as a result, disappear. And since the shift in thinking eventually would also produce insight into the connection between sexual intercourse and pregnancy, "magical" pregnancy through wish-fulfilling prayer to statuettes of maternal females was no longer viable. Hence these statuettes, too, would disappear.

This change indeed happened during the final Cro-magnon civilization in Europe, the Azilian (10,000-8,000 BCE). The great animal paintings on cave walls gradually ceased, as portable art no longer was expressed in statuettes, but became characterized by engraved or painted pebbles, and bones decorated with various signs.[119]

This is not to say that Cro-magnon men and women no longer inhabited caves and rock shelters, or that they no longer painted on walls. Azilian rock paintings in open-air sites in eastern Spain show that these artists no longer focused on the animals in their world, but were putting a new and revealing emphasis on humans. This was a dramatic change because human figures had been extremely rare and sketchy in Paleolithic art,[120] while they became for Azilians the center of artistic preoccupation.[121] Since the Azilians in France and Spain still had a hunting-gathering lifestyle,[122] they demonstrate that the change from pre-logical to concrete, logical thinking preceded, rather than went hand in hand, with the agricultural revolution.

The evolution of 7–D

Although the thinking of modern youngsters in elementary school is internalized, it still has an important limitation. They cannot yet think speculatively in the abstract, or self-observe their own thinking, since it is still hooked entirely into the visible and tangible 4–D world. They can find a solution to a problem only by trial and error, rather than first working through different hypothetical solutions in their head and then verifying the assumed solution in 4–D. The shift to thinking in the abstract requires adding a final experiential dimension that is one step removed from one's concrete mentation in 5–D, namely 7–D. 7–D enables us not only to manipulate our concrete mentation in 5–D, but also allows us to erect a ladder of abstractions in 7–D itself. In modern youngsters, 7–D and abstract thinking do not emerge until adolescence.

When did this final step in our intellectual maturation, 7–D, emerge in our evolution? Tracing the origin of the most highly developed use of 7–D in scientific thinking may help answer this question (I already mentioned in Chapter 8 how alpha and beta scientists and alpha and beta laymen develop different thinking styles).

Scientific thinking, which is abstract thinking in 7–D *par excellence,* made its first appearance simultaneously in both the West and the East. It appeared in Ancient Greece and in Ancient China between 600 and 500 BCE.[123] My focus is on the emergence of scientific thinking in the West.

The foundation of western civilization was the middle of its ancient world, the Mediterranean. Following in the footsteps of Mesopotamia and Egypt, Ancient Greece was its center between 600 and 300 BCE. During this period, the groundwork was laid for philosophy, logic, biology, medicine, mathematics, and many other basic features of western thought.

People of earlier civilizations had a completely different mentality from our own.

Prior to the sixth century BCE, the Ancient Greeks did not think of themselves as having a mind. To them, words that later acquired a mental meaning initially referred only to physical things. For example, in Homer's famous epic about the Trojan War, the Iliad, written around 900 BCE, the word "psyche" usually meant blood or breath, a life-substance: a dying warrior bled out his psyche or breathed it out in his last gasp. It was not until Pythagoras (c. 580-c. 500 BCE) that the "life matter" that permeates the person while alive became the "immortal soul matter" that survives the person after death.[124]

Meanwhile, Ionian philosophers from Milete, Turkey, moved beyond their preoccupation with the appearance of things (observations of the world in 4–D) toward speculating about the ultimate nature beyond ("meta") the appearance ("physis") of things. Hence, this philosophical thinking became referred to as "metaphysics." Thales (c.624-c. 546 BCE) thought that was made up of water; Anaximander (c.610-c. 545) claimed the primal matter of the universe was "unlimited stuff;" and Anaximenes (c.545) thought that the universe was basically made up of "air." These alternative explanations meant that philosophers were criticizing each other's thinking. Such critical thinking became the earmark of Greek scientific thinking as it is of our own.[125]

Notwithstanding the above evidence of emerging abstract thinking in 7–D, Ancient Greeks had yet to discover a word for "self-awareness" (thinking in 7–D about oneself in 5–D). Plato (427-347 BCE) became the first to recognize that what we call "conscious mental functioning" has two major aspects: the conscious experience of the material world of atoms or "perceiving"; and the conscious experience of the immaterial world of ideas, or "thinking." He believed that outside one's sensorium (one's awareness), the material world of atoms and the immaterial world of ideas existed side-by-side, independent of humans. They only meet in the human awareness.

His pupil, Aristotle (384-323 BCE) elaborated this by stating that immaterial ideas are immaterial forces that direct formless matter toward its potential form, the "goal" of this formless matter. Plato's immaterial ideas thus became the built-in goal of matter or what he called its "entelechy." In plants this immaterial force was the vegetative soul that brought about life with nutrition and reproduction. Animals possessed in addition an animal soul that allowed for sensory impressions, memories, and emotional desires that pass over into action. In animals and humans, the vegetative and animal souls were interwoven with their material body. But humans possessed also a uniquely human soul, or "nous," which was purely immaterial and enabled them to think. Thus the question arose: where is this immaterial human soul located in the material body, if at all?[126] In due course, Aristotle's body-thinking split grew from a crack (body-thinking) into a canyon (the metaphysical body-mind problem) that Descartes (1596-1650) created.[127]

Plato's and Aristotle's self-reflections (in 7–D) on aspects of mental functioning (in 5–D) were still vague and confusing. They did not yet recognize the world of imagination in 5–D. But their formulations were the first to indicate a basic difference between the perceptual world in 4–D and the abstract world of thinking in 7–D.

That Plato and Aristotle testify to the evolution of abstract thought in 7–D is even more evidenced by Dr. J. T. Fraser, the much-published, world-authority on the study of time. He pointed out to me:

> "For Plato, time was a 'moving image of eternity.' That moving image is the rotation of the heavens. It is continuous, seamless. It does not single out a preferred instant. Future and past are, so to say, continuously in mind. A clock or watch with a dial display, (with the small hand adjusted to take 24 hours for a rotation) makes that dial a model of the heaven and makes the clock Plato's moving image of eternity. All our dial displays represent time as understood by Plato. We [nowadays] call such a representation an analog display.

> For Aristotle, time was 'the number of motion with respect to before and after' referenced to the present. A clock or watch which displays numbers, one at a time, makes that display represent time as understood by Aristotle. In this, you recognize [to-day] a digital watch.

> Your beta people live with the flow of time as identified by Plato. Your alpha people live with the present instants of Aristotelian time, which they count by number."[128]

Although Plato's and Aristotle's views do not necessarily reflect implicitly the basic difference between alphas and betas, they unquestionably demonstrate that the evolution of 7–D itself had been accomplished.[129] This is strongly supported by the fact that, by the time of Aristotle's death in 322 BCE, many areas of scientific knowledge, built on abstract rules and laws and thus requiring 7–D, had been mapped out (such as geometry, mathematics, logic, astronomy, physics, and biology).

The evolution of silent self-talk

In contemporary children, the internalization of language leads also to "silent self-talk," an internalized discussion between I_1 (ego or Inner Child) and an "I" analog, I_2 (superego or Inner Parent). Eventually, this silent self-talk importantly regulates the child's, and later the adult's social behavior and reflects how one emotionally relates to oneself. It is in this context of interest to consider the nature of a Cro-magnon's internalized discussions and how they reflected upon her or his key relationships with other tribe members.

The late Julian Jaynes, Princeton professor of psychology, spoke in his book *The Origin of Consciousness in the Breakdown of the Bicameral Mind* of one of the internalized, silent voices of Ancient Greeks as "auditory hallucinations," in which a God was instructing them how to behave. These voices of Gods represented an internalized social interaction and played a significant role in regulating individual behavior.[130] The absence of 7–D precluded the Ancient Greeks from experiencing both silent voices as two sides of the self.

Although the thinking of these Ancient Greeks occurred at a concrete, pragmatic, logical level, it makes sense to trace the origin of these "auditory hallucinations" to the Cro-magnon, even if the latter still functioned at a pre-logical level. Given the mammalian-hierarchical power structure among the Cro-magnon, it is likely that one of the silent inner voices was experienced as belonging to the tribe's leader, a maternal female, or mythological tribe member, who was telling them what to do. This silent self-talk would not have reflected a single system of dos and don'ts, nor would it have allowed for a fused, single image of the imaginary person who spoke. Depending on the 4–D situation in which the Cro-magnon found her or himself, it would in each situation have reflected an appropriate set of dos and don'ts. In other words, the inner (silent) discussions which the Cro-magnon experienced had nothing to do with how modern people relate to themselves.

With the arrival of the agricultural revolution, the shift from pre-logical to concrete, logical thinking influenced the nature of the inner silent voices of the Cro-magnon. Julian Jaynes pointed in this context to the Natufians, nomadic hunting tribes in the Levant in the Middle East, who around 10,000 BCE were still living in the mouths of caves in groups of about twenty. Not only were they skillful in working bone, antler and stone, but also had artists among them who drew animals almost as well as the Cro-magnon artists of Lascaux. These Natufians became agricultural a thousand years later, at which time they were living in villages of at least 200 persons. They obviously had shifted from pre-logical to concrete, logical thinking. As their communities were growing in size and were becoming more complex, they required an organized and definite rule system of how to behave within these communities. Gradually, their rulers enunciated more comprehensive, rather fixed, if not relatively absolute rules which the Natufians readily accepted.

The need for a system of definite rules arising hand in hand with the shift from pre-logical to concrete, logical thinking is also demonstrated by contemporary youngsters. By age six, the child can play a game with simple rules without adult supervision and shows an acceptance of a wide variety of parental codes of behavior.[131] This means that the child responds to the silent inner voice of the Inner Parent or superego. At this stage, the child believes rules are absolute. When asked: "Do people always play like that?" the child will answer: "Yes, always." Asked: "Why?" the child will say something like "'Cause you can't play any other way." Even as late as 10, a child may believe it impossible to change the rules because "that would be cheating."[132]

Julian Jaynes wrote in detail about how the Natufians internalized the rather organized system of absolute rules that their rulers had enunciated. They identified the inner voice in their silent thinking as that of their ruler, no matter whether he or she had actually instructed them what to do.[133] This means that the ruler's silent voice was functioning as a modern superego, except that it was not yet recognized as "part of me." As successive rulers traditionally continued to enunciate the same (fixed) rules, their commands became a single system of rules that was voiced to the Natufians from where the ruler and his predecessors had been buried. Gradually these voices of the rulers became fused into a single voice of a living god. Thus, the ruler's tomb gradually became the house of the god and the source of the commands that controlled the world of the Natufians. Over the millennia, this belief system continued as a feature of many civilizations, particularly in Egypt. More often, throughout Mesopotamia for example, the burial site was replaced by a temple, and the corpse of the ruler-god by a statue which enjoyed even more worship and reverence, since it did not decompose.[134]

The fact that people in earlier civilizations heard their gods directing their lives means that their mentality was profoundly different from our own. As Jaynes pointed out, from the ninth millennium to the second millennium BCE, people did not have a free will of their own. They were not responsible for their actions because a carefully established hierarchy of divine inner voices ordered them about like slaves.[135] Homer's famous epic about the Trojan war, the Iliad, shows that the early Greeks did not think of themselves as having a will of their own. Actions and speeches of gods initiated their behavior, rather then their own conscious plans and motives. When toward the end of the Trojan war Achilles reminded King Agamemnon of how he had robbed him of his mistress, the king responded that it was not he, but Zeus and other gods who had made him do it, which is not unlike our contemporary saying: "The Devil made me do it!" Achilles, who also was obedient to his gods, fully accepted this explanation.[136]

Julian Jaynes rightly wrote that during the civilizations that followed the Cro-magnon, from Natufians until Ileadic men, people did not yet know of subjectivity as we do. Instead of recognizing their own free will and responsibility for their own actions, they heard the "hallucinated" voice of their god, or one of their gods, telling them what to do.[137] Jaynes realized that the ancient experience of listening to the silent voice of the gods was a forerunner of the modern silent self-talk between, in modern terms, ego and superego. This means that with the evolution of abstract thinking in 7–D and the ability to self-reflect, the Greek culture quickly gave rise to a literature of self-awareness. While the listening I_1 in 5–D (the ego or Inner Child) remained, the silent voice of gods in 5–D was taken over by another analog self, I_2 (the superego or Inner Parent or Voice of Conscience). In due course a third analog self appeared, I_3 (the paraego or Inner Adult or Voice of Reason in 7–D), the enabler of the new self-awareness. Thus subjective consciousness began.[138]

Jaynes advanced the interesting proposition that the evolutionary development that led to the disappearance of the divine auditory hallucinations in 5–D had a profound and widespread consequence. Since the world had long known rules that were divinely ordained and humanly obeyed, the disappearance of the divine voices induced a belief that the gods were forsaking their human slaves because of offenses they had committed. Only then did the mighty themes of the religions of the world sound for the first time that the gods had abandoned their people because of their offenses; that their misfortunes are their punishments for these; and that they have to go down on their knees, begging for forgiveness and seeking redemption.[139]

Jaynes traced the earliest evidence of the change in internalized silent talk to Assyria, Mesopotamia, around 1,200 BCE. He felt that the literature on the loss of the gods represents a change in Mesopotamia's history that cannot be questioned. This change can be recognized in Assyrian psalms up until the first millennium BCE. He considered these psalms the song of the Assyrians and the wailing of the Hebrews which expressed "the groping of newly conscious men to narratize what has happened to them, the loss of divine voices and assurances in a chaos of human directives and selfish privacies." This, he thought, was the source and first premise of the world's great religions.[140]

Since the disappearance of divine inner voices apparently emerged well before the sixth century BCE when the Greeks began to show evidence of scientific thinking, it may be that the disappearance of the divine voices came first and the emergence of abstract scientific thought followed later.

NOTES

1   There are a few exceptions: for example, the evolution of some mental functions that express right versus left brain functioning [Dimond and Blizard (1977)], and the evolution of language [Harnad, Steklis and Lancaster (1976)].
2   Gore (2003), p. 16.
3   The classification of living primates is a matter of some dispute [Tattersall (1993)].
4   Wells (2002), p. 33, 67.
5   Wells (2002), p. 88-89.
6   Richard Leaky quoted by Morgan (1982), p. 14.
7   Some recent finds may push this time line further back to about 7 million years ago [Gore (2003), p. 31].
8 . Wells (2002), p. 67.
9   Lemonick (1994), p. 57.
10   The aquatic ape theory was first propounded by Professor Alister Hardy [Morgan (1982)].
11   Like the alleged aquatic, the elephant went into the water for a prolonged period of time and subsequently readapted to terrestrial life [Morgan (1982), p. 157-159].
12   Morgan (1982).
13   La Lumiere Jr. (1982).
14   Lemonick (1994, 1994a, 1999)].
15   Wilford (2002) quoting Bernard Wood, paleontologist at George Washington University (paraphrased).
16   Lemonick (1994), p. 54; Gorman (1995), p. 42.
17   Isaac (1976), p. 285.
18   Steklis and Harnad (1976), p. 448.
19   Howells (1959), p. 206.
20   Isaac (1976), p. 283, 285.
21   Raven and Johnson (1989), p. 439; Lemonick (1994), p. 42, 44.

22   Steklis and Harnad (1976), p. 448; LeMay, (1976), p. 349.

23   Wells (2002), p. 38.

24   Raven and Johnson (1989), p. 439.

25   Howells (1959a), p. 249-250.

26   Wells (2002), p. 119.

27   de Lumley (1986), p. 197-199.

28   Wells (2002), p. 119, 123, 129.

29   Raven and Johnson (1989), p. 440.

30   Campbell (1959), p. 371.

31   Wells (2002), p. 125.

32   Isaac (1976), p. 283, 286.

33   de Lumley (1986), p. 197-199; Putman (1988), p. 453.

34   Brandon (1966), p. 144-145; Rappoport (1972), p. 18; Eccles (1977), p. 171.

35   Hawkes (1965) quoted by Eccles (1977), p. 171; Constable et al. (1973), p. 97.

36   Prideaux et al. (1973), p. 139.

37   Goudsmit et al. (1966), p. 11.

38   Campbell (1959), p. 371.

39   Gimbutas (1991), p. 324, quoting J. J. Bachofen (1815 - 1887).

40   Constable et al. (1973) p. 40; Howell et al. (1968), p. 175)

41   Constable et al. (1973), p. 100.

42   Jaynes (1976), p. 319.

43   Hartmann (1967), p. 15; Dement and Kleitman (1957).

44   Tanner and Zihlman (1976), p. 475.

45   The German biologist, Ernst Heinrich Haeckel (1834-1919) formulated that the development of the individual is a recapitulation of the development of the species. The American psychologist, Granville Stanley Hall (1846-1924) and others extended this to mental development. While there certainly are some problems with this, it remains useful to compare potential parallels between stages of individual development in the modern child with stages of development in the evolution of humans [Stern and Stern (1931)]. The principle of parallelism has gained support from Piaget's claim that children develop through the same stages in the same order in spite of vast differences in their cultural milieu, educational training, and personal experiences; in North Slope Eskimos of Alaska, Mexicans, Costa Ricans and Koreans, Rwandese, French-speaking Canadians, Iranians, Norwegians, Hungarians, for example [Green (1989), p. 188].

46   Pos (1980).

47   Terr (1991), p. 12.

48   Constable et al. (1973), p. 71, 81, 104.

49   Campbell (1959), p. 342; Constable et al. (1973), p. 98, 101, 148; Marshack (1976), p. 295.

50   Lieberman and Crelin quoted by Constable et al. (1973), p. 132.

51   Jaynes (1976), p. 316-317.

52   Constable et al. (1973), p. 38.

53   Wang (1976), p. 61-63].

54   Campbell (1959), p.339-341, 344-345, 348.

55   Constable et al. (1973), p. 104-105.

56   Campbell (1959), p. 373.

57   Constable et al. (1973), p. 114; Marshack (1976), p. 296-297.

58   Isaac (1976), p. 283.

59   At about age 3, youngsters move onto the creation of six diagrams -- Greek cross, square, circle, triangle, odd-shaped area and diagonal cross -- and, thereafter begin to produce combinations and permutations of the six diagrams. Only after the child has these patterns clear in its mind, does it proceed, around age 4, to use them in a pictorial way, in that they become suns, buildings, vehicles, plants, animals, and humans. Kellogg (1965), quoted by Harlan (1970), p. 32-33; Harlan (1970), p. 32-33.

60   Svante quoted by Wells (2002), p. 122; Wells (2002), p. 125.

61   White et al. (2003).
62   Wells (2002), p. 83.
63   Stringer (2003); Wells (2002), p. 14, 30, 33, 49].
64   Wells (2002), p. 60, 83, 98-99, 107-108.
65   Wells (2002), p. 68-69.
66   Constable et al. (1973), p. 133.
67   Bar-Yosef and Vandermeersch (1993), p. 94, 100.
68   Wells (2002), p. 77.
69   Bar-Yosef and Vandermeersch (1993).
70   Wells (2002), p. 85, 93, 100.
71   Isaac (1976), p. 286.
72   Wells (2002), p. 85, 87.
73   Savage-Rumbaugh, Shanker and Taylor (2001).
74   Jaynes (1976), p. 315, 323; Wescott (1976), p. 104-105.
75   Berk (1994), p. 78.
76   Binford (1968) quoted by Marshack (1976), p. 295. Compare Steinen (1894), quoted by Werner (1957), p. 302-303. (
77   Hallowell (1937).
78   Campbell (1959).
79   Wells (2002).
80   Wells (2002), p. 59].
81   Wells (2002), p. 72, 75.
82   Wells (2002), p. 69, 78-79.
83   For example, Proto-Elamite, Proto-Dravidian, Proto-Indo-Uralic, Proto-Afro-Asian, and Proto-Congo-Kordofanian [Wescott (1976), p. 108-112].
84   Gallant (1990), p. 34.
85   de Lumley (1986), p. 197-199.
86   Two schemes gained successive popularity: the first scheme by the French cleric abbé Henri Breuil, who was superseded by the French prehistorian André Leroi-Gourhan. For further details see the comparable section of Chapter 12 in the unabridged e-book version [Pos (2004)].
87   Ruspoli (1986), p. 18, 44; de Lumley (1986), p. 197-199.
88   Chauvet, Brunel Deschamps and Hillaire (1996), p. 122.
89   Clottes (1996), p. 124-126.
90   Clottes & Courtin (1996), p. 186.
91   Clottes and Courtin (1996), p. 175.
92   Campbell (1959), p. 304 - 306; Brandon (1966).
93   Hallowell (1937).
94   Hallowell (1937).
95   Clottes & Courtin (1996), p. 173.
96   Bray and Trump (1986), p. 54.
97   Chauvet, Brunell Deschamps, Hillaire (1996), p. 10.
98   Bray and Trump (1986), p. 147)],.
99   Campbell (1959), p. 21.
100   Jaynes (1976), p. 138.
101   Campbell (1959), p. 311.
102   Putman (1988), p. 448.
103   Ruspoli (1986), p. 162.
104   Clottes and Courtin (1996), p. 177
105   Butzer (1979).
106   Clottes and Courtin (1996), p. 175.

107   de Lumley (1986), p. 197-199; Bahn (1996), p. 10-11.

108   Gimbutas (1991), p. 222.

109   Prideaux et al. (1973); Gimbutas (1991), p. 222.

110   Gallant (1990), p. 38.

111   Smith (1998), p. 169.

112   Prideaux et al. (1973), p. 46-49.

113   Smith (1998), p. 28.

114   Johnson (1997).

115   Check (2005), p. 266.

116   Smith (1998), p. 12-13.

117   Smith (1998), p. 16, 19, 209, 213-214.

118   Gimbutas (1991). p.324, 331, 349, 351-352

119   de Lumley (1986), p. 197-199

120   Chauvet, Brunell Deschamps, Hillaire (1996), p. 10.

121   "...for the first time in the history of art [these so-called Spanish Levantine paintings from between 11,400 - 4,500 years ago] depict men, women and children in social groups..." [Prideaux et al. (1979), p. 146].

122   Prideaux et al. (1979), p. 146.

123   Fraser, Lawrence and Haber (1986).

124   Pos (1963), p. 35.

125   The philosopher Denis Corish pointed in this context to the difference between scientific thinking and technological thinking. The purpose of technology is entirely practical; technological thinking is involved in how to make things. Techniques may be very simple, as in hunting or gathering, or they may be highly organized and elaborate as in building Egyptian pyramids which emerged long before Greek scientific thinking. A highly skilled, practical technology can be achieved without 7–D. Beavers can construct magnificent dams, and bees complicated hives. Technology does not imply the kind of speculative thinking that is characteristic of 7 D thinking in general, and of scientific thinking in particular. Speculative thinking involves reasoning that moves beyond the visible, tangible and finite reality in 4–D to arrive at general rules and laws. The thinking in Ancient Greece was scientific rather than technological because it represented for the first time in the West organized abstract knowledge such as geometry, rather than the rule-of-thumb land-measuring practices of the Egyptians [Corish (1986), p. 69-70]. At the time, Denis Corish was Chairman of the Department of Philosophy, Bowdoin College, Brunswick, Maine.

126   Pos (1963), p. 41.

127   Pos (1963). For further details see the relevant footnote in Chapter 12 of the unabridged e-book version [Pos (2004)].

128   Fraser (2005).

129   Corish (1986), p. 71.

130   Jaynes (1976). p. 137, 140.

131   Robson and Minde (1977).

132   Piaget (1932).

133   Jaynes (1976), p. 139.

134   Jaynes (1976), p. 142-144, 150-151.

135   Jaynes (1976), p. 202.

136   Jaynes (1982), p. 69-73.

137   Jaynes (1976), p. 75.

138   Jaynes (1976), p. 81-83.

139   Jaynes (1976), p. 223, 226-227.

140   Jaynes (1976), p. 223 - 226, 253, 444.

APPENDIX 1

The Research Sample

Over the four-year period 1987-1991 I assessed 405 people. To evaluate whether the method of time gender assignment as well as the research sample itself remained stable, I divided the research cohort into an early group (August 1, 1987-July 31, 1989: 273 subjects) and a late group (August 1, 1989-July 31, 1991: 132 subjects) and examined the distributions of time gender and sexual gender in both groups.[537] It turned out that the proportions of men and women in the early group (45.8% versus 54.2%) and late group (49.2% versus 50.8%) did not significantly differ statistically (p=0.514),[538] nor did the proportions of alphas and betas in the early group (59.0% versus 41.0%) and late group (62.1% versus 37.9%) (p=0.545).[3]

In the early group, I extracted from each subject's file a number of additional variables with the aid of a scoring sheet of 128 individual items. Originally, these data were transferred to a computerized data bank (Appleworks GS-Claris Data Base), but later these data were entered into a statistical program for Macintosh (Systat 5.2.1) to facilitate their statistical analyses. Since I am not a professional statistician, I attempted to satisfy professional statistical standards as best as I could,[4] and sought the opinions and assistance of professional statisticians.

In the beginning, the potential importance of the time gender duality made me wonder whether it was a figment of my imagination, but in due course the statistical analyses resulted in an impressive coherence of statistical data that supported the time gender model. The first scientific confirmation of the alpha-beta duality appeared, however, when I plotted the men and women of my early group and its alphas and betas in 5-year-age groups to indicate to which age group these subjects belonged when first seeking my assistance.[5] The resulting figure Appendix 1.1 demonstrates that these *age groups* did not significantly differ in their distributions of men and women (p=0.078),[6] but that they significantly differed in their distributions of alphas and betas (p<0.001).[7] While alphas peaked in the 25-34 year old group, betas peaked ten years later, that is in the 35-44 year old group. Although in the latter age group of 35-44 equal amounts of alphas and betas looked for help, prior to that (during the ages of 20-34), more alphas than betas were inclined to seek help and after age 45 more betas than alphas.

Figure Appendix 1.2 is even more dramatic in showing the reality of the alpha-beta duality. The top section demonstrates that the distributions of alpha females and alpha males in these age groups did not significantly differ (p=0.704),[8] while the bottom section shows that the same applies to beta females and beta males (p=0.345).[9]

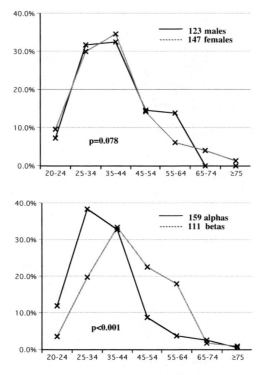

Figure Appendix 1.1: The difference in age distribution of 270 subjects of age ≥20 who sought help, broken down by sexual gender (above) and time gender (below)

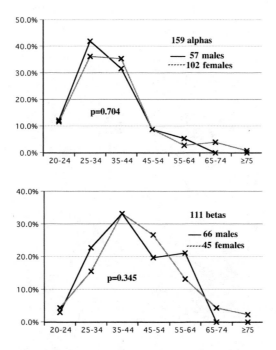

Figure Appendix 1.2: The difference in age distribution of 159 alphas (top) and 111 betas (bottom) of 270 subjects of age ≥20 who sought help, broken down by sexual gender

Reinforcing these findings was the difference in the *average age* at which men and women, and alphas and betas, sought help with their problem. Statistically speaking, men sought help at the same average age (39.4 years) as women (39.1 years) (p=0.789),[10] but alphas (36.4 years) tended to do so almost 7 years earlier than betas (43.3 years), a highly significant difference (p<0.001).[11] But the statistical difference between alpha females (36.8 years)[12] and alpha males (35.8 years)[13] was not significant (p=0.506);[14] neither was the one between beta females (44.2 years)[15] and beta males (42.6 years)[16] (p=0.668).[17]

The important conclusion is that men and women are not necessarily homogenous categories on studied variables as there may be significant differences between alpha men and beta men, and between alpha women and beta women between such variables.

Potential implications of the time gender distribution in the sample

Figure Appendix 1.3 (top section) shows that the *sex distribution* in my four-year sample of 405 subjects (53% females-47% males) was similar to that in the general population of Greater Vancouver BC (52% females-48% males).[18] Therefore the sample was, at least in regards to, reflecting the general population from which it derived. But the bottom section of figure Appendix 1.3 indicates that, although the *time gender distribution* in the entire sample was 60% alphas and 40% betas, this ratio was different for the men (almost 50% alphas-50% betas) and the women (about 70% alphas-30% betas).

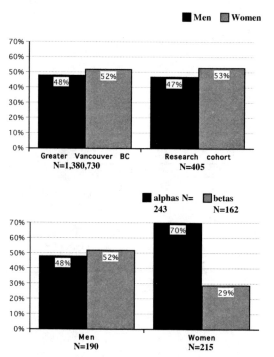

Figure Appendix 1.3: The *sex distributions* in Greater Vancouver BC and in our 4-year sample (above), and the *time gender distributions* among men and women in that sample (below)

In other words, among the male-female ratio among alphas and betas was more or less inversed, namely almost 1:2 among alphas and close to 2:1 among betas, as figure Appendix 1.4 demonstrates. This reflected a strong and stable statistical connection between time gender and sexual gender.

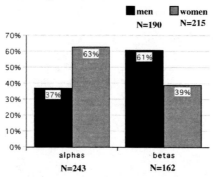

Figure Appendix 1.4: The sexual gender distributions
among the alphas and betas in my 4-year sample

The significant question in this context is whether the time gender distribution among the men and women of my 4-year research cohort applies, like their sex distribution, to the almost 1.4 million general population of Greater Vancouver, BC, if not beyond. Since the sample represents my 1987-1991 psychiatric private practice in Vancouver, BC, people could argue this not to be so as my practice cohort might have represented a pre-selected group of mentally disordered people rather than a randomly selected general population sample. In other words, the alpha-beta ratio I found might be valid for a particular psychiatric practice but not for the general population from which these clients were drawn.

About being a psychiatric patient

Since I am a psychiatrist, the 405 subjects of my research cohort were by definition 'psychiatric patients.' However, being a 'psychiatric patient' means no more than that one is seeing a psychiatrist, since the reason for doing so may vary greatly with the particular psychiatrist one is visiting. Some psychiatrists are 'generalists;' they will accept any referrals 'in need of psychiatric assessment or help,' as defined by either the patient, or the referral source, or both. Other psychiatrists, particularly in large population centers, specialize in distinct problem areas or therapeutic techniques. Some are child, or adolescent, or geriatric psychiatrists. Others specialize in psychotic patients such as those suffering from schizophrenia, or alcohol and drug addictions, anxiety disorders, mood disorders, sleep problems, difficulties in sexual functioning, eating disorders, marital difficulties, forensic psychiatry, and so on. Furthermore, some psychiatrists concentrate on analyzing health care professionals who are preparing for a future career in counseling, and analyze also people who choose analysis and self-reflection as a way toward understanding themselves and functioning more efficiently. In this context I am thinking, for example, of the American film director and actor Woody Allen.

In short, speaking of someone being a 'psychiatric patient' means very little. On one end of the continuum it may mean that one is representative of persons with a particular psychiatric diagnosis. On the other end it may reflect people who seek help in coping with one of the many problems of living, or who simply want to understand themselves better. These latter are more 'normative' than mentally disordered.

How the subjects were assembled for the study

For all practical purposes my catchment area for the subjects of my research cohort turned out to be Greater Vancouver, BC since 97% resided in Greater Vancouver BC. However, what were the pathways by which these subjects entered the study sample, and were the referrals more or less random and therefore approximating the general population, or was there a sampling bias?

Referral source	total	%-age
29 GPs @ 1 client	29	10.6%
21 GPs @ 2-10 clients	104	38.1%
3 GPs @ >10 clients	79	28.9%
53 GPs (*)	212	77.7%
Other psychiatrists	18	6.6%
Lawyers	13	4.8%
Other client/friends	12	4.4%
Women's agency	10	3.7%
Other sources	8	2.9%
Other sources (**)	61	22.3%
TOTAL	273	100.0%

(*) : GP=general practitioner
(**): Referral via GP
Table Appendix 1.1: Referral source of 273 subjects

Table Appendix 1.1 provides details about the referral sources of the first 273 subjects (1987-1989) of the research cohort. Just over three quarters (78%) were directly referred by 53 general practitioners. Although the remaining subjects (22%) were also referred by their general practitioners they actually constituted indirect referrals from various other sources in the community. Of the direct referrals from general practitioners (78%), twenty nine physicians made a single referral, and twenty four made more than one, with only three making more than 10 each during the 2-year period. In short, there was considerable mix in the referral sources.

I accepted all referrals with three exceptions:

1) primary referrals of children and adolescents (since I am not qualified in these subspecialties). However, when it was deemed helpful to include a child or adolescent of an adult referral in the treatment process, this was done.

This necessitated that, when making comparisons of my sample with the population of Greater Vancouver BC, the age distribution of the general population had to be adjusted accordingly;

2) subjects involved in the Criminal Justice system. My reasoning was that these people could be looked after more properly by the staff of the Forensic Services Commission of British Columbia;[19] and

3) referrals with the specific request for treatment of a sexual deviation (because of certain professional opinions I hold in this area).

These three types of referrals were re-referred to colleagues active in those particular areas. Even so, exclusions sub 2 and sub 3 constituted a negative referral filter bias which might, or might not have influenced the time gender distribution of my sample, albeit minimally so.

However, a general sampling bias was implicitly possible. This relates to the argument that, since my research cohort came out of my psychiatric practice, a high concentration of mental disorders, particularly serious mental illnesses, could have invalidated the assumption that this sample might in many aspects be representative of the general population of Greater Vancouver BC.[20] For example, a mixed inpatient-outpatient group of psychiatric patients in a 1989 US study had 18.0% of the subjects diagnosed as suffering from schizophrenia and 32.9% as having a major depressive episode.[21] However, in my catchment area chronically, seriously mentally ill people are dealt with by a network of government-sponsored community mental health teams. As a result, such patients tend not to show up in private psychiatric practices. This created in my sample an implicit negative diagnostic access bias toward serious mental disorders, resulting in prevalence rates for these disorders that are compatible with those in the general population.[22] For example, in my 273 consecutive clients (1987-1989), only 1.5% were diagnosed as suffering from schizophrenia which reflects its prevalence in the general population.[23] And only 1.1% ere diagnosed as occasionally suffering from manic attacks (the so-called bipolar disorders), with only 3.7% as suffering from serious major depressive episodes, the latter two numbers once again reflecting the prevalence of these mental illnesses in the general population.[24] Furthermore, my sample did not have any patients with organic brain diseases causing dementia. Apparently, patients who need the assessment of organic brain problems in Greater Vancouver tend to avail themselves of the full inpatient and outpatient psychiatric facilities of the University of British Columbia. Similarly, only 2% of my clients were referred because of suicidal feelings, since acutely suicidal people tend to end up in the emergency ward of a hospital for admission to their psychiatry department. The diagnosis of mental retardation was made in only 0.7% of subjects which reflects, once again, its prevalence of approximately 1% in the general population.[25] Finally, the 8% of subjects who were referred because of legal problems were not suffering from a type of a mental illness which may get a person into criminal activities. In British Columbia these people are dealt by facilities of the

Provincial Forensic Psychiatric Services Commission.

A third referral bias, centripetal in nature, was present in 22 subjects (8.1%) who had initiated the referral because they had heard about, and were seeking my particular expertise and interest: practicing holistic medicine and, if need be, long term therapy, while acknowledging the time gender duality, and dealing accordingly with their problems of living. This bias added to prevalence rates of mental disorders that were similar to those in the general population.

Finally, a fourth referral bias, also centripetal and also contributing to rather normative prevalence rates of mental disorders, occurred because some referral sources became aware of my interest in the conjoint counseling of marital partners. Hence it is no surprise that 48 (18%) of the 273 subjects were referred because of 'marital problems' and that the clinical diagnosis of 'marital problem' was made in 51 (19%) of the referred subjects.

The psychiatric profile of the sample

If the 1987-1989 sample of 273 consecutive clients did not yield a concentrated group of seriously mentally ill people, what then was its psychiatric configuration? In the first place I looked at four psychiatric indicators, namely 1) the reason for referral (the client's presenting problem); 2) the distribution of clinical diagnoses; 3) the severity of psychosocial stressors (DSM-III-R's Axis IV); and 4) the global level of functioning (DSM-III-R's Axis V). Next, I reviewed six factors that in psychiatric samples may be found, or assumed to be found to deviate from corresponding ones in the general population, namely 5) the mean age of first sexual intercourse; 6) the prevalence of abortions among females; 7) the prevalence of marital infidelity; and the prevalence of a history of 8) parental alcohol abuse, 9) childhood sexual abuse, and 10) childhood physical abuse.

1. *The reason for referral or the client's presenting problem.* Table Appendix 1.2 documents the most frequently given reasons for referral (N=210).

Presenting problem (reason for referral)	Number of clients	Percentage (N=273)
Depression with or without anxiety	74	27%
Problem with marital partner	48	18%
Legal problem	23	8%
Moodswings	18	7%
Panics, anxiety, phobias	17	6%
Requesting psychotherapy, hypnosis, support, follow up, advice	17	6%
Violence toward family or others	8	3%
Feeling suicidal	5	2%
Total number of clients	210	77%

Table Appendix 1.2: The most frequently given reasons for referral for 210 out of 273 subjects

62% came with some symptom, while 38% came to settle some specific issue, such as a marital problem, employability assessment, legal assessment, pressure from a parent or friend, welfare assessment, and so on.

2. *The distribution of clinical diagnoses* according to the third, revised edition of the American Psychiatric Association's Diagnostic and Statistical Manual (DSM-III-R), which became available in 1987. I did not use the subsequent DSM-IV or DSM-IV-R because these became available only in 1994 and 2000, well after my data collection had been concluded in 1991. The results in table Appendix 1.3 provide any diagnosis made in ≥5% of the subjects.

Diagnoses	Number of clients	Percentage (N=273)
Depressive disorder NOS(*)	113	41%
Panic disorder	60	22%
Marital problem	51	19%
Alcohol abuse/dependence	43	16%
Drug abuse/dependence	27	10%
Parent-child problem	15	5%
Total number of diagnoses (**)	309	N/A

(*): Depressive Disorder Not Otherwise Specified indicates that the person has depressive symptoms but does not meet criteria for any specific Mood Disorder or Adjustment Disorderr with Depressed Mood.
(**): The average number of diagnoses per client was 1.5

Table Appendix 1.3: Clinical diagnosis made in ≥5% of the subjeccts (N=273)

One out of five subjects was diagnosed as having a marital problem. However, high separation and divorce rates in the general population testify to the fact that marital problems occur much more frequently than only in 19% of marital unions. Indeed, of the 140 married subjects in my sample, 85% saw their marriage as problematic (see figure Appendix 1.8). That 5% of the subjects had a parent-child problem for their diagnosis is also well below what one would expect in the general population. As I will also show later, of the 127 subjects with children, 43% experienced parenthood problems (see figure Appendix 1.8).

The overall distribution of the more typical clinical diagnoses does not vary a great deal from their prevalence in the general population. Having depressed feelings is, as anyone knows, quite common. The prevalence of panic disorder also is common in the general population.[26] As far as the 16% of referrals diagnosed as alcohol abuse or dependence is concerned, a 1981-1983 community study in the United States indicated that approximately 13% of the adult population would meet the criteria for alcohol abuse or dependence at some time in their lives.[27] Concerning the 10% of referrals who suffered from drug abuse or dependence, the same US community study indicated that approximately 1.1%

of the adult population had abused, or where dependent on, sedatives, hypnotics or anxiolytics during some time in their lives,[28] 0.7% on opioids,[29] 0.2% on cocaine,[30] 4% on cannabis,[31] and 2% on amphetamines.[32] Although these drug abuses or dependencies may overlap, the 10% of my subjects so diagnosed does not appear extravagant in comparison with the general population.

3. *The severity of psychosocial stressors according to DSM-III-R's Axis IV.* I took into account the average severity of psychosocial stressors in my sample, according to DSM-III-R's Axis IV which is indicated in table Appendix 1.4.[33] I had relevant information on 262 out of the 273 subjects (96%).

Code	Term	Examples of stressors	
		Acute events	**Enduring circumstances**
1	None		
		No acute events that may be relevant to the disorder	No enduring circumstances that may be relevant to the disorder
2	Mild		
		Broke up with boyfriend or girlfriend; started or graduated from school; child left home	Family arguments; job dis-satisfaction; residence in high-crime neighborhood
3	Moderate		
		Marriage; marital separation; loss of job retirement; miscarriage	Marital discord; serious financial problems; trouble with boss; being a single parent
4	Severe		
		Divorce; birth of first child	Unemployment; poverty
5.	Extreme		
		Death of spouse; serious physical illness diagnosed; victim of rape	Serious chronic illness in self or child; ongoing physical or sexual abuse
6.	Catastrophic		
		Death of child; suicide of spouse; devastating natural disaster	Captivity as hostage; concentration camp experience

Table Appendix 1.4: DSM-IIIR's Axis IV: Severity of psychosocial stressors: (adults)

Figure Appendix 1.5 demonstrates the distribution of stress level from none (1) to catastrophic (6) as defined by table Appendix 1.4. It shows that 68% of the sample fell in the mild and moderate categories, testifying to the reasonable normalcy of the sample.[34]

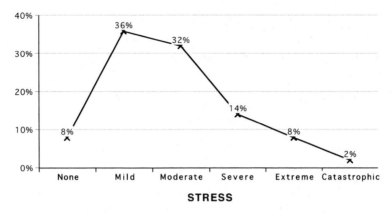

Figure Appendix 1.5: Stress level distribution in the 1987-1989 sample (N=262)

4. *The global level of functioning according to DSM-III-R's Axis V.* Finally, I assessed the average level of functioning according to DSM-III-R's Axis V as per table Appendix 1.5.[35]

Code	
90-81	**Absent or minimal symptoms** (e.g. mild anxiety before an exam), **good functioning in all areas, interested and involved in a wide range of activities, socially effective, generally satisfied with life, no more than everyday problems or concerns** (e.g. an occasional argument with family members).
80-71	**If symptoms are present, they are transient and expectable reactions to psychosocial stressors** (e.g. difficulty concentrating after family arguments); **no more than slight impairment in social, occupational, or school functioning** (e.g. temporarily falling behind in school work).
70-61	**Some mild symptoms** (e.g. depressed mood and mild insomnia) **OR some difficulty in social, occupational, or school functioning** (e.g., occasional truancy, or theft within the household), **but generally functioning pretty well, has some meaningful interpersonal relationships.**
60-51	**Moderate symptoms** (e.g., flat affect and circumstantial speech, occasional panic attacks) **OR moderate difficulty in social, occupational, or school functioning** (e.g., few friends, unable to keep a job).
50-41	**Serious symptoms** (e.g., suicidal ideation, severe obsessional rituals, freqent shoplifting) **OR any serious impairment in social, occupational, or school functioning** (e.g., no friends, unableto keep a job).
40-31	**Some impairment in reality testing or communication** (e.g., speech is at times illogical, obscure, or irrelevant) **OR major impairment in several areas, such as work or school, family relations, judgment, thinking, or mood** (e.g., depressed man avoids friends, neglects family, and is unable to work; child frequently beats up younger children, is defiant at home, and is failing at school).
30-21	**Behavior is considerably influenced by delusions or hallucinations OR serious impairment in communication or judgment** (e.g., sometimes incoherent, acts grossly inappropriately, suicidal preoccupation) **OR inability to function in almost all areas** (e.g., stays in bed all day; no job, home, or friends).
20-11	**Some danger of hurting self or others** (e.g., suicide attempts without clear expectation of death, frequently violent, manic excitement) **OR occasionally fails to maintain minimal personal hygiene** (e.g., smears feces) **OR gross impairment in communication** (e.g., largely incoherent or mute).
10-1	**Persistent danger of severely hurting self or others** (e.g. recurrent violence) **OR persistent inability to maintain minimal personal hygiene OR serious suicidal act with clear expectation of death.**
0	**Inadequate information.**

Table Appendix 1.5: DSM-IIIR's Axis V: Global assessment of functioning scale

I had relevant information on 271 out of the 273 subjects (99%). The average functioning level of my sample as defined by table Appendix 1.5 was 70.6,[36] that is a level with some mild symptoms or with some difficulty in social, occupational, or school functioning, but generally functioning pretty well, and having some meaningful interpersonal relationships. The distribution of the functioning levels in my sample is shown in figure Appendix 1.6 which demonstrates that 70% of these subjects functioned at a level higher than 61 and 45% at a level above 71 which, once again, does not sound very abnormal.

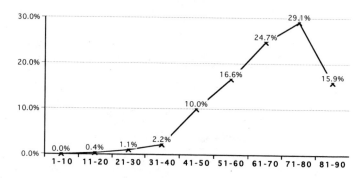

FUNCTIONING LEVEL

Figure Appendix 1.6: Distribution of functioning levels in the 1987-1989 sample (N=271)

5. *Age of first sexual intercourse.* Subjects in my Vancouver group had their first sexual intercourse at an average age of 18.0 which is in line with the overall American statistics.[37] Again in line with data in several American reviews,[38] the males in my sample tended to experience their first sex during adolescence somewhat earlier than girls. I found, however, no significant difference in the average age at which females and males, generally speaking, experience their first sex because my statistics include also the subjects who first experienced genital sex in adulthood unlike the American statistics which, because of the AIDS danger, focused predominantly on adolescents.

6. *Abortions.* My group of 145 women, whose data I collected during 1987-1989, showed a prevalence rate of 252 abortions per 1000 life birth. This appears not out of line with relevant statistics for the general population of the Province of British Columbia, Canada. For example, in the ten years between 1971-1980 the average annual incidence of abortions/1000 life births there increased from 202 in 1971 to 316 in 1980, for a ten year average of 283/1000. And in the US. there were 239 abortions/1000 life births in 1973, and in 1996 379/1000.[39]

7. *Marital fidelity.* In my group of heterosexual subjects in marital-type unions, 84% stated they had been faithful. This is in line with a number of American surveys. The 1992 *Sex in America* study, for example, found that, among married people of age 18-59, more than 80% of women and 65-85% of men had only one partner; and that those who are unmarried and living together were almost as likely to be

faithful.[40] In other words, a significant majority of people who get married or start living together restrict their sexual activity to their primary partner.

8. *Parental alcohol abuse.* I found that parental alcohol abuse occurred in 27% of the 263 subjects on whom relevant information was available. Comparing this prevalence rate with that in the general population causes a difficult problem. Firstly, one cannot be sure about the general prevalence of alcohol abuse because definitions of abuse and sources of information vary. Various definitions of problem drinkers, clinical syndromes and hazardous consumption are used, while tax and population data, population surveys, and catastrophe counts (death rates, hospital admissions, arrests, car accidents, etc.) also render different prevalence rates.[41] Population surveys in the United States have suggested that 13% drink several times a month, though usually no more than three or four drinks per occasion, and 12% are heavy, almost daily drinkers.[42] Later studies have yielded similar results.[43] However, population surveys may underestimate alcohol use by up to 50%. For example, annual consumption of beer, wine and distilled spirits based on house hold surveys do not account for the alcohol consumption reported in tax-population data.[44] If assuming that a prevalence of 12% heavy, almost daily drinkers is correct, it is even less clear how many of these abusers are in a parental role. So, it is difficult to assess whether my prevalence of parental alcohol abuse of 27% is, or is not out of line with what one may expect in the general population.

9. *Childhood sexual abuse.* An increased prevalence of maltreatment during childhood (notably physical and sexual abuse) has been well recognized in psychiatric clinical populations,[45] as compared with the general population samples. Even so, a rather wide range of childhood sexual abuse in women was found in general population samples with prevalence rates of 27-51%.[46] My prevalence rate of 14% in women was considerable lower. That this rate does not match the one in clinical psychiatric populations, let alone in general population samples, suggests either that the members of my sample were more shielded in this regard or that the reporting of sexual abuse by women in general population samples and, perhaps in clinical samples, might have been exaggerated. On the other hand, my male rate of 8% for sexual abuse in childhood, while below that of clinical population samples, may be in line with at least some rates found in general populations, such as the 6% prevalence in the 1984 Boston survey.[47]

10. *Childhood physical abuse.* In my group of 271 subjects with relevant information, 10% claimed to have experienced childhood physical abuse. The prevalence of physical abuse I found in my sample is, generally speaking, below that of clinical psychiatric populations, but in line with the 9% rate of physical abuse found among a group of male and female college students.[48]

Comparing the 1987-1989 sample with the 1986 Census of Greater Vancouver BC

Before comparing my sample with the 1986 Census of Greater Vancouver BC, and thus considering its time gender distribution as the one in the general population from which it was derived, a few remark on the sexual orientation of my cohort and its distribution of birth order is in order .

Sexual orientation. Male homosexuals accounted for 14% of the male sample and 7% of all 273 subjects. Although prevalence estimates of male homosexuality are in general about 4-6%,[49] my sample's 14% was not out of line with what one would expect in a city like Vancouver BC, which, as San Francisco and New York City, has a large gay community. Prevalence estimates of female homosexuality are about 2%,[50] and downtown Vancouver has quite an active lesbian community, my sample did not include exclusively lesbian women for reasons stated in Chapter 7. As a result, heterosexual women were slightly over-represented in my sample, and the *total* group of exclusive homosexuals under-represented. However, since the time gender distribution among homosexual men was similar to that of the heterosexual men, and I assume the same for heterosexual and homosexual women, sexual orientation probably does not account for the sample's time gender distribution.

Birth order. Of the 268 of my 273 subjects for whom information was available, 112 (42%) were first-born, 75 (28%) second born, 46 (17%) third born and 35 (13%) fourth-tenth born. This came very close to the results of a large North American sample of close to 12,000 people,[51] according to which 46% were first born (versus 42% in my sample), 26% second born (versus 28% in my sample) and 28% beyond that rank (versus 30% in my sample). In terms of birth order my sample does not appear to deviate from a large North American population sample.

In order to compare the 273 subjects from my 1987-1989 private psychiatric practice in downtown Vancouver BC with the general population, I first had to define which general population they belonged to. While just over 60% lived within the City of Vancouver where my office was located, 97% or almost all of them were living within the boundaries of so-called Consolidated Vancouver,[52] a well-defined census area in Greater Vancouver with a population of close to 1.4 million people at the time.[53] The population of this census area as polled in 1986 is therefore tailor-made for comparison with our cohort of 273 subjects.

1. *Sexual gender distribution.* The proportion of women in psychiatric patient populations is usually considerably higher than the proportion of men, as exemplified by a US study of a mixed inpatient-outpatient group of psychiatric patients which consisted of 64% women.[54] By contrast Table Appendix 1.6 demonstrates that the sexual gender distribution of the population of Greater Vancouver of ≥age 20 was within the 95% confidence levels of the one in my 1987-1989 sample of 270 subjects of age ≥20.[55] In other words, in terms of sexual gender distribution my sample was representative of the population of Greater Vancouver BC.

	Females	Males	Total
Greater Vancouver	533,325	499,185	1,032,510
%-age	51.7%	48.3%	100.0%
Research cohort (N=270)	147	123	270
%-age	54.4%	45.6%	100.0%
95% ConfL.	51.5%-57.4%	42.6%-48.7%	

Table Appendix 1.6:
Comparing the sexual gender distribution of the Greater Vancouver population ≥age 20 (Census 1986) with that of the research sample (N=270)

2. *Age distribution.* Figure Appendix 1.7 compares the age distribution (≥20 and ≤74) in the population of Greater Vancouver (Census 1986) (left side) and in the research cohort (1987-1989) (right side). To make this comparison reasonable, 3 subjects below the age of 20 and 2 subjects above the age of 74 were omitted from the research cohort.

Figure Appendix 1.7 shows that the proportion of subjects between ages 25 and 45 in my sample well exceeded that in the general population; that the proportions in the age group 45-54 were similar; and that beyond the age of 55 the proportion of subjects of the research cohort dropped well below that of the general population. This emphasizes that for subjects in the general population who at one point or another need counseling support, the greatest need for such assistance apparently occurs in the age range of 25-45, which is the one in which career and family building figure a great deal and which therefore presents a potential for psychological bruising. In this respect I specifically screened my cohort where applicable for the presence of problems in marriage (N=140),[56] parenting (N=127),[57] full-time work (N=146)[58] or physical health (N=273).[59]

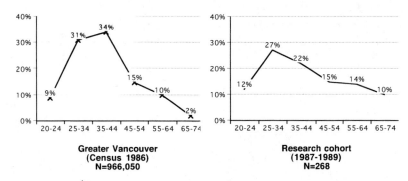

Figure Appendix 1.7: Age distribution (≥20 and ≤74 years of age) in the population of Greater Vancouver (Census 1986) (left side) and the research cohort (1987-1989) (right side)

Figure Appendix 1.8 shows that 85% of marital partners verbalized marital problems, 43% of parents mentioned problems in the relationship with their children, 52% of the fully employed subjects articulated problems at work, and 35% of the entire sample of 273 subjects voiced one or more physical complaints as, for example, headaches, diarrhea or a clear physical illness.

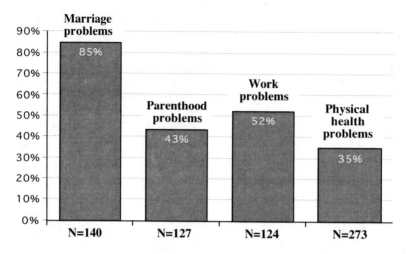

Figure Appendix 1.8: Proportion of subjects in my sample with
problems in marriage, parenting, work, or physical health

3. *Canadian-born versus foreign born.* Table Appendix 1.7 compares the ratio of
Canadian born to foreign born subjects in my sample (on whom I had relevant data
available) with the population of almost 1.4 million people of Greater Vancouver,
BC (Census 1986). It shows that the proportions of Canadian and non-Canadian
born subjects in each group is exactly the same, so that the research sample is a
precise representative of the general population of Greater Vancouver. albeit that
the Canadian province or territory of birth among Canadian-born subjects and
the country of birth among non-Canadian subjects do not necessarily coincide.

	Greater Vancouver 1986 Census		Research cohort 1987-1989		
	N	%-age	N	%-age	95% Conf.L
Canadian born:					
British Columbia	616,065	45.2%	103	38.3%	
Other Canadian provinces	354,530	26.0%	90	33.5%	
Total Canadian born	970,595	71.2%	193	71.7%	69.3%, 74.1%
Non-Canadian born					
U.S.A.	23,925	1.8%	10	3.7%	
U.K.	90,695	6.7%	22	8.2%	
Other Europe	108,980	8.0%	25	9.3%	
Other world	168,240	12.3%	19	7.1%	
Total non-Canadian born	391,840	28.8%	76	28.3%	25.9%, 30.7%
TOTAL	1,362,435	100.0%	269	100.0%	

Table Appendix 1.7: Country of birth: comparing the population of Greater Vancouver BC
(Census 1986) with the Research Cohort (1987-1989)

4. *Education.* I previously compared (Chapter 9) the educational level of 269 of
my sample on whom I had relevant data with that of the population of Greater
Vancouver BC (Census 1986). When categorizing achieved educational levels into
three groups (education below grade 9, education of grade 9-13, and having attended

college and/or university), the educational level of my subjects was very similar to that of the general population. However, a more detailed analysis of those with an educational level of grade 9 and beyond showed that in my group the proportion of those who had completed high school was higher than in the general population, and the proportion of drop-outs therefore lower; furthermore that among those who had continued their education beyond high school the proportion with a university degree was higher in my group than in the general population. In short, my sample slightly under-represents the ones who dropped out of high school and somewhat over-represents those who attained a university degree.

This tendency may well be related to the fact that most of my subjects sought professional counseling when facing problems of living and therefore apparently exhibited an inclination toward psychological sophistication that not everyone in the general population possesses.

5. *Employment status.* Table Appendix 1.8 compares the employment status of the population ≥age 15 of Greater Vancouver BC (Census 1986) with that of my 1987-1989 research sample.[60] The table indicates that the proportion that did not participate in the labor market was much higher in the general population (31.7%) than in my sample (13.9%). By contrast, the unemployment rate of the actual labor force in the general population (11.4%) was lower than among my subjects (18.7%). However, whether through unemployment or by being non-participating in the labor force, 30% of my sample was not employed, while this number was almost 40% in the general population.[61]

	Greater Vancouver 1986 Census		Research cohort 1987-1989		
	N	%-age	N	%-age	95% Conf.L
Total employed	670,805	60.5%	191	70.0%	67.5%, 72.5%
Unemployed	86,715	7.8%	44	16.1%	
Total labor force	757,525	68.3%	235	86.1%	84.7%, 87.5%
Total non-participating	351,070	31.7%	38	13.9%	12.5%, 15.3%
Total subjects	1,108,595	100.0%	273	100.0%	
Total labor force	757,525	100.0%	235	100.0%	
Unemployed	86,715	11.4%	44	18.7%	16.8%, 20.6%

Table Appendix 1.8
Employment status: comparing the population of Greater Vancouver BC
≥ age 15 (Census 1986) with the Research Cohort (1987-1989)

6. *Marital status.* I was unable to compare the marital status of the general population of Greater Vancouver ≥age 15 of 1,126,680 (1986 Census) with the relevant 1978-1989 sample (N=271). This was because my sample was denoting only 'currently married, common-law (heterosexual or homosexual), divorced or separated' and 'single subjects, rather than, as the BC Census 1986 did, 'single and never married' subjects. Furthermore, unlike my sample, the BC 'married' category did not include common law unions but included separations.

Concluding remarks

I began this Appendix with reporting the early data on the age distribution of men and women in my sample of 273 subjects because these data were for me the first dramatic proof of the reality of the alpha-beta duality. Whereas the graphs demonstrated that the group of men and of women behaved the same, they showed scientifically that the group of alphas and of betas did not, with the alpha men and women behaving the same as did the beta men and women.

The central issue in this Appendix was, however, whether the time gender distribution I found in the four-year sample of 405 consecutive referrals, as well as the various statistical analyses on the first 273 subjects, have implications for the population of Greater Vancouver BC from which these subjects derived, if not beyond.

The sample reflected a sex distribution which was similar to that of the general population of Greater Vancouver BC. Furthermore, the 1987-1989 sample of 273 subjects mirrored in many aspects the general population of Greater Vancouver BC. True, in my sample heterosexual women were slightly over-represented, and the total group of exclusive homosexuals under-represented. Also, the sample slightly under-represented those who dropped out of high school and somewhat over-represented those who attained a university degree. And the sample featured more participants in the labor market than the general population, albeit a higher unemployment rate. What appears significant, however, is the fact that the sample's proportion of subjects between ages 25 and 45 well exceeded that of the general population, for this age range has a significant potential for psychological bruising since career and family building figure a great deal during this period.

In large-scale community surveys in such North American centers as Stirling County, Baltimore, Midtown Manhattan and New Haven, it was found that just under 25% of the general population were experiencing serious problems due to the wide spectrum of psychiatric disorders. Similar European studies arrived at estimating a percentage ranging from 16-25% of the population.[62] In other words, about 25% of the North American population experiences trouble of one kind or another at any given time, so that one out of four people may be in circumstances that might require psychiatric help. This emotionally troubled quarter of the population does not reflect a steady, fixed configuration but is in constant flux.

In my view, the 273 subjects of my sample were often people who had problems in their marriage, or with their children, or job, as well as with their own personality. They frequently suffered from depressed feelings, or anxiety, or had mood swings, or drank too much, or had problems with using drugs. Some were getting into legal issues. They frequently went through stressful circumstances and had problems adjusting to this and came for some advice or emotional support. Others just wanted to find out more about themselves.

Thus these 273 subjects appeared to have constituted a reasonable sample of the fluctuating problem-ridden quarter of the general population from which they derived. As a result, the study provides strong support for the assumption that the stable distribution of time gender among the sexes which I found over the four years of data collecting applies in significant measure to the population of Greater Vancouver BC in 1986. At that time, the time gender distribution in the general population of Greater Vancouver could therefore have been 60 % alphas and 40% betas, with an alpha-beta ratio among men of 50%-50% and among women of 70%-30%.

When I previously discussed the immigration factor (Chapter 11), I noted that these data testify to a remarkable stability in the alpha-beta distribution in the four sub-groups of Canadian-born subjects (60% alphas and 40% betas) of the Vancouver sample and its four sub-groups of foreign-born subjects (58% alphas and 42% betas). This may lend some credence to the assumption that the time gender distribution of the 1987-1991 Vancouver sample may not be just a local phenomenon, but might well have significance for Canada, if not beyond.

In light of recent genetic studies, it is likely that the strong statistical connection I found between sexual gender and time gender is based on the theory that time gender is linked to the X-chromosome of which women have two (one from their father and one from their mother) and men only one (from their mother) with the alpha gene being dominant and the beta gene being recessive.

NOTES

1   The early group of 273 clients included some whom I had assessed prior to August 1, 1987 and who were still in counseling at the beginning of the intake period. Some clients in the late group of 132 clients continued counseling with me after the conclusion of my intake on July 31, 1991.

2   Pearson chi-square value=0.426, DF=1, p=0.514.

3   Pearson chi-square value=0.367, DF=1, p=0.545.

4   For example, wherever it appeared reasonable to do so, I have mentioned mean, p and t, df, 95% confidence intervals [Gardner and Altman (1989), p. 14, quoted by Morgan (1989), p. 882.] and N and variation, properly expressed [Morgan (1989), p. 881)], i.e. as standard deviation (average deviation from the mean) or standard error (for the distribution of means) [Norman and Streiner (1986), p. 20].

5   I left out three subjects below the age of 20 in order to later facilitate a comparison with the adult population of Greater Vancouver, BC, Canada, from which virtually all my clients were drawn (see later in this Appendix). Thus I was plotting 270 of my subjects in 5-year age groups from age 20 on.

6   Pearson chi-square value=11.367; DF=6; p=0.078.

7   Pearson chi-square value=35.170; DF=6; p<0.001.

8   Pearson chi-square value=3.797; DF=6; p=0.704.

9   Pearson chi-square value=6.742; DF=6; p=0.345.

10 Independent samples t-test on 123 males (mean=39.4, SD=10.99) and 147 females (mean=39.1; SD=12.72); separate variances T=0.267; DF=267.7; p=0.789; pooled variances T=0.264; DF=268; p=0.792.

11 Independent samples t-test on 159 alphas (mean=36.4, SD=10.97) and 111 betas (mean=43.3; SD=12.18); separate variances T=-4.713; DF=220.7; p<0.001; pooled variances T=-4.801f; DF=268; p<0.001.

12 102 alpha females; SD=11.709.

13 57 alpha males; SD−9.576

14 Independent samples t-test: separate variances T=-0.569; DF=136.0; p=0.570; pooled variances T=-0.537; DF=157; p=0.592.

15 45 beta females; SD=13.516.

16   66 beta males; SD=11.232.

17   Independent samples t-test: separate variances T=-0.668; DF=82.8; p=0.506; pooled variances T=-0.691; DF=109; p=0.491.

18   Of the 405 subjects (1987 - 91) 53% were female (215) [95% Confidence level 50.6% - 55.4%], and 47% male (190) [95% Confidence level 44.6% - 49.4%]. The general population of Greater Vancouver, age 20 and over (like my sample), consisted in 1986 [*Selected Characteristics for Census Tracts,* Canadian Census (1986] of 52% females, 48% males.

19   For some years I had been spending one half day per week as a jail psychiatrist serving the prisoners in the Vancouver Pre-Trial Service Centre, Vancouver, BC., Canada. These subjects were not included in the research sample.

20   This is not to say that the time gender distribution among mentally disordered persons is different from the time gender distribution of people without mental disorder. I have no information about this matter.

21   Skodol and Shrout (1989).

22   With 'general population' I mean the 'non-institutionalized population of Greater Vancouver.'

23   For example, Bland (1988) wrote that the 6 months prevalence of schizophrenia in the general population of Edmonton, Alberta, Canada, was 0.3% with, and in the Epidemiological Catchment Area (ECA) program in the US, had a low of 0.5% and a high of 1.4%.

24   For example, Bland (1988) wrote that the prevalence rate for bipolar disorder in the general population of Edmonton, Alberta, Canada, was 0.1% with, in the Epidemiological Catchment Area (ECA) program in the US, a low of 0.2% and a high of 0.9%. The prevalence rate for major depressive episodes was 3.2% in Edmonton and in the US's ECA. program a low of 2.0% and a high of 3.7%.

25   DSM-III-R (1987), p. 31.

26   DSM-III-R (1987), p. 237.

27   DSM-III-R (1987), p. 174.

28   DSM-III-R (1987), p. 185.

29   DSM-III-R (1987), p. 183.

30   DSM-III-R (1987), p. 179.

31   DSM-III-R (1987), p. 177.

32   DSM-III-R (1987), p. 176.

33   DSM-III-R (1987), p. 11.

34   The variance was 1.328 and the S.D. 1.152.

35   DSM-III-R (1987), p. 12.

36   The variance was 197.73 and the S.D. 14.062.

37   Michael, Gagnon, Laumann and Kolata (1994), p. 90.

38   For example, the 1992 *Sex in America* review [Michael, Gagnon, Laumann and Kolata (1994), p. 91, Figure 7].

39   Church (1996), p. 20.

40   Michael, Gagnon, Laumann, Kolate (1994), p.101, 105-106. They added: "These findings are confirmed by data from the General Social Survey, which reported virtually identical figures for extramarital sex." See also Smith (1991); Billy, Tanfer, Grady, Klepinger (1993).

41   Blume (1981).

42   Cahalan, Cisin and Crossley (1969)

43   Blume (1981), p. 11.

44   Blume (1981), p. 11-13; Ferrence (1980).

45   For example Browne & Finkelhor (1986); Bryer et al. (1987); Chu & Dill (1990); Brown and Anderson (1991); Paris,(1994); Paris (1996); McCauley et al. (1997).

46   See, for example: Pope Jr. and Hudson (1992). They mention prevalence rates among females in the general population of 27 - 51%.

47   Finkelhor (1984).

48   Berger et al. (1988).

49   Meyer (1985), p. 1058.

50   Meyer (1985), p. 1058.

51 Gonzalez and Zimbardo (1985), p. 22 (in excess of 95% came from North America).

52 To be precise 169 out of the 273 subjects (61.9%) lived within the City of Vancouver, 96 (35.2%) outside of the City of Vancouver but still within Greater Vancouver, while only 8 clients (2.9%) came from with British Columbia outside of Greater Vancouver.

53 Consolidated Vancouver includes the City of Vancouver, North Vancouver, West Vancouver, Burnaby, Richmond, Delta, New Westminster, Surrey, White Rock, Coquitlam, Port Coquitlam, Pitt Meadows, Maple-Ridge and the two Langleys [*Selected Characteristics for Census Tracts,* Canadian Census (1986].

54 Skodol and Shrout (1989).

55 Here the sexual gender distribution of the Greater Vancouver population ≥age 20 of 1,032,510 (1986 Census) is compared with the sexual gender distribution of the 1987-1989 research sample of 270 subjects. In the upper section of figure Appendix 1.3 the sexual gender distribution of the total population of Greater Vancouver of 1,380,730 (1986 Census) is compared with the sexual gender distribution of the 1987-1991 research sample of 405 subjects.

56 There were 144 subjects who were married (exclusive of separated subjects) or living common law, but relevant information was missing in 4 subjects); 119 subjects (85%) were verbalizing marital problems and 21 (15%) did not.

57 127 subjects had natural and/or adopted children and/or step children. Of these 55 (43%) verbalized problems in the relationship with their children and 72 (57%) did not.

58 Not included were 28 part-time employed subjects and 6 subjects on sick leave. There were 146 fully employed subjects, but relevant information was lacking in 22 (15%). Of the 124 subjects with relevant information, 65 (52%) verbalized work-related problems and 59 (48%) said they had no problems in this area.

59 Information on physical health was available on all 273 subjects; 96 (35%) had physical complaints, 177 (65%) said they did not.

60 The 191 'total employed' (70.0%) in the research cohort (1987-1989) consisted of 28 part-time employed (10.3%), 146 full-time employed (53.5%) and 17 on sick leave (6.2%). The 38 subjects who are non-participating in the labor market (13.9%) consisted of 10 students (3.7%), 10 retirees (3.7%), and 18 homemakers (6.6%).

61 To be precise, 39.49%.

62 Bland (1988).

APPENDIX 2

The Chronologic Biographic Interview[1]

1. *Introduction* (about 5 minutes): initial talk about the reason for seeing me without, however, going into the history of the presenting problem;

2. *Personal calendar* (25-30 minutes): constructing a framework of successive personal milestones. This is the backbone of my chronologic, biographic history. It is based on a series of questions, the answers to which are re-arranged into a *personal calendar*, involving the following four steps:

2.1. *Columnizing:* setting up *three* parallel columns, as follows:

2.1.1. *calendar column:* the *calendar year* in which a personal event took place, because people remember some events as *calendar-related*— *"this happened in 1945, that in 1934,"* for example. In addition, the *calendar year* may also define the society at the time; the 1930s were depression years, 1939-1945 World War II, the mid 1950s until 1975 the Vietnam War, 1956 the year of the Hungarian uprising against the Soviets, the 1960s the years of the flower children, and so on.

2.1.2. *age column:* the *biological age* of the client at the time; since people remember some events as *age-related: "I was 18 when that happened"* or *"I was just turning forty."* It indicates at the same time the stage in the lifecycle in which the personal milestone occurred (e.g. puberty, midlife);

2.1.3. *milestone column:* a *description of the personal milestone.* This column also accommodates that people may remember some milestones *not* as calendar-, or age-related, but in a sequence with other personal milestones; *"this happened in the year father died,"* for example, or *"that took place during the time we were living in Yonge Street;" "that occurred when I was working at the bank;"* or *"when that happened our second child was born already."*

2.2. *Questioning:* translating the circumscribed answers to the following seven groups of questions into this *three-column personal calendar* format (generally leaving any detailed information for later):

> The art of the game is to unfold this calendar on paper in such fashion that one does not get crammed for space. On the average, ten years of life per page works out reasonably well, particularly when only using one side of the paper, leaving the opposite side free in case more space is needed.

2.2.1. *place and year of birth;* "Where were you born, when were you born?" and

"How long did you live there? Where did you move then? " If the birthplace is unfamiliar, ask for some descriptive details (big or small city, rural, etc.).

2.2.2. *religious history;* In which religion were you born, if any? Is it still important? Did they quit? When and why? Any changes in religion and how so? How important is religion to them now? What does this involved? Are they actively involved? Do they pray? When?

> Mental health workers rarely explore their clients' *religious history.* I added it because, for in the cultural matrix in which the client grew up, the religious background and early programming — Roman Catholic, Orthodox Jewish, fundamentalist protestant, Sikh, Moslem, Hindu, Ismali, Bahai, for example — is of major significance. Changing one's religious attitude indicates a major change and one should inquire what triggered this. If presently active in a religious group it is important to know what this involves. Faith healing? Predestination?

2.2.3. *family history (parents, siblings).* The *family history* is a succinct discussion of the members and nature of the family they were born into and grew up in, including relations with parents, siblings and significant others, if any. Was there fostering, adoption, a step-parent? As to the *father:* "Is father still alive?" and if so "Is he healthy, what is his age" If he died, "when did he die, at what age, what was the cause of death, how long was he ill?" Also, "what is (was) his job?" "How do you describe him as a person?" "How close are (were) you to him?" As to the *mother:* repeat same questions as to the father. Note the age difference between father and mother, i.e. Mother (-2 years). "Try to describe the kind of marriage your parents had." List *siblings* and client in birth order (No. 1, 2, 3 etc.), nothing for each their first name, gender, how much older (e.g. +3) or younger (e.g. -2) than patient they are, their state of health, dates of death and cause; whether they are married with children; their general area of residence, their job; and a short indication of their personality and how close to the client each of them is.

2.2.4. *educational history;* I ask about Kindergarten and elementary school(s): when started-when finished; grades reached and repeated. The same about high school(s) or alternative(s) and higher education or alternative(s), including diplomas, degree(s).

2.2.5. *occupational history;* I asked about which job(s) they held and now hold; when these started and finished; promotions; periods of unemployment.

2.2.6. *marriage & children;* When married or common-law? Divorce(s), separations? When did they first meet? Age difference with partner(s)? When were children born? Sex, first name? When did they leave home; what are they doing? Where living now? Grandchildren?

2.2.7. *residential history;* beginning at birth and ending in the present: where and when did they live for how long, including cities with residences in that area, and countries? How long?

Mental health professionals often omit the *residential history* but I consider it very significant, for it is the only stream of life events that cuts across all others and, therefore, is important in establishing a personal time frame.

Table Appendix 2.1 demonstrates how answers to the preceding seven groups of questions translate into the personalized, three-column personal calendar of a 73 year old man whom I saw in 1978.

A calendar year	B biological age	C personal milestones with personal sequencing as applicable
1905	0 (now 73)	Born in London, UK; Anglican
		F.(+2):*1875; died age 75, 1950 (ca. bowel); retired bookkeeper; aloof, strict, short with money, not close to client
		M.(-2);*1873; died age 46, 1919 (typhoid fever); housewife,; warm, affectionate, close to client
		S.: 1. male (+2); John; x, 3 kids, healthy7, engineer, Toronto; outgoing; rather close.
		2. Client
		3. female (-3), Mary, died age 24, accident; secretary, single; rather shy; not close.
		4. male (-7), William; alive, healthy; x, 2 kids; chemist; rather moody, nervouse; relation with client so-so.
1908	3	Mary (-3) born
1910	5	To Kindergarten
1911	6	To public school
1912	7	William (-7) born
1917	12	To high school
1919	14	Mother died (typhoid fever); loses faith in Anglican Church.
1920	15	gr.9; family London->Toronto, Canada; Yonge Street x 6 yrs with father and sibs
1923	18	grade 12 -> University of Toronto (general arts); at home
1926	21	B.A..->teaching 1 yr in public school (Toronto); own aprtmt on Jarvis Street
1927	22	University of Toronto (MA English); living in residence
1929	24	Mary (-3) died (accident); meets future wife, June (-2), also teacher
1930	25	M.A.; high school teacher, english, school (A), Toronto x 6 yrs; marries June (-2) ->aprmnt on Ave Road x 3 yrs; June working
1931	26	1st child Michael; now age 47, x 2 kids; insurance salesman; in Saskatchewan; good relation, writes often, occasionally visits; June stops working
1933	28	Buys own house at Flat Street x 10 yrs; 2nd child John, now age 45, x, divorced; 2nd marriage, 3 kids; high school teacher, Hamilton; relation distant
1936	31	To school B (Head, English Dpt), Toronto, x 3 yrs; Peter born (No.3); now age 41, single, at CBC, Toronto; visits often; a bit argumentative
1939	34	4th child, Theresa; now age 39, x and divorced, one child; advertising agency; Toronto; regular contact, "has her own mind". Joins Army (Tank brigade, 2nd Lieutenant -> UK.
1943	38	1st Lieutednant -> Italy, France, Holland
1945	40	->Captain ->to school B, Toronto (Head English Dpt); to own home at Riddel Street (x 25 yrs)
1948	43	Father sick (ca. bowel)
1950	45	Father died (ca. bowel); Michael, age 19 (No.1) leaves home ->university
1951	46	Vice-principal School B
1953	48	John, age 20 (No.2) leaves home (marries)
1954	49	Principal School C, Toronto x 16 yrs
1958	53	Theresa, age 19 (No. 4) leaves home; secretary
1960	55	Peter, age 24 (No. 3) leaves home (under pressure)
1970	65	Retired, involved in farm (Collingwood, ON); service clubs

Table Appendix 2.1: An example of a complete personal calendar

2.3. *Window-sorting:* delineating in a completed *personal calendar* of *milestones* a meaningful succession of circumscribed *life-periods* or *time windows.*

Table Appendix 2.2 reflects an example of sub-dividing the personal calendar of a 73-year-old male I saw in 1978 into time windows.

calendar years	age	time window of personal calendar of milestones
1905-1911	0-6	Preschool years
1911-1917	6-12	Elementary school years
1917-1920	12-15	High school years in London, UK
1920-1923	15-18	High school years in Toronto, Canada
1923-1930	18-25	University years
1930-1939	25-34	Pre-war high school teacher and early marriage years
1939-1945	34-40	War years
1945-1953	40-49	Post-war years at school B
1953-1970	49-65	Years as principal at school C
1970-1978	65-73	Retirement

Table Appendix 2.2: An example of sub-dividing a personal calendar into time windows

2.4. *Lifecycling:* The sequence of personal *time windows* naturally unfolds against the background of the *life cycle* — the developmental progression from infancy (0-2) to early childhood (2-6), middle childhood (6-12), adolescence (12-18), early adulthood (18-25), adulthood (24-40), midlife (40-55) and maturity (>55). Each phase of the life cycle defines its own bodily state; level of intellectual, emotional and interpersonal functioning; and imposes its own social expectations. A four-year old, for example, uses a different kind of logic and way of organizing the reality, and has different emotional needs and ways of relating to the environment and has to grapple with different social expectations than an eleven or twenty-four year old or a person in the fifties.

Table Appendix 2.3 shows how inserting the life cycle supplements the time windows in the personal calendar of my given example.

calendar years	age	personal calendar with life cycle in mind	
1905-1911	0-6	Preschool, including	
		0-2	*infancy*
		2-6	*early childhood*
1911-1917	6-12	*middle childhood*	
		6-12	Elementary school years
	12-18	*adolescence,*	including
1917-1920		12-15	High school years in London, UK
1920-1923		15-18	High school years in Toronto, Canada
1923-1930	18-25	*early adulthood,*	including
		18-25	University years
	24-40	*adulthood,*	including
1930-1939		25-34	Pre-war high schoo teacher at school A and early marriage years
1939-1945		34-40	War years
	40-55	*midlife,*	including
1945-1953		40-49	Post-war years at school
1953-1970		49-65	Years as principal at school C
	> 55	*maturity,*	including
1970-1978		65-73	Retierment

Table 2.3: An example of the time windows of a personal calendar with the life cycle in mind

3. *Stress and strain history* (25-30 minutes): it completes the integrated life history by taking the client from birth until the history of the present problem through a *window-by-window review* of a *stress-and-strain-grit* of questions, inserting emerging

data as we go along:

I use the empty page opposite the personal calendar as needed.

3.1. *unfocused, spontaneous memories;* In other words, encouraging in a time window an *unfocused* mode of autobiographic recall. For example, "Do you have any memories whatever from the days before you went to school, anything at all?" Or "What sort of memories come to mind when you think back to your days in the Army?"

3.2. *focused memories:*

3.2.1. *elaborating on relevant milestones;* for example, when encountering *educational* milestones, how well did they do in public school, for example, or high school, with higher education? Any learning problems? Did they have to study hard? Did it come milestones, where they happy in their work? How did they get along with their peers and superiors? Did they climb the ladder? If there were there frequent job changes, why? If there was unemployment between jobs, how did this affect them? In meeting *residential* milestones, why the move? Did they like it? In encountering *children,* what is each child like and what kind of relationship do they have with them? What is the story of their health and happiness or lack thereof?

3.2.2. *significant interpersonal relations;* for example, in the earlier school days, how was the relation with father and mother and siblings? Who was the favorite of whom? Who the villain? How did they get along with the boys and girls in the neighborhood, and with teachers? During high school days: did they date, have many friends or were they loners? Were they leaders, followers? In job situations: how did they get along with the people above and below them and with their peers? In their marriage: what is their relationship with their marital partner, their children, in-laws, their siblings and parents? And so on.

Throughout successive time windows we may begin to see some patterns emerging which began in childhood and are being carried forward into intimate relations, the parent-child relation, the work situation, and so on.

3.2.3. defining external historic circumstances; for example, how did the depression years affect them? How the war years? Or questions related to any turmoil in the country they were living in during this time window, as the Soviet invasion of Czechoslovakia (presently the Czech and Slovak Republics), for instance. If they were in their teens during the 1960s, did they use any drugs? And so on.

This reflects the impact of a dysfunctional society, if any; as in the depression years, World War II, the Vietnam war, for example.

3.2.4. *relevant life cycle issues* that have not yet been touched on. For example, during the *preschool period* and thereafter did they have a bedwetting problem? In the teens, with girls: when did they begin to menstruate; had she been prepared? How did she react? With boys: had they been told they would have nocturnal emissions? Was it frightening, reassuring? For boys and girls: how did they obtain their sexual knowledge? This is a good place to extend the *sexual history* somewhat *backward:* what are their first memories of solitary or shared sexual experiences? What are the earliest memories having anything to do with sexuality? Any sexual childhood play? Any traumatic stuff? And *forward:* What kind of solitary and interpersonal sexual experiences including dating evolved during adolescence and later in adulthood? Any premarital experience? Any unforeseen pregnancies, any abortions? What is the history and are the positive and negative aspects of their present and preceding heterophile or homophile intimate partnerships, if any. And what is or was the personality of their partner? Any extra-marital involvement?

3.2.5. *emotional and physical state* at the time with reasons. Concerning *physical* well-being: was there in this time window any major illnesses, hospitalization, operation? What was the experience like? What about alcohol and drugs, or brushes with the law? Concerning *emotional* well-being: was the time window generally happy or unhappy? Why? In the most recent time window, the history of the presenting problem will thus unfold as an inseparable, interwoven part of the client's entire life rather than as an isolated subject-compartment.

This section of the stress-and-strain grit provides how the client's defines psychosocial factors that provide need satisfaction and those that create stress and strain. It also provides information about the relation between psychosocial distress and physical illness, if any. Clients are often unaware of their vulnerabilities and resiliences and what favors their well-being and what promotes ill health. The Cornell Medical Project Study showed that clusters of ill physical health in given time windows suggest a high probability of emotional maladjustment during such phase.[2] The Yale Medical Center Study showed that just before a surgical-medical illness become apparent, patients have a significant increase in psychological symptoms compared with the general population.[3] Others supported that observation, concluding that physical illness of any kind can be preceded by psychological distress that produces a "giving up reaction," a response of despair and apathy.[4]

NOTES

1   Pos (1978).
2   Hinkle (1961).
3   Duff and Hollingshead (1968).
4   Engel (1968).

APPENDIX 3

Summary Of Time Gender Features

This Appendix summarizes and compares most behavioral and experiential tendencies of alphas and betas. This may assist one in viewing one's own or someone else's personality through the paradigm of the time gender model, as depicted in Figure Appendix 3.1.

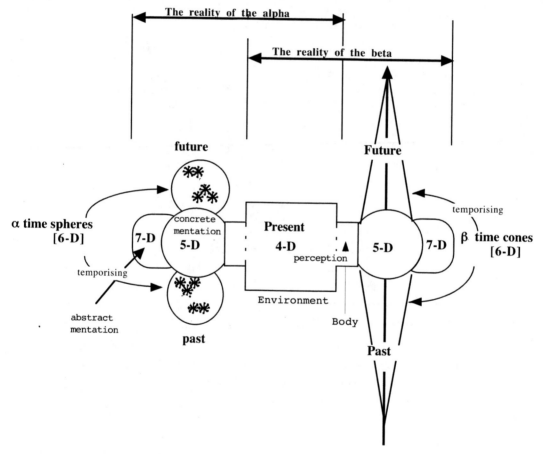

Figure Appendix 3.1:The complete time gender model with it's four attention modes:
4-D, 5-D, 6-D, and 7-D

SUMMARY OF FEATURES OF THE ALPHA TIME GENDER

The fundamental time gender difference between alphas and betas originates in the different structure of their 6-D, as follows.

274

1. experiencing time:

1.1. timestructure: alphas experience time as a succession of discontinuous events or time fragments;

1.2. timeexperience: for alphas only the present is real, the past ("once upon a time") and future ("one day") are mythological;

1.3. life story: their autobiography has a flexible time order with alpha amnesia (a greater memory decay of life vignettes), while retained life vignettes often are unemotional.

2. preferred attention mode: 4-D (the here-and-now)

2.1. dynamismof renewal: alphas live a day at a time.

2.2. vulnerability and resilience: over time, alphas are relatively vulnerable to the consequences of in-attending to what happened in the past, or to what may happen in the future. And they are relatively vulnerable to negative present circumstances. If their 4-D varies a great deal between being positive and negative, they are prone to mood swings; if the present is predominantly negative, they are subject to a situational depression. They are relatively resilient in the face of past traumatic or rewarding experiences, or future promises and threats;

2.3. need for control: alphas tend to maintain a continuous vigilance in 4-D, and a relentless pursuit toward their best possible control of 4-D;

2.4. motivation: they are externally driven, rather than internally by past rewards or traumas, or future promises or threats. They tend to have few future-oriented forethoughts and often little foresight, and they devote little afterthought to what they have done or what happened before; they use little hindsight. In other words, alphas are time-blind, so to speak. Taking pleasure in the subject or activity they are currently involved in motivates them ("do I like what I am doing?"), as does the potential for improving their control over their 4-D, or for obtaining situational self esteem in the here-and-now. Indeed, their craving for external situational self esteem is strong.

2.5. curiosity: because alphas are not constantly distracted by their 6-D, they have space in their head, so to speak, and therefore crave in their work and recreation varied, if not exciting, input. This presents them not only as restlessly curious by nature, and rather intolerant of prolonged familiar situations, but also as having more vitality.

2.6. thinking: the 7-D thinking of alphas is 4-D-oriented (extroverted) and therefore takes its lead from 4-D, rendering their thinking fact oriented, pragmatic, empirical, experimental, deductive, and a posteriori in nature. Furthermore, because of the discontinuity of their intellectual 6-D, their 6-D contents need not be intellectually coherent and integrated, which leaves alphas with a tolerance for cognitive dissonance in their 6-D. This, in turn, leaves lots of room for variety of input to satisfy their natural curiosity. Hence, they are accumulators of a broad range of facts, particularly if they are highly intelligent and therefore tend toward intellectual restlessness. Unless they really like a subject, they soon become bored with it, and therefore do not necessarily pursue in depth the quality of relevant knowledge.

2.7. tacticalapproach toward 4-D: alphas are specialists in dealing with the immediacy of 4-D, the here-and-now. Their social perceptiveness tends to be broadly inclusive. Because they are contextually highly sophisticated, they are born actors who are good at manipulating 4-D. Since they tend to be more action-oriented, if not more impulsive, than deliberate and thoughtful, they are natural tacticians, so to speak. Sometimes they become bold and high-risk taking, competent entrepreneurs. Frequently, their life style is crisis-oriented.

3. identity structure: the identity of alphas is equally contextually partitioned, that is context-bound and multifocal, based on their contextually partitioned, time-wise discontinuous 6-D;

3.1. personality: the paradigm according to which alphas think, feel, and act in one context is different from the paradigm they use to do so in another. As a result, they have a contextual perspective on their reality. If self-aware of this, their tolerance for cognitive dissonance between contexts usually shows: "This is how the world is." Sometimes, however, their partitioned, context-bound, multifocal identity, becomes disturbing to them, and their central existential problem then becomes: "Who is the real me?"

3.2. socialvalue system: Conscious preoccupation with their value system—their set of internalized rules about the social desirability or undesirability of potential behaviors—usually does not play a major role in the life of alphas. Because of their partitioned 6-D, their Ideal Self, which personifies their value system (and which, in the beginning largely represents the values of their superego, voice of conscience, or inner parent), is situational, and therefore contextually partitioned and multifocal in nature. This presents a natural potential for significant inconsistency between the values alphas apply in different contexts. In the absence of a timescape, alphas (that is, their paraego) usually remain unaware of this, but if they gain insight into this matter through external feedback, for example, alphas usually, and understandably, accept it as a normal fact of life.

The fact that, when alphas move from one context to another, they make intuitive adjustments to their values and thus their Ideal Self, demonstrates a conspicuous flexibility in their value system is. Given this flexibility, and their corresponding freedom from an overall, systematized internal structure of rules, alphas frequently do not mind having to rely upon a system of external rules in their environment. Indeed, they often prefer to do so. Once the social value system in a particular context is settled, however, alphas tend to be rather inflexible, if not intolerant, toward others, who apply different values in that situation. Indeed, alphas then often attack those others on their ethics, rather than on their actions. For, although they consider their own values superior to, and therefore taking precedence over, the "deviating" values of others, exhibiting values contrary to their own constitutes a personal threat in that it questions the rationale of their own values.

This is, however, not always the case. As a result of persistent external criticism, combined with self reflection (as sometimes happens to mid-adolescents, for example), alphas sometimes may begin to experience a particular dominant contextual value system in a negative way. Or they may, indeed, become troubled by the inconsistencies in their overall value system. Thus they may be left to wonder: "Which values do, or should, I really stand for?" By joining in those circumstances a group with an outspoken, rigid value system, a particular religious sect, for example (or in younger people, even a gang), some go through a wholesale exchange of values and lifestyle. For, this group provides them not only with a ready-made value system which, in their view, unquestionably holds precedence over the value system of "outsiders," but also provides them with an entity-derived identity that sets them apart from "outsiders." In those cases, some indeed end up feeling genuinely reborn. Yet their new identity and value system do not dissolve the preceding partitioned nature of their identity and Ideal Self, of course, but simply overlay the old ones, at least for the time being.

3.3. <u>thinking</u>: the partitioned, contextual nature of their 7-D thinking gives alphas not only a tolerance for cognitive dissonance between contexts, but also provides any particular contextual thinking with its 6-D-paradigm which makes only context-specific intellectual 6-D contents available and, as a result, supplies the thinking of alphas with its contextual perspective.

4. **planning for the future:** alphas do not relate emotionally to the future in a sustained fashion and, as a result, do not follow through on working persistently toward any future goal they may have set at some point. Nor are they motivated to struggle to overcome any obstacles in the way of their goal. When obstacles appear, they often shift to some other goal, or simply give up. In other words, when left to their own resources, realistic planning for the future, including the various steps involved, and follow through, is not their strong suit, unless they like whatever they are doing and have enough innate ability to do so with relative ease. Otherwise, to actually achieve any goal they pursue, alphas need ongoing external backing and intercession to keep them from derailing. The latter is why they usually do well in a social structure, as in a corporation or private boarding school, for example, which has built-in goals and reinforces, if not imposes, its future goals on a day to day basis. Occasionally, however, alphas may develop a persistent strategic vision of

their future, and pursue this vision persistently and with considerable energy, as if following a Star of Bethlehem, so to speak, rather than following realistic, step-by-step planning. As a result, they may follow highly unorthodox ways and, if their environment allows for this, and their luck holds out, they may be very successful. Since this approach lacks precise and realistic planning, their dream for the future misfires, however, more often than not.

5. social behavior:

5.1. theneed for solitude versus interaction: in alphas, the need for social interaction outweighs their need for solitude.

5.2. theneed for individuality versus group membership: In terms of I-consciousness versus We-consciousness, the need to be part of an emotionally significant group with which alphas can identify exceeds their need to experience themselves, and be seen as and behave as, an individual. Belonging to a group or institution which, in their eyes, is highly respected, contributes ongoingly to their situational self esteem and thus to their well-being and their protection against alienation. Institutional or group objectives and rules are therefore more important than allowing for individual initiatives. In the final analysis, the group or organization provides them with a secure and respectable identity which sets them apart from outsiders. Membership in the group or organization should therefore outweigh the individual needs of its members. This is the price one should be willing to pay for belonging to that group.

5.3. extrovertedinterpersonal style.

5.4. authoritarian-competitiveinterpersonal style: power is first and foremost to be enjoyed, to guarantee one's sense of security of mind (giving one control over one's 4-D) and to provide one with ongoing situational self esteem. Alphas enjoy the role of power-broker.

5.5. blame-assigning: given their 4-D-orientation, alphas in interpersonal conflicts tend to assign blame to the other party, rather than to themselves. They tolerate criticism poorly.

5.6. time gender linguistics: these extroverts use flexible, situational, alpha speak with context-related word meanings, which is audience-oriented, and tends to make them into expert communicators who, at a given occasion, use the right word at the right time. This, together with their vitality, sometimes gives them a charismatic quality.

5.7. empathydeficiency: they readily alphacize betas. Because their primary need to belong, based on their extroverted orientation, makes individuality only secondary to group identity, it is harder for them to recognize the behavior pattern of the opposite time gender than it is for betas to do so.

SUMMARY OF FEATURES OF THE BETA TIME GENDER

The fundamental time gender difference between alphas and betas originates in the different structure of their 6-D, as follows.

1. experiencing time:

1.1. time structure: betas experience the imminence of a past-present-future continuity;

1.2. time experience: for betas time is enduring and past and future are therefore historic;

1.3. lifestory: their autobiography has a chronological time order, based on personal milestones, with beta hypermnesia (a greater memory retention of life vignettes), and their life vignettes are often emotionally charged.

2. preferred attention mode: 6-D (their timescape)

2.1. dynamismof stability: betas live in their timescape (their imminent past-present-future);

2.2. vulnerability and resilience: over time, betas are relatively vulnerable to the consequences of in-attending to what has been happening in the present. And they are relatively vulnerable if their timescape reflects a negative past or future. They are relatively resilient, however, in the face of a negative present, provided they can see light at the end of the tunnel. Given that their dominant mood, whether positive or negative, is often timescape-related, their dominant mood tends to be stable. When their mood is negative it may reflect a timescape-oriented depression;

2.3. need for control: betas tend to maintain a continuous vigilance in 6-D, and a relentless pursuit toward their best possible control of 6-D;

2.4. motivation: they are internally driven by future promises or threats, as well as past rewards or traumas, rather than externally by what is happening in their 4-D. As a result, their motivation is usually interwoven with future-oriented forethoughts, while recollections about what they have done or what happened before (hindsight) may also play an important role. That is, betas have time distance perception, so to speak. Their motivation depends far less on whether the activity they are currently involved in is pleasurable or not, but rather on the potential for improving their control over their 6-D and obtaining global self esteem ("Is what I am doing good for me?"). Rather than craving for external situational self esteem, their craving for internal global self esteem is strong.

2.5. curiosity: the fact that betas are constantly distracted by their 6-D leaves them with less space in their head, and tends to put a brake on their 4-D input. They therefore look in their recreation for quiet enjoyment, generally speaking, rather than for varied and excitement-producing input (unless they seek to counteract their preoccupation with 6-D). Their inclination toward continuous involvement with familiar situations in their work renders them less curious toward 4-D, and makes them appear more reserved.

2.6. <u>thinking</u>: the 7-D thinking of betas is 6-D-oriented (introverted) and therefore takes its lead from their timescape, particularly its intellectual aspects. This renders their thinking idea-oriented, rational, theoretical, inductive, and a priori in nature. Because of their intellectual timescape, their 6-D contents furthermore need to be intellectually coherent and integrated, which leaves betas with an intolerance for cognitive dissonance in their 6-D, puts a brake on the variety of subject matter they want to be concerned with and, if they are highly intelligent, gives their thinking a unifying and integrating quality, making them pattern builders. Since they are able to maintain their intellectual focus, their knowledge tends to be more in depth than broad-based.

2.7. <u>strategicapproach toward 4-D</u>: betas are specialists in dealing with the future in 6-D. Their social perceptiveness is focused accordingly, and therefore selective, which may leave them somewhat uncomfortable and awkward in contexts they do not view in line with their future goals. This lack of overall contextual sophistication makes them poor actors. Since their lifestyle is, as a rule, future-oriented, they tend not to be action-oriented, let alone impulsive. Rather, their actions in 4-D come across as thoughtful and deliberate and they are, generally speaking, risk averse. In short, they are natural strategists.

3. identity structure: based on their timescape in 6-D, the identity of betas is contextually unified (trans-contextual), and monofocal, rather than context-bound;

3.1. <u>personality</u>: betas tend to think, feel, and act in all contexts in a relatively systematic fashion. As a result, they have a global perspective on their reality with an intolerance for cognitive dissonance: "one should be consistent in how one views the world." When betas become aware of their identity as being global and continuous, their central existential problem is: "How can I make myself more consistent?"

3.2. <u>socialvalue system</u>: Conscious preoccupation with their value system—their set of internalized rules about the social desirability or undesirability of potential behaviors—usually plays an important role in the life of betas. Because of their timescape their Ideal Self, which personifies their value system (and which, in the beginning largely represents the values of their superego, voice of conscience or inner parent), becomes progressively more global and monofocal in nature over time. For as the timescape of adolescent betas gradually grows and they become self-reflective, they (their paraego, that is) may become aware of inconsistencies between the values they apply in different contexts, that is in their overall value system. These conscious value conflicts in their timescape (between their superego and paraego) detract from their global self esteem, and they experience this as a personal problem which they can deal with only by amending their future actions in line with their global Ideal Self, that is by incorporating aspects of their paraego (or voice of reason) in their Ideal Self. Seeking a solution for these value conflicts by joining, and identifying with, a group with an outspoken, rigid value system, never solves them, for it would mean a wholesale exchange of values and lifestyle, a rebirth, so to speak, which is at odds with the enduring reality of their timescape and the sense of individuality it represents.

The intolerance for value conflicts in their timescape betas exhibit over the years naturally increases their consistency in overall values. This is also, however, accompanied by an increasing tendency toward inflexibility, if not rigidity, in adhering to these values, leaving them with little leeway for adjustment when facing environs with values that conflict with their own. This is why betas do not like external rules in their social environment (their work place, for example) since these are often bound to conflict with their own overall value system. Anyway, typical for betas is to hang onto their values for better or worse, sometimes making them heroes, sometimes leaving them abandoned dysfunctionals. However, since betas hold their own individuality in high regard they tend, by extension, to respect the individuality of others and are therefore, despite their inflexible attitude toward their own values, rather tolerant of others who have different value systems.

Their rigid adherence to their own values does not necessarily mean, however, that betas do not make changes in their value system as they grow older. They certainly may benefit from considerable self-reflection, life experience, and eventually appreciating that progression in the life cycle from childhood to maturity naturally should include changes in values. This may help their Voice of Reason, their paraego, to mature and gain more and more influence in their Ideal Self and the evolving value system it personifies, so that, eventually, their paraego comes to outweigh the influence over their superego on their Ideal Self.

3.3. <u>thinking</u>: because the 7-D thinking of betas is oriented toward their singular, unpartitioned timescape, particularly its intellectual contents, it does not remain contextually focused, but soon moves beyond its immediate starting context toward a wider, more global perspective. This makes their thinking not only intolerant of cognitive dissonance between contexts, but may also give it a historic perspective.

4. **planning for the future:** their timescape enables them to relate emotionally to the future in a sustained fashion and, as a result, betas usually follow through spontaneously on working persistently toward any future goal, so that they are motivated to struggle to overcome any obstacles in their way. Their need for ongoing external backing and intervention is negligible. They may, indeed, view

a social structure that imposes future goals which deviate from their own as just another obstacle they must overcome. In short, realistic planning for the future, including the various steps involved, and follow-through, is one of their strong suits. Although betas may have strategic visions, they soon underpin such visions with a realistic, step-by-step planning process.

5. social behavior:

5.1. the need for solitude versus interaction: in betas, the need for solitude outweighs their need for social interaction.

5.2. the need for individuality versus group membership: In terms of I-consciousness versus We-consciousness, betas are typical individualists. Given their timescape, experiencing themselves (and by extension others) as individually unique and wanting to act and be treated as an individual in one's own right, exceeds their need to be part of an emotionally significant group with which they can identify. Although betas may be very proud of a group or institution they belong to, institutional or group objectives and rules should not interfere with their individual initiatives and success, which are more important to their global self esteem than belonging to the group or institution itself. For in the final analysis, their individualism, not the group, is what gives them their identity. For betas, the price of belonging to the group has therefore its limits. This naturally sets them apart from alphas within that group or organization.

5.3. introverted interpersonal style.

5.4. authoritarian-competitive interpersonal style may be present; egalitarian-cooperative interpersonal style is optional; power is there to facilitate the realization of future goals and is, as such, a responsibility which, in itself, does not contribute a great deal to one's global self esteem. In leadership positions, betas tend to be consensus builders.

5.5. blame-assigning in interpersonal conflicts: given their 6-D-orientation, betas tend to assign blame to themselves, rather than to the other party. They may accept criticism, albeit often defensively so.

5.6. time gender linguistics: since their beta speak has fixed word meanings which are not context-related, and their introverted language is usually more self-directed, and therefore rather idiosyncratic (instead of audience-oriented) they are, as a rule, mediocre communicators. To change this for the better is not impossible, but may require major effort.

5.7. empathy deficiency: they readily betacize alphas. Because of their adherence to individualism, based on their monofocal identity, they are more open to recognizing the behavior pattern of the opposite time gender than it is for alphas to do so.

BIBLIOGRAPHY

Addison, P.: *Churchill on the Home Front, 1900-1955.* London: Cape, 1992.

Allport, G. W. *Pattern And Growth In Personality.* New York: Holt, Rinehart and Winston, 1961.

Ames, L. B.: "The development of the sense of time in the young child." *J genet Psychol,* 68 (1946): 97-125

Andreasen, N. C., D. S. O'Leary, T. Cizadlo, S. Arndt, K Rezai, G. L. Watkins, L. L. Boles Ponto and R. D. Hichwa: "Remembering the past: two facets of episodic memory explored with positron emission tomography." *Am J Psychiatry* 152 (1995), 11: 1576-1585.

Anthony, E. J.: "Piaget." *Brit Med Psychol* (29) (1956): 1.

Argyle, M.: *The psychology of happiness.* London: Methuen & Co, 1987.

Aris, D. J. B.: "Wet and wetshandhaving: sociaal gedrag." Utrecht: *Unpublished paper,* 1998 (a).

————: Personal communication (2000).

————: *Hersenspinsels: bouwstenen voor de psychologie.* CD v.0.01, 21 Augustus 2002.

Arnstein, R. L.: "The adolescent identity crisis revisited. In: S. C. Feinstein and P. L. Giovacchini (eds): Adolescent Psychiatry (volume 7). Chicago, IL: The University of Chicago Press, 1979: 71-84.

Attlee, C. "The Churchill I knew." in: *Churchill by His Contemporaries.* London: Hodder and Stoughton (1965)

Azari, N. P., K. D. Pettigrew, P. Pietrini, D. G. Murphy, B. Horwitz and M. D. Shapiro: "Sex differences in patterns of hemispheric cerebral metabolism: a multiple regression/discriminant analysis of positron emission tomographic data. *Int J Neurosc.* 1995 Mar; 81 (1-2): 1-20.

Baddeley, A.: *Working Memory.* Oxford: Oxford University Press, 1986.

Bahn, P. G.: "Foreword" in: J-M. Chauvet, E. Brunel Deschamps and C. Hillaire: *Dawn of Art: The Chauvet Cave; The oldest known paintings in the World.* New York: Harry N. Abrams, Incorporated, 1996; p. 7-12.

Bar-Yosef, O. and B. Vandermeersch: "Modern humans in the Levant." *Scientific American,* April 1993: 94-100.

Barnett, L.: *The Universe and Dr. Einstein.* New York: The New American Library of World Literature, Inc., 1958.

Baumgartner, P. and F. S. Perls : *Gifts from Lake Cowichan and legacy from Fritz.* Palo Alto, Ca.: Science & Behaviour Books Inc., 1975.

Beahrs, J. O.: *Unity and Multiplicity: Multilevel Consciousness of Self in Hypnosis, Psychiatric Disorder and Mental Health.* New York: Brunner/Mazel, 1982.

Beard, R. M.: *An Outline of Piaget's Developmental Psychology For Students and Teachers.* New York: The New American Library, Inc., 1972.

Becker, E.: *The Denial of Death.* New York: The Free Press, 1973.

Bengtsson, S., H. Berglund, B. Gulyas, E. Cohen and I. Savic: "Brain activation during odor perception in males and females." *Neuroreport.* 2001 Jul 3; 12(9): 2027-2033.

Berger, A. M., J. F. Knutson, J. G. Mehm and K. A. Perkins: "The self-report of punitive childhood experiences of young adults and adolescents." *Child Abuse Negl* 1988; 12:251-262.

Berk, L. E.: "Why children talk to themselves." *Scientific American,* 271 (1994), 5: 78-83.

Berne, E.: *Transactional Analysis in Psychotherapy.* New York: Grove Press, 1961.

Bettelheim, B.: "Obsolete youth." In: S. C. Feinstein, P. L. Giovacchini and A. A. Miller (eds): *Adolescent Psychiatry (volume 1).* Chicago, IL: The University of Chicago Press, 1971: 14-39.

Billy, J. O., K. Tanfer, W. R. Grady and D. H. Klepinger: "The sexual behavior of men in the United States." *Fam Plann Perspect* 25(1993):52-60.

Binford, S. R.: "A structural comparison of disposal of the dead in the Mousterian and the Upper Paleolithic." *Southwestern J. Anthropol.* 24(1968): 139-154.

Bland, R. C.:"Psychiatric Epidemiology." *Can J Psychiatry* 33 (1988): 618-625

Block, J. A.: "A contrarian view of the five-factor approach to personality description." *Psychol Bull* 117 (1995): 187-215.

Blotkey, M. and J. Looney: "Normal female and male adolescent psychological development help to clarify Jung's argument." In: S. C. Feinstein, P. L. Giovacchini, J. G. Looney, A. Z. Schwartzberg and A. D. Sorosky (eds): *Adolescent psychiatry (volume 8).* Chicago IL: The University of Chicago Press, 1980: 184-199.

Blume, S.: "National patterns of alcohol use and abuse." In: R. B. Millman, P. Cushman, Jr., J. H. Lowinson (eds): Research developments in drug and alcohol use. *Annals of the New York Academy of Sciences.* New York: New York Academy of Sciences, 1981: ANYAA 362, 1, p. 4-15.

Boernstein, W. S.: "Perceiving and thinking: their interrelationship and organismic organization." pp. 673-681 in E. Harms and M. E. Tresselt (Eds): "Third conference on the fundamentals of psychology: various approaches to the study of perception." *Annals New York Academy of Sciences:* 169 (1970), 3: 595-738.

Boule, M. and H. V. Vallois: "Fossil monkeys and apes" in *Human Evolution,* eds. N. Korn and H. Reece Smith, 227-230, New York: Henry Hold and Company, 1959.

Bowman, M. L.: "Individual differences in posttraumatic distress: problems with the DSM-IV model." *Can J Psychiatry,* 44 (1999): 21-33).

Brady, J. V.: "The paleocortex and behavioral motivation." In *Biological and biochemical bases of behavior,* eds H. F. Harlow and C. N. Woolsey, 193-235. Madison: The University of Wisconsin Press, 1958.

Bragg, M.: *Richard Burton: A Life.* Boston: Little, Brown & Company, 1989.

Brandon, S. G. F.: "Time and the destiny of man" in *The Voices of Time,* ed. J. T. Fraser, 140-157, New York: George Braziller, 1966.

Bray, W. and D. Trump: *The Penguin Dictionary of Archaeology,* 2nd edition. New York, N.Y.: Viking Penguin Inc., 1986.

Brechner, G. A.: "Die Entstehung und Biologische Bedeutung der Subjektiven Zeiteinheit des Momentes." Zeitscr. für vergleichende Physiologie. 18 (1932-33): p. 204.

Britannica CD. Encylopedia Britannica, Inc., 1999.

Browne, A. and D. Finkelhor: "Impact of child sexual abuse: a review of the research." *Psychol Bull* 1986; 99:66-77.

Brown, G. R. and B. Anderson: "Psychiatric morbidity in adult inpatients with childhood histories of sexual and physical abuse." *Am J Psychiatry* 1991; 148: 55-61.

Bryer, J. B., B. A. Nelson, J. B. Miller, P. A. Krol: "Childood sexual and physical abuse as factors in adult psychiatric illness." *Am J Psychiatry* 1987; 144: 1426-1430.

Busby, H.: "Reflections on a leader." In: Thompson, K. W.,(ed.): *The Johnson Presidency: Twenty Intimate Perspectives Of Lyndon B. Johnson. Portraits Of American Presidents, Vol. V.* Lanham, New York, London: University Press of America, 1986:251-270.

Buss, A. H.: *Psychopathy.* New York: Wiley, 1966.

Butzer, K. W.: "Prehistoric People" in: *World Book,* volume 15: 666-675, Chicago: World Book-Childcraft International, Inc., 1979.

Cahalan, E., I. H. Cisin and H. M. Crossley: *American drinking practices; a national study of drinking behavior and attitudes.* New Brunswick, N. J.: Rutgers Center of Alcoholic Studies, 1969.

Campbell, J.: *The Masks of God: Primitive Mythology.* New York: The Viking Press: 1959.

Cannon, L.: *President Reagan: The Role of a Lifetime.* New York: Public Affairs, 1991.

Caro, R. A.: *The Path To Power: The Years Of Lyndon Johnson.* New York: Alfred A. Knopf, 1982.

Carr, A. C.: "Grief, mourning, and bereavement." In *Comprehensive Textbook Of Psychiatry IV,* eds. H. I. Kaplan & B. J. Sadock, 1287-1293. Baltimore, London, Los Angeles, Sydney: Williams & Wilkins, 1985.

Carrel, L. & H. F. Willard: "X-inactivation profile reveals extensive variability in X-linked gene expression in females." *Nature* 434 (2005): 400-404..: "X-inactivation profile reveals extensive variability in X-linked gene expression in females." *Nature* 434 (2005): 400-404.

Chamberlain, C. G.: "Adolescence and young adulthood" in S. E. Greben, R. Pos, V. M. Rakoff, A, Bonkalo, F. H. Lowy and G. Voineskos G (eds): *A Method Of Psychiatry:* 33-42 Philadelphia: Lea & Febiger, 1980.

Chan, W-T: "Chinese Philosophy." in P. Edwards (Ed): *The Encyclopedia of Philosophy, vol.2,* New York: Macmillan Publish Co., Inc. & The Free Press, 1967: 87-96.

Chauvet, J-M, E. Brunel Deschamps and C. Hillaire: *Dawn of Art: The Chauvet Cave; The oldest known paintings in the World.* New York: Harry N. Abrams, Incorporated, 1996.

Check, E.: "The X factor"; *Nature* 434 (2005),: 266-267.

Choy, T. and F. de Bosset: "Post-traumatic stress disorder: an overview." *Can. J. Psychiatry,* 1992: 37, 8: 578-584.

Chu, J. A. and D. L. Dill: "Dissociative symptoms in relation to childhood physical and sexual abuse." *Am J Psychiatry* 1990; 147: 887-892.

Church, G.J.: "Are they living better?" *Time,* February 5, 1996:18-22.

Clottes, J.: "Epilogue: Chauvet Cave today." in J-M Chauvet, E. Brunel Deschamps and C. Hillaire: *Dawn of Art: The Chauvet Cave; The oldest known paintings in the World.* New York: Harry N. Abrams, Incorporated, 1996, p. 89-127.

Clottes, J. and J. Courtin: *The Cave Beneath the Sea; Paleolithic Images at Cosquer.* New York. Harry N. Abrams, Inc., Publishers, 1996.

Coen, E.: *The art of genes.* New York: Oxford University Press, 1999.

Cohen, J.: "Subjective time." In: *The Voices Of Time,* ed. J. T. Fraser, 257-275. New York: George Braziller, 1966.

Coles, E. M.: *Personal communication* (2000).

Constable, G. and the Editors of Time-Life Books: *The Emergence of Man: The Neanderthals.* New York: Time-Life Books, 1973.

Corish, D.: "The mergence of time: a study in the origins of Western Thought." in J. T. Fraser, N. Lawrence and F. C. Haber (eds): *Time, science, and society in China and the West.* Amherst: the University of Massachusetts Press, 1986.

Costa, P. T. and R. R. McCrae: *Revised NEO Personality Inventory (NEO-PI-R) and the NEO Five-Factor Inventory (NEO-FFI) professional manual.* Odessa (FL): Psychological Assessment Resources, Inc.; 1992.

———: "Domains and facets: hierarchical personality assessment using the Revised NEO Personality Inventory." *J Pers Assess* 64 (1995): 21-50.

———: "Six approaches to the explication of facet-level traits: examples from conscientiousness." *European J of Personality* 12 (1998): 117-134.

Cowdry, R. W., D. L. Gardner, K. M. O'Leary, E. Leibenluft, D. R. Rubinow: "Mood variability: a study of four groups." *Am J Psychiatry,* 148 (1991): 1501-1511.

DeLisi, L. E., S. H. Shaw, T. J. Crow, G. Shields, A. B. Smith, V. W.Larach, N. Wellman, J. Loftus, B. Nanthakumar, K. Razi, J. Stewart, M. Comazzi, A. Vita, T. Heffner and R.Sherrington: "A genome-wide scan for linkage to chromosomal regions in 382 sibling pairs with schizophrenia or schizoaffective disorder." *Am J Psychiatry* 159 (2002), 5: 803-812.

Del Parigi A, K. Chen, J. F. Gautier, A. D. Salbe, R. E. Pratley, E. Ravussin, E. M. Reiman and P. A. Tataranni: "Sex differences in the human brain's response to hunger and satiation." *Am J Clin Nutr.* 2002 Jun; 75(6): 1017-1022.

De Lumley, H.: "Chronology of the Palaeolithic." pp 197-199 in: M. Ruspoli: *The Cave of Lascaux.* New York: Harry N. Abrams, Inc., Publishers, 1986.

Dement, W. and N. Kleitman: "Cyclic variations in EEG during sleep and their relation to eye movements, body motility and dreamingl." *Electroencephalog Clin Neurophysiol* 9 (1957): 673.

Depue, R.A. and P.F. Collins: "Neurobiology of the structure of personality: dopamine, facilitation of incentive motivation, and extraversion." *Behav Brain Sci* 22 (1999): 491-569.

Dimond, S. J. and D. A. Blizard, eds.: "Evolution and lateralization of the brain." *Annals of the New York Academy of Sciences* 299 (1977).

Division of Vital Statistics: *Vital statistics of the Province of British Columbia, 118th Annual Report.* 1989.

Drury, A.: *Into What Far Harbor?* New York: William Morrow and Company, Inc., 1993.

DSM-III-R: Diagnostic and Statistical Manual of Mental Disorders, Third Edition-Revised. Washington, D.C.: American Psychiatric Association, 1987.

DSM-IV: Diagnostic and Statistical Manual of Mental Disorders (Fourth Edition). Washington, D.C.: American Psychiatric Association, 1994.

Duff, R. S., and A. B. Hollingshead: *Sickness and Society.* New York: Harper & Row, 1968.

Eccles, J. S.: "Evolution of the brain in relation to the development of the self-conscious mind." in Evolution and Lateralization of the Brain, eds S. J. Dimond, D. A.Blizard. *Annals of New York Academy of Sciences,* 299 (1977):161-179.

Edelman, G. M.: *The Remembered Present: A Biological Theory Of Consciousness.* New York: Basic Books, Inc., 1989.

Edwards, A.: *Early Reagan: The Rise to Power.* New York: William Morrow & Company, 1987.

Eisenberg, L.: "The Social Construction of the Human Brain.: *Am. J. Psychiatry,* 152: 11, 1995, p. 1563-1575.

Ellenberger, H.: *The Discovery of the Unconscious.* New York: Basic Books, 1970.

Engel, G. L.: "A life setting conducive to illness: the giving-up complex." *Arch. Int. Med.* 69 (1968): 293.

Engelberg, S.: " Poland faces choices on economic austerity and the character of the State." *New York Times,* 1990.

Erikson, E. H.: *Childhood and Society.* New York: W. W. Norton $ Company, 1950, 1963

————: "Identity and the life cycle." *Psychol Issues* vol 1 (1959).

————: "The problem of ego identity" in M. R. Stein, A. J. Vidich and D. M. White (eds): *Identity and Anxiety: Survival of the Person in Mass Society:* 37-87. Glencoe, Ill.: The Free Press, 1960

————: "The problem of ego-identity." *J of American Psychoanalytic Association* 4 (1964): 56-121.

————: *Identity: Youth and Crisis.* New York: WW Norton, 1968.

Escalona, S.: *Roots of Individuality.* Chicago: Aldine, 1968.

Escalona, S. and G. Heider: *Prediction and Outcome.* New York: Basic Books, 1959.

Escalona, S. and M. Leitch: *Early Phases of Personality Development.* Evanston: Child Development Publications, 1953.

Eysenck, H. J.: *The Structure of Human Personality.* London: Routledge and Kegan Paul, 1960.

————: *The Biological Basis of Personality.* Springfield: C. C. Thomas, 1967.

————: "Genetics and personality." Pp 163-179 in: J. M. Thoday and A. S. Parkes (Eds): *Genetic and environmental influences on behaviour.* New York: Plenum Press, 1968.

————: *Crime and Personality.* London: Routledge Kegen Paul, 1977.

————: "Comments on 'the orthogonally of extraversion and neuroticism scales'" *Psychological Reports* 612 (1987): 50.

————: "Four ways five actors are not basic." *Pers and Ind Diff* 13 (1992): 667-673.

Eysenck, H. J. and S. B. G. Eysenck: *The Eysenck Personality Inventory.* London: University of London Press, 1965.

————: "On the unitary nature of extraversion." *Acta Psychologica* 26 (1967): 383-390.

Eysenck, H. J. and M. W. Eysenck: *Personality and Individual Differences: a Natural Science Approach.* New York: Plenum, 1985.

Farber, E. A. & B. Egeland: "Invulnerability among abused and neglected children." Chapter 10 in: E. J. Anthony & B. J. Cohler: *The invulnerable child.* New York, London: The Guilford Press, 1987: 254-5.

Ferrence, R. G. P.: "Sex differences in the prevalence of problem drinking." In: U. J. Kalent (Ed.): *Research advances in alcohol and drug problems, Vol. 5.* New York: Plenum Press, 1980.

Ferris, P.: *Richard Burton.* New York: Coward, McCann & Geoghegan, 1981.

Festinger, L.: *A Theory of Cognitive Dissonance.* Stanford University Press, Palo Alto, Calif. 1957.

Finagrette, H.: *The self in transformation: Psychoanalysis, philosophy, and the life of the spirit.* New York: Harper & Row, 1977.

Finkelhor, D.: *Child sexual abuse-New theory and research.* New York, Free Press, 1984.

Flavell, J. H.: *The Developmental Psychology Of Jean Piaget.* Princeton, New Jersey: D. van Nostrand Company, Inc., 1963.

Flor-Henry, P.: "Gender, hemispheric specialization and psychopathology." *Soc Sci & Med,* 12B (1978): 155-162.

Fordham, F.: *An Introduction to Jung's Psychology;* New York, NY: Penguin Books, second edition (1959), reprinted in 1978.

Fortas, A.: "Portrait of a friend. In: K. W. Thompson, (ed.): *The Johnson Presidency: Twenty Intimate Perspectives Of Lyndon B. Johnson. Portraits Of American Presidents, Vol. V.* Lanham, New York, London: University Press of America, 1986, 3-20

Fraisse, P.: The psychology of time. New York: Braziller, 1966: 277-280.

Frank, J. D., and F. B. Powdermaker: "Group psychotherapy." Chapter 67 (1362-1374) in S. Arieti (Ed): *American Handbook of Psychiatry,* vol. 2. New York: Basic Books, Inc., 1959.

Fraser, J. T. (ed): *The Voices of Time,* New York: George Braziller, 1966.

————: *Personal communication* (2005, August 18).

Fraser, J. T., N. Lawrence and F. C. Haber, eds: *The Study of Time V: Time, Science, and Society in China and the West.* Amherst: The University of Massachusetts Press, 1986.

Freud. S.: (1899, 1900) *The Interpretation of Dreams;* New York: Macmillan, 1913.

————: "Ansprache an die Mitglieder des Vereins B'nai B'rith" (1926) [Erikson (1960), p. in *Gesammelte Werke, XVII.*49-53. London: Imago Publishing Col, 1941.

————: *An Autobiographical Study* (translation by James Strachey), fifth impression. London: Hogarth Press and the Institute of Psycho-analysis, 1950.

————: *Collected Papers,* vol. 1-5; New York: Basic Books, Inc., 1959.

————: "The aetiology of hysteria (1896)," in: *Complete Psychological Works, standard ed, vol.3.* London: Hogarth Press, 1962.

Friedman, M. and R. Rosenman: "Association of specific overt behavior pattern with blood and cardiovascular findings." *JAMA* 169 (1959): 1286.

Galin, D.: "Lateral specialization and psychiatric issues: speculations on development and the evolution of consciousness." in S. J. Dimond, D. A. Blizard (Eds): Evolution and Lateralization of the Brain. *Annals of New York Academy of Sciences,* 299 (1977):397-411.

Gallant, R. A.: *The peopling of Planet Earth: Human Population Growth Through the Ages.* New York: MacMillan Publishing Company; London: Collier MacMillan Publishers, 1990.

Galsworthy, J.: "Swan Song," pt. II, ch.6., 1928. Quoted from J. Bartlett: *Familiar Quotations,* ed. E. Morison, p. 893. Boston, Toronto: Little, Brown and Company, 1969.

Gardner, H.: *Frames Of Mind,* New York: Basic Books, Inc., 1985.

Gardner, M. J. and D. G. Altman (eds): "Statistics with confidence-confidence intervals and statistical guidelines." *Brit Med J* London, 1989.

Gazzaniga, M. S.: "Consistency and diversity in brain organization." In: Dimond, S. J. and D. A. Blizard, eds.: "Evolution and lateralization of the brain." *Annals of the New York Academy of Sciences* 299 (1977): :415-423.

Gesell, A., et al.: *The First Five Years of Life: A Guide to the Study of the Preschool Child.* New York: Harper & Row, 1940.

Gilbert, A. M., B. O. Gilbert and D. G. Gilbert: "Fears as a function of gender and extraversion in adolescents." *J of Social Behavior and Personality* 9 (1994), 1:89-94, p. 92).

Gilbert, M.: *Churchill, A Life.* London: Heinemann, 1991.

Gimbutas, M.: *The Civilization Of The Goddess,* ed. J. Marler. San Francisco: Harper. 1991.

Goldman-Rakic, P.S.: "Working Memory and the Mind." *Scientific American,* 267, 3 (September 1992): 111-117.

Goldschneider, G. and J. Elffers: *The secret language of birthdays: personology profiles for each day of the year.* New York NY: Viking Penguin, 1994.

Golombek, H., P. Marton, B. Stein and M. Korenblum: "A study of disturbed and non disturbed adolescents: the Toronto Adolescent Longitudinal Study, I." *Can J Psychiatry,* 31 (1986): 532-535.

Gonzalez, A. and P. G. Zimbardo: "Time in perspective: the time sense we learn early affects how we do our jobs and enjoy our pleasures." *Psychology Today* (1985): 21-26.

Gore, R.: "The rise of mammals." *National Geographic* 203 (2003), 4: 2-37.

Gorman, C.: "On its own two feet." *Time,*146 (1995), 9: 40-42.

Goudsmit, S. A., R. Claiborne, R. Dubos, H. Margenau, C. P. Snow (eds): *Time. Life Science Library.* New York: Time Incorporated, 1966

Gray, J.: *Men are from Mars, women are from Venus.* New York: Harper Perennial, 1994.

Green, H. B.: "Aging: temporal stages in the development of the self" in J. T. Fraser and N. Lawrence (eds): *The Study of Time II.:* 1-19. New York: Springer-Verlag, 1975.

Green M.: *Theories Of Human Development: A Comparative Approach.* Englewood Cliffs, New Jersey 07632: 1989.

Greenspan, S. I.: "Normal Child Development" in: *Comprehensive Textbook Of Psychiatry/IV,* eds. H. I. Kaplan and B. J. Sadock, 1592-1607, Baltimore Md: Williams & Wilkins, 1985.

Groesbeck, C. J.: "Carl Jung." In *Comprehensive Textbook Of Psychiatry IV,* eds H. I. Kaplan, B. J. Sadock, 433-440. Baltimore, London, Los Angeles, Sydney: Williams & Wilkins. 1985.

Guantao, J., F. Dainian, F. Hongye, L. Qingfeng: "The evolution of Chinese science and technology." In: J.T. Fraser, N. Lawrence and F. C. Haber (eds): *Time, science, and society in China and the West.* Amherst: the University of Massachusetts Press, 1986: 170.

Gur, R. C., L. H. Mozley, P. D. Mozley, S. M. Resnick, J. S. Karp, A. Alavi, S. E. Arnold and R. E. Gur: "Sex differences in regional cerebral glucose metabolism during a resting state." *Science.* 1995 Jan 27; 267 (5197): 528-31.

Hall, C. S. and G. Lindzey: Theories of Personality. New York: John Wiley & Sons, Inc., 1957.

Hall, J. A.: *Clinical Uses of Dreams: Jungian Interpretations and Enactments.* New York, San Francisco, London: Grune & Stratton, 1977.

Hallowell, A. I.: "Temporal orientation in Western Civilization and in a pre-literate society." *American Anthropologist,* 36 (1937): 647-670.

Hamburg, D. A.: "Toward a strategy for healthy adolescent development." *Am J Psychiatry,* 154 (June 1997), *Festschrift Supplement*: 6-12

Hamilton, N.: *JFK: Reckless Youth.* New York: Random House, 1992.

Harlan C.: *Vision and Invention, a Course in Art Fundamentals,* Englewood Cliffs, New Jersey: Prentice-Hall, Inc. 1970.

Harnad, S. R., H. D. Steklis and J. Lancaster, eds: "Origins And Evolution Of Language And Speech." *Annals of the New York Academy Sciences,* 280 (1976): 1-914.

Hartmann, E.: *The Biology Of Dreaming.* Springfield, Ill.: Charles C. Thomas, 1967.

Hawkes, J.: *Prehistory in History of Mankind, Cultural and Scientific Development,* Vol. 1, Part 1.UNESCO, London: New English Library Ltd., 1965.

Hillman, J.: *Anima: an Anatomy of a Personified Notion.* Dallas: Spring, 1985.

Hinkle, L. E.: "Ecological observations of the relation of physical illness, mental illness, and the social environment." *Psychosom. Med.* 23 (1961): 289.

Hofstede, G.: "Motivation, leadership and organization: do American theories apply abroad?" pp. 42-63 in: *Organizational Dynamics,* AMACOM, a Division of American Management Associations, summer 1980.

Howell, F. C. et al.: *Early Man,* New York: Time-Life Books, 1968.

Howells, W.: "The Pleistocene" in *Human Evolution,* eds. N. Korn and H. Reece Smith, 210-209, New York: Henry Hold and Company, 1959.

————: "Pithecantropus and Sinanthropus" in *Human Evolution, Readings in Physical Anthropology,* eds. N. Korn and H. Reece Smith: 236-250, New York: Henry Holt and Company, 1959a.

————: *Mankind in the Making.* Garden City, NY: Doubleday, 1967.

Innis, B.: "Cast your own horoscope." Insert in *Man, Myth & Magic,* 3, Published by Purnell for BPC Publishing Ltd.: London, 1970: p.1-4, 13-16.

Isaac, G. L.: "Stages of cultural elaboration in the Pleistocene: possible archaeological indicators of the development of language capabilities " in Harnad, S. R., H. D. Steklis and J. Lancaster, eds: "Origins And Evolution Of Language And Speech." *Annals of the New York Academy Sciences,* 280 (1976): 275-288.

Jacobi, J.: *The Psychology of C. G. Jung.* Revised edition; New Haven: Yale University Press, 1951.

Jacoby, M.: *Individuation and Narcissism, The Psychology of the Self in Jung and Kohut.* London and New York: Routledge, 1990 (first published in German; München: Verlag J. Pfeiffer, 1985).

Jaffé, A.: Introduction. In *Memories, Dreams And Reflections,* Carl Jung, v-ix. New York: Vintage Books, 1965.

James, R. R.: Churchill: a study in failure, 1900-1939. World Publishing Company, 1970.

James, W.: *Principles of Psychology.* New York: Holt, 1890.

————: *Pragmatism: A New Name for Some Old Ways of Thinking.* London and Cambridge, Mass., 1907.

————: *Psychology: American Science Series, Briefer Course.* New York: Henry Holt and Company, 1910.

————: *Psychology: The Briefer Course* (G. Allport, ed.); New York: Harper & Brothers, 1961.

Jang, K. L., P. A. Vernon and W. J. Livesley: "Behavioural-genetic perspectives on personality function." *Can J Psychiatry* 46 (2001): 234-244.

Jaynes, J.: "The evolution of language in the late pleistocene" In: Harnad, S. R., H. D. Steklis and J. Lancaster, eds: "Origins And Evolution Of Language And Speech." *Annals of the New York Academy Sciences,* 280 (1976): 312-325.

————: *The Origin Of Consciousness In The Break-Down Of The Bicameral Mind.* Boston: Houghton, Mifflin Company, 1982.

Jenkins, R.: *Churchill; A Biography.* Ferrar, Straus and Giroux; 2001.

Jespersen, O.: *Language, Its Nature, Development And Origin.* New York: W.W. Norton and Co, 1964.

Johnson, G.E.: *Psycho-Asthenics* 2 (1997) 26-32.

Jones, E.: *The Life And Work of Sigmund Freud, volume 1.* New York: Basic Books, 1953.

————: *The Life And Work of Sigmund Freud, volume 2.* New York: Basic Books, 1955.

Jones, M. E.: *How to learn astrology; a beginner's manual.* Stanwood, Washington: Sabian Publishing Society, 1970.

Jonides, J., E. E. Smith, R. A. Koeppe: "Spatial working memory in humans as revealed by PET." *Nature* 363 (1993): 623-625.

Jung C. G.: *The Collected Works of C. G. Jung (1953-78),* ed. H. Read, M. Fordham and G. Adler; London: Routledge; New York: Pantheon Books, 1953-1960; New York: the Bollingen Foundation, 1961-1967; Princeton: Princeton University Press New Jersey (1967-1978).

————: "A psychology theory of types" in *Collected Works,* vol. 6, 1928.

————: "Psychological factors determining human behaviour" in *Collected Works,* vol 8, 1936.

————: *Commentary on the Secret of the Golden Flower,* translated by C. F. Baynes. London: Collins and Routlege & Kegan Paul, 1962.

————: *Civilization in Transition.* (from the Collected Works of C. G. Jung, vol. 10, Bollingen Series XX). Princeton: Princeton University Press, 1964.

————: *Memories, Dreams And Reflections,* New York: Vintage Books, 1965.

————: *Psychology and alchemy.* 2nd Edition. Princeton, N. J.: Princeton University Press, 1968(b).

————: *Two Essays on Analytical Psychology* (translated by R. F. C. Hull). Cleveland and New York: Meridian Books, The World Publishing Company, 1970.[originally published in Switzerland as "Ueber die Psychologie des Unbewussten (1943) and "Die Beziehungen zwischen dem Ickhund dem Unbewussten (1945). Also contained in the Collected Work, Vol. 7]

————: *Psychological Types.* Vol. 6 of the Collected Works. Bollingen Series XX. Princeton, N. J.: Princeton University Press; translated by H. G. Baynes as revised by R. F. C. Hull (1971); third printing: 1977.

Jung, C. G. and A. Jaffé: *Memories, Dreams, Reflections.* London: Collins, London: Routledge & Kegan Paul, 1963.

Junor, P.: *Burton: The Man Behind the Myth.* London: The Leisure Circle, 1985.

Kagan, J.: *Galen's prophecy: temperament in human nature.* New York: Basic Books, 1994.

Kalmus, H.: "Organic evolution and time" in *The Voices Of Time,* ed. J. T. Fraser, ed., 330-352, New York: G. Braziller, 1966.

Kastenbaum, R.: "Time, Death and Ritual in Old Age " in *The Study of Time II,* eds J. T. Fraser and N. Lawrence, 20-38. New York: Springer-Verlag, 1975.

Kellogg, R.: Form-similarity between phosphenes of adults and preschool children's scribblings, *Nature,* 208 (1965): 1129-1130.

Kernberg, O.: "Neurosis, psychosis, and the borderline states." Chapter 14.4 in H. I. Kaplan and B. J. Sadock (Eds): *Comprehensive Textbook of Psychiatry/IV;* 621-630. Baltimore Md, Williams & Wilkins, 1985.

Kerwin, C. and the Editors of Time-Life Books: *The Emergence Of Man: The First Men.* New York: Time-Life Books, 1973.

Kimbrell, T. A., M. S. George, P. I. Parekh, T. A. Ketter, D. M. Podell, A. L. Danielson, J. D. Repella, B. E. Benson, M. W. Willis, P. Herscovitch and R. M. Post: "Regional brain activity during transient self-induced anxiety and anger in healthy adults." *Biol Psychiatry.* 1999 Aug 15; 46 (4): 454-65.

Knoll, M.: "Transformations of science in our age." In: Joseph Campbell, Ed.: *Man and Time. Papers from the Eranos Yearbooks; Bollingen Series XXX.* Princeton: Princeton University Press, 1983; p. 271-272.

Kohut, H. : *The Restoration of the Self.* New York: International Universities Press, 1977.

————: "Reflections." in *Advances in Self Psychology,* ed. A. Goldberg, 473-554. New York: International Universities Press, 1980.

Kretschmer, E.: *Physique and Character, 2nd ed.* revised by Miller (originally in German: *Körperbau und Charakter* 1921), London, 1936

Kristof, N. D.: "On language." *The New York Times Magazine,* August 18, 1991: 8-10.

Kristofferson, A. B.: *A Time Constant Involved In Attention And Neural Information Processing. N.A.S.A. CR-427. Washington, D.C.: National Aeronautics and Space Administration,* April 1966.

Kübler-Ross, E.: *On Death and Dying,* 1969.

La Lumiere, Jr., L. P.: "Danakil Island" in E. Morgan: *The Aquatic Ape,* New York: Stein and Day, 1982: pp. 123-135.

Lamendella, J. T.: "Relations between the ontogenesis and phylogenesis of language: a neo-recapitulationist view." In Origins And Evolution Of Language And Speech, eds S. R. Harnad, H. D. Steklis and J. Lancaster. *Annals of the New York Academy Sciences,* 280 (1976): 396-412.

Leacock, E: "Three social variables and the occurrence of mental disorder." Chapter 10 in: A. L. Leighton, J. A. Clausen, R. N. Wilson (Eds): *Explorations in social psychiatry.* New York: Basic Books, Inc., 1957: 321-329.

LeMay, M.: "Morphological cerebral asymmetries of modern man, fossil man, and nonhuman primate" in: Origins and evolution of language and in speech, eds S. R. Harnad, H. D. Steklis and J. Lancaster; *Annals of the New York Academy of Sciences* 280 (1976):349-366.

Lemonick, M. D.: "How man began." *Time,* 143 (1994), 11:38-45.

————: "Lucy's grandson" *Time,* 143 (1994a), 15:51.

————: "The first butcher." *Time,* 155 (1999), May 3, 50-51.

Leutwyler, K.: "Depression's double standard. Clues emerge as to why women have higher rates of depression." *Sci Am.* 1995 Jun; 272 (6): 23, 26.

Lewin, T.: "Virgins outnumber sexually active teenagers, study reports. High school students say they are waiting longer to have intercourse." *The New York Times* CLII, Nr. 52256, National Edition, September 29, 2002, p. 26.

Lief, A., ed.: *The Commonsense Psychiatry Of Dr. Adolf Meyer.* New York, Toronto, London: McGraw-Hill Book Company, Inc., 1948

Linn, L.: "Clinical manifestations of psychiatric disorders." Chapter 13 in H. I. Kaplan and B. J. Sadock (Eds): *Comprehensive Textbook of Psychiatry/IV.* Baltimore Md, Williams & Wilkins, 1985: 550-590.

Littman, S. K. and G. Shugar: "The examination: history." Chapter 8 (81-90) in S. G. Greben, R. Pos, V. M. Rakoff, A. Bonkalo, F. H. Lowy and G. Voineskos (Eds): *A Method of Psychiatry.* Philadelphia: Lea & Febiger, 1980.

Loat, C. S., Asbury, K., Galsworthy, M.J., Plomin, R & Craig, J. W.: *Twin Res.* 7 (2004): 54-61.

Mahler, M. S., F. Pine and A. Bergman: *The Psychological Birth of the Human Infant.* New York: Basic Books, 1975.

Mair, M.: "The community of self" in D. Bannister (ed.) *New Perspectives in Personal Construct Theory.* London: Academic Press, 1977.

Maraniss, D.: *First in His Class; The Biography of Bill Clinton.* New York: Simon & Shuster, 1995.

Marshack, A.: "Some implications of the paleolithic symbolic evidence for the origin of language" in: Origins and evolution of language and in speech, eds S. R. Harnad, H. D. Steklis and J. Lancaster; *Annals of the New York Academy of Sciences,* 280 (1976): 289-311.

Masler, E. G.: "The subjective perception of two aspects of time: Duration and timelessness." *International J. of Psychoanalysis,* 1973, 54: 426-429.

Maslow, A. H.: *Toward a Psychology of Being.* New York: Van Nostrand, 1968.

———: *Motivation and Personality* (3rd edn), New York: Harper and Row, 1987.

McAdams, D. P.: "The 'Imago': a key narrative component of identity" in P. Shaver (ed) *Self, Situations and Social Behaviour.* Beverly Hills, Ca.: Sage, 1985.

McCauley, J., D. E. Kern, K. Kolodner, L. Dill, A. F. Schroeder, H. K. DeChant, J. Ryden, L. R. Derogatis, and E. G. Bass: "Clinical characteristics of women with a history of childhood abuse: unhealed wounds." *JAMA,* 1997; 277: 1362-1368.

McCrae, R. R., and P. T. Costa: "Validation of the five-factor model of personality across instruments and observers." *J Pers Soc Psychol* 52 (1987): 81-90.

———: *Personality in adulthood.* New York: Guilford; 1990.

McPherson, H.: "Johnson and Civil Rights." In: K. W. Thompson, (ed.): *The Johnson Presidency: Twenty Intimate Perspectives Of Lyndon B. Johnson. Portraits Of American Presidents, Vol. V.* Lanham, New York, London: University Press of America, 1986: 43-58.

Meissner, W. W.: "Theories of personality and psychopathology: Classical Psychoanalysis." Chapter 8 (p. 337-418) in H. I. Kaplan and B. J. Sadock (Eds): *Comprehensive Textbook of Psychiatry/IV.* Baltimore Md, Williams & Wilkins, 1985.

Merritt, C.: "Researchers, physicians paying more attention to weather's impact on health." *Can Med Assoc J* 148 (1993): 436-439.

Meyer, J. K.: "Ego-dystonic homosexuality." Chapter 23.4 (p. 1056-1065) in: H. I. Kaplan and B. J. Sadock (Eds): *Comprehensive Textbook of Psychiatry/IV.* Baltimore Md, Williams & Wilkins, 1985

Michael, R. T., J. H. Gagnon, E. O. Laumann, G. Kolata: *Sex in America: a definitive survey.* Boston, New York, Toronto, London: Little, Brown and Company, 1994

Michon, J. A.: "Time experience and memory processes." In: *The Study of Time II*, eds J. T. Fraser and N. Lawrence, 302-313. New York: Springer-Verlag, 1975.

———: Timing your mind and minding your time. In: *Time and Mind, the Study of Time VI*, ed. J. T. Fraser, 17-39. Madison, Connecticut: International Universities Press, Inc., 1989.

Morgan, E.: *The Aquatic Ape*. Scarborough House, Briarcliff Manor, N.Y. 10510 : Stein and Day, 1982

Morgan, P.P.: "Confidence intervals: from statistical significance to clinical significance" CMAJ vol. 141, Nov 1, 1989: 881-883

Mowrer, O. H.: *Learning Theory and Behavior*. New York, London: John Wiley & Sons, Inc. 1960

Murphy, L. B., et al.: *The Widening World of Childhood*. New York: Basic Books, 1962.

Murphy, L. B., and A. E. Moriarty: *Vulnerability, Coping and Growth*. New Haven: Yale University Press, 1976.

Muske, C.: "I Married the Ice-Pick Killer. Scenes from the life of an actor's wife." *The New York Times Magazine*, March 19, 2000, Section 6: 116.

Muuss, R. E.: "The philosophical and historic roots of theories of adolescence." In: R. E. Muuss (ed): *Adolescent behavior and society (2nd ed)*. New York: Random House, 1975: 90-124.

Myers, D. G. *The pursuit of happiness: who is happy-and why*. New York: Avon, 1993.

Nakamura, H.: *Ways of Thinking of Easter Peoples: India-China-Tibet-Japan*, ed. P. P. Wiener. Honolulu, Hawaii: East-West Center Press, 1964.

———: "Time in Indian and Japanese thought" in *The Voices Of Time*, ed. J. T. Fraser, 77-91. New York: G. Braziller, 1966.

Nishizawa, S., C. Benkelfat, S. N. Young, M. Leyton, S. Mzengeza, C. de Montigny, P. Blier and M. Diksic: "Differences between males and females in rates of serotonin synthesis in human brain." *Proc Natl Acad Sc USA*. 1997 May 13; 94 (10): 5308-13.

Norman, G. R. and D. L. Streiner: *PDQ Statistics*, Toronto, Philadelphia: B.C. Decker Inc. 1986.

O'Connor, E.: *Our Many Selves: a Handbook for Self-Discovery*. New York: Harper and Row, 1971.

Orasanu, J., M. K. Slater and L. L. Adler: "Introduction" in: *Language, Sex and Gender*, eds. J. Orasanu, J., M. K. Slater and L. L. Adler. New York: New York Academy of Sciences, 327 (1979): vii-x.

Orwell, S. and I. Angus (Eds): *The Collected Essays, Journalism and Letters of George Orwell, Volume 4, In Front of Your Nose, 1945-1950*, Harcourt, Brace: 1968, pp. 491-495.

Osler, Sir W.: *A Way of Life*, address at Yale, spring 1913, quoted from L. Eichler Watson: *Light from many lamps*, New York: Simon and Schuster, 1951, 214.

Ostwald, F. W.: *Grosse Männer*. Leipzig, 1910; 3/4 ed, 1919

Paris, J.: *Borderline personality disoder: a multidimensional approach*. Washington (DC): American Psychiatric Press, 1994.

———: *Social factors in the personality disorders*. New York: Cambridge University Press; 1996.

———: "Does childhood trauma cause personality disorders in Adults?" *Can J Psychiatry*, 43, 1998: 148-153.

———: "Why behavioural genetics is important for psychiatry." *Can j Psychiatr* 46 (2001): 223.

Parker, D. and J. Parker: *The New Complete Astrologer*. New York NY: Crown Publishers, 1990.

Pasternak, B.: *Doctor Zhivago* (Translated from the Russian by Max Hayward and Manya Harari); London: Wm. Collins Sons and Co. Ltd, 1958.

Paulesu, E, C. D. Frith and R. S. J. Frackowiak: "The neural correlates of the verbal component of working memory." *Nature* 1993; 362: 342-345.

Paykel, E. S.: "Contribution of life events to causation of psychiatric illness." *Psychological Med.* 1978: 8: 245-253.

Perls, F. S.: *Gestalt Therapy Verbatim.* Moab, Utah: Real People Press, 1969.

Person, E. S.: "Manipulativeness in entrepreneurs and psychopaths." In: *Unmasking the Psychopath: Antisocial Personality and Related Syndromes,* Eds. W. H. Reid, D. Dorr, J. I. Walker and J.W. Bonner, III. New York, London: W. W. Norton & Company, 1986.

Peters, T. J. and R. H. Waterman: *In search of excellence.* New York: Harper & Row, 1982.

Piaget, J.: *The Language And Thought Of The Child.* London: Routledge & Kegan Paul, 1926.

————: *The Child's Conception Of The World.* London: Routledge & Kegan Paul; 1929.

————: *The Child's Conception Of The World.* New York: Harcourt, Brace and Company; 1929a.

————: *The Moral Judgment Of The Child.* London: Kegan Paul, 1932.

————: *The Origin of Intelligence in Children.* New York: International Universities Press, 1952.

————: *Psychology of Intelligence.* Totawa, N. J.: Littlefield, Adams, 1966a

Pollex, R., B. Hegele and M. R. Ban: "Celestial determinants of success in research." *Canad Medical Ass J* 165 (2001), 12:1584

Pope, Jr., H. G. and J. I. Hudson: "Is childhood sexual abuse a risk factor for bulimia nervosa?" *Am J Psychiatry,* 1992: 149, 4: 455-463.

Pos, R.: *The Psyche-Soma Complex: Its Psychology And Logic.* Doctoral Thesis, Rijksuniversiteit, Utrecht, the Netherlands. The Hague: Lankhout & Immig, 1963.

————: *The Informational Underload Theory Of States Characterized By The Freudian Primary Process (Psychotic Decompensation, Primary Process Dreaming And The Earliest Phase Of Life): A Multi-Disciplinary Research Effort Using Neurophysiological Data Of Experimental Animals (Cats) And Human Subjects With The Application Of Mathematical Pattern Extraction Techniques Realized Through Digital Computers: A Summary And A Survey Of The First Four And A Half Years Of Research.* Toronto: Department of Psychiatry, University of Toronto, 1969.

————: *History taking.* Unpublished lecture, Toronto: Department of Psychiatry, Toronto General Hospital, 1964; second ed. Owen Sound General & Marine Hospital, Owen Sound, Ont., 1978.

————: "Sleep disorders." In *A Method Of Psychiatry*, eds S. E. Greben, R. Pos, V. M. Rakoff, A. Bonkalo, F. H. Lowy, G. Voineskos, 163-169. Philadelphia: Lea & Febiger, 1980.

————: *The Gender Beyond Sex: Two Distinct Ways of Living in Time*; e-book (2004); obtainable via <http://robertpos.info>.

Pratkanis, A. and E. Aronson: *Age of Propaganda: The Everyday Use and Abuse of Persuasion.* New York: W. H. Freeman and Company, 1992.

Pribram, K. H.: "Neocortical function in behavior" in *Biological and Biochemical Bases of Behavior,* eds H. F. Harlow and C. N. Woolsey, 151-172. Madison: The University of Wisconsin Press, 1958.

Prideaux, T. and the Editors of Time-Life Books: *The Emergence of Man: Cro-Magnon Man.* New York: Time-Life Books, 1973.

Prigerson et al.: "Complicated Grief and Bereavement-Related Depression as Distinct Disorders: Preliminary Empirical Validation in Elderly Bereaved Spouses." *Am J Psychiatry* 152 (1995), 1.

Putman, J. J.: "The search for modern humans" *National Geographic*, 174 (1988):438-477.

Rae-Grant, N., B. H. Thomas, D. R. Offord, M. H. Boyle: "Risk, protective factors, and the prevalence of behavioral and emotional disorders in children and adolescents." *J. Am. Acad. Child Adolesc. Psychiatry,* 1989; 28,2,: 262-268.

Ragland, J. D., A. R. Coleman, R. C. Gur, D. C. Glahn and R. E. Gur: "Sex differences in brain-behavior relationships between verbal episodic memory and resting regional cerebral flood flow." *Neuropsychologia.* 2000; 38(4): 451-61.

Rappoport, H. and K. Enrich: "Relation between ego identity and temporal perspective." *J Personality Social Psychology* 48 (1985), 6: 1-12.

Rappoport, H., K. Enrich and A. Wilson: "Ego identity and temporality: psychoanalytic and existential perspectives." *J Humanistic Psychology,* 22 (1982): 53-70.

Rappoport, L.: *Personality Development. The Chronology Of Experience.* Glenview, Illinois, London: Scott, Foresman and Company, 1972.

Raven, P. H. and G. B. Johnson: *Biology.* St. Louis, Toronto, Boston, Los Altos: Times Mirror/ Mosby College Publishing, 1989.

Reason, P. and J. Rowan (eds): *Human Inquiry: a Sourcebook of New Paradigm Research.* Chichester: John Wiley, 1981.

Ridley, M.: *Genome: The Autobiography of a Species in 23 Chapters.* New York NY: Harper Collins Publishers, 2000.

Robson, B. and K. Minde: "Normal child development" in: P.D. and Q.Rae-grant eds. *Psychological Problems of the Child and His Family.* Toronto: Macmillan of Canada, 1977.

Ross, M.T. et al.: "The DNA sequence of the human X-chromosome" *Nature* 434 (2005), 325-337.

Rowan, J.: *Subpersonalities, The People Inside Us.* London, New York: Routledge, 1990.

Rulon, P. R.: *The Compassionate Samaritan: The Life Of Lyndon Baines Johnson.* Chicago: Nelson-Hall, 1981.

Ruspoli, M.: *The Cave of Lascaux.* New York: Harry N. Abrams, Inc., Publishers, 1986.

Rutter, M.: Psychosocial resilience and protective mechanisms. Chapter 9 in: J. Rolf, A. S. Masten, D. Cicchetti, K. H. Nuechterlein, S. Weinraub: *Risk and protective factors in the development of psychopathology.* Cambridge, New York, Port Chester, Melbourne, Sydney: Cambridge University Press, 1990, 182-3.

Rutter, M., A. Cox, C. Tupling, M. Berger, W. Yule: Attainment and adjustment in two geographical areas. Brit. J. Psychiat., 1975: 126, 493-509.

Rutter, M. and B. Maughan: "Psychosocial adversities in psychopathology." *J. Personal Disorder* 1997; 11: 4-18.

Sadato, N., V. Ibanez, M. P. Deiber and M. Hallett: "Gender difference in premotor activity during active tactile discrimination." *Neuroimage.* 2000 May; 11(5 Pt 1): 532-40.

Sadock, B. J.: "Group psychotherapy, combined individual and group psychotherapy, and psychodrama." Chapter 29.5 (1403-1427) in H. I. Kaplan and B. J. Sadock (Eds): *Comprehensive Textbook of Psychiatry/IV.* Baltimore Md, Williams & Wilkins, 1985.

Safran, C.: "The road to self-esteem." *Ladies' Home Journal,* 110 (1993): 50-57.

Sanders, S. A. and J. Machover Reinisch: "Would You Say You 'Had Sex' If...?" *JAMA,* 281 (1999), 3: 275-277.

Savage-Rumbaugh, S., S. G. Shanker and T. J. Taylor: *Apes, Language, and the Human Mind.* New York: Oxford University Press Inc. 2001.

Schama, S.: "Rescuing Churchill." Review of Roy Jenkins' *Churchill;* Ferrar, Straus and Giroux; *The New York Review of Books.* XLIX, 3 (February 28, 2002): 15-17.

Schwartz, R. C.: "Our multiple selves: applying systems thinking to the inner family." *Networker* (March/April 25-31):80-83, 1987.

Selected Characteristics for Census Tracts, Census of Canada. Ottawa: Statistics Canada, 1986.

Seton, P. H.: "The psychotemporal adaptation of late adolescence." *J. of the American Psychoanalytic Association,* 1974, 22: 795-819.

Shapiro, S. B.: *The Selves Inside You.* Berkeley, Ca.: Explorations Institute, 1976.

Shaw, G. B.: *Selected Prose.* New York: Dodd, Mead and Col, 1952.

Shaywitz, B. A., S. E. Shaywitz, K. R. Pugh, R. T. Constable, P. Skudlarski, R. K. Fulbright, R. A. Bronen, J. M. Fletcher, D. P. Shankweiler, L. Katz and J. C. Gore: "Sex differences in the functional organization of the brain for language." *Nature* 1995; 373: 607-609.

Sherrington, C.:*The Integrative Action of the Nervous System.* Cambridge, England: Cambridge University Press, 1947.

Sivin, N.: "On the limits of empirical knowledge in the traditional Chinese sciences." In: J. T. Fraser, N. Lawrence and F. C. Haber (eds): *Time, science, and society in China and the West.* Amherst: the University of Massachusetts Press, 1986: 151-169.

Skodol, A. E. and P. E. Shrout: "Use of DSM-III Axis IV in Clinical Practice: Rating Etiologically Significant Stressors." *Am J Psychiatry* 146 (1989):1, 61-66.

Smith, B. D.: *The emergence of agriculture.* New York: Scientific American Library, 1998.

Smith, T. W.: "Adult sexual behavior in 1989; number of partners, frequency of intercourse, and risk of AIDS. *Fam Plann Perspect* 23(1991): 102-107.

Stanislavski, C.: *An Actor Prepares.* Methuen Publishing Ltd., 1980

Stein, B. A., H. Golombek, P. Marton and M. Korenblum: "Consistency and change in personality characteristics and affect from middle to late adolescence." *Can J Psychiatry,* 36 (February 1991): 16-20.

Stein, E.: *On the Problem of Empathy.* The Hague: Martinus Nijhoff, 1964.

Stein, M. R. and A. J. Vidich: "Identity and history: an overview" in M. R. Stein, A. J. Vidich and D. M. White (eds): *Identity and Anxiety: Survival of the Person in Mass Society:* 17-33. Glencoe, Ill.: The Free Press, 1960.

Steinen, K. v.d.: *Unter den Naturvölkern Zentral-Brasiliens,* 1894, quoted by (1957), p. 302-303.

Steinhauer, P. D.: "Infancy and childhood" in *A Method of Psychiatry,* eds. S. E. Greben, R. Pos, V. M. Rakoff, A. Bonkalo, F. H. Lowy, G. Voineskos, 9-32, Philadelphia: Lea & Febiger, 1980.

Steklis, H. D. and S. R. Harnad: "From hand to mouth: some critical stages in the evolution of language" in: Origins and evolution of language and in speech, eds S. R. Harnad, H. D. Steklis and J. Lancaster; *Annals of the New York Academy of Sciences* 280 (1976): 445-455.

Stern, C. and W. Stern: Erinnerung, Aussage unde Lüge. 1931 [Quoted by Werner (1957), p.24].

Stevens, A.: *On Jung.* London, New York: Routledge, 1990.

Stodghill II, R.: "Where'd you learn that? American kids are in the midst of their own sexual revolution, on leaving many parents feeling confused and virtually powerless." *Time* 151(1998), 23: 38-45.

Stone, I.: *The Origin.* Bergenfield, NJ: New American Library Penguin Inc., 1982.

Stringer, C.: "Human evolution: out of Ethiopia." *Nature,* 42 (June 2003): 692-695.

Sullivan, H. S.: *The Interpersonal Theory of Psychiatry.* New York: W. W. Norton & Company, 1953.

Tanner, N. and A. Zihlman: "Discussion paper: The evolution of human communication: what can primates tell us?" In: Origins and evolution of language and in speech, eds S. R. Harnad, H. D. Steklis and J. Lancaster; *Annals of the New York Academy of Sciences* 280, 2-3 (1976): 467-480.

Tattersall, I.: "Primates" in *Academic American Encyclopedia*, on line edition, Danbury, CT.: Grolier Electronic Publishing, 1993.

Tellegen, A., D. T. Lykken, T. J. Bouchard, K. J. Wilcox, N. C. Segal, S. Rich: "Personality similarity in twins reared apart and together." *J Pers Soc Psychol* 54 (1988): 1031-1039.

Terr, L. C.: "Childhood traumas: an outline and overview." *Am. J. Psychiatry,* 148 (1991): 10-20.

Thomas, A. and S. Chess: *Temperament and Development.* New York: Brunner/Mazel, 1977.

Thomas, A., S. Chess and H. G. Birch: *Behavioral Individuality in Early Childhood.* New York: New York University Press, 1963.

————: *Temperament And Behavior Disorders In Children.* New York: New York University Press, 1968.

Thompson, K. W. (ed.): *The Johnson Presidency: Twenty Intimate Perspectives Of Lyndon B. Johnson. Portraits Of American Presidents, Vol. V.* Lanham, New York, London: University Press of America, 1986

Tichener, E.: *Experimental psychology of the thought processes.* New York: Macmillan, 1909.

Time: "New Worlds of Discovery." Special Issue: The New Age of Discovery, Winter 1997-1998.

Twombly, R. C.: *Frank Lloyd Wright: An Interpretive Biography;* Harper, 1973.

U.S. Department of Energy: "Primer on Molecular Genetics." *DOE Human Genome 1991-92 Program Report.* Washington, DC 20585, June 1992.

Valenti, J.: "Managing the White House, leading the country." In: K. W. Thompson, (ed.): *The Johnson Presidency: Twenty Intimate Perspectives Of Lyndon B. Johnson. Portraits Of American Presidents, Vol. V.* Lanham, New York, London: University Press of America, 1986:21-39.

Van Laere, K. J. and R. A. Dierckx: "Brain perfusion SPECT: age-and sex-related effects correlated with voxel-based morphometric findings in healthy adults." *Radiology.* 2001 Dec; 221(3): 810-17.

Vaughan, F.: *The Inward Arc.* Boston: New Science Library, 1985.

Vaughn, S.: *Ronald Reagan in Hollywood: Movies and politics (Cambridge studies in the history of mass communications).* New York: Press Syndicate of the University of Cambridge, 1994.

Viederman, M.: "Grief: Normal and Pathological Variants." *Am J Psychiatry* 152 (1995): 1-4.

————: "Personality change through life experience: III. Two creative types of response to object loss." In *The Problem of Loss and Mourning: Psychoanalytic Perspectives* (D. Dietrich and

P. Shabad, Eds); New York: International Press, 1989.

Wang, W. S-Y.: "Language change" in: Origins and evolution of language and in speech, eds S. R. Harnad, H. D. Steklis and J. Lancaster; *Annals of the New York Academy of Sciences* 280, 2-3 (1976): 61-72.

Weigel, G.: *Witness to Hope: The Biography of Pope John Paul II.* Cliff Street Books / Harper Collins, 1999.

Weisman, A. D.: "Thanatology." Chapter 28.2 in: A. M Freedman, H. I. Kaplan, B. J. Sadock (Eds):*Comprehensive textbook of psychiatry II.* Baltimore: The Williams & Wilkins Company, 1975, p. 1754.

Wells, S.: *The Journey of Man: a Genetic Odyssey.* Princeton and Oxford: Princeton University Press, 2002.

Werner, E. M.: High-risk children in young adulthood. A longitudinal study from birth to 32 years. *Amer. J. Orthopsychiat*, 1989: 59, 1: 72.

Werner, H.: *Comparative Psychology of Mental Development,* Revised Edition, Second Printing, New York: International Universities Press, Inc, 1957.

Wescott, R. W. : "Protolinguistics: the study of protolanguages as an aid to glossogonic research" in Harnad, S. R., H. D. Steklis and J. Lancaster, eds: "Origins And Evolution Of Language And Speech." *Annals of the New York Academy Sciences,* 280 (1976): 104-116.

Wessman, A. E. and B. S. Gorman: "The emergence of human awareness and concepts of time" in *The Personal Experience of Time,* eds. B. S. Gorman and A. E. Wessman, 3-55. New York: Plenum Press, 1977.

Whissell, C., M. Fournier, R. Pelland, D. Weir and K. Makarec: "A dictionary of affect in language: IV. Reliability, validity, and applications." *Perceptual Motor Skills* 62 (1986): 875-888.

White, T. D., B. Asfaw, D. Degusta, H. Gilbert, G. D. Richards, G. Suwa & F. C. Howell: "Pleistocene Homo sapiens from Middle Awash, Ethiopia." *Nature,* 42 (June 2003): 742-747.

Whorf, B. L.: *Language, Thought, and Reality.* New York: The Technology Press of Massachusetts Institute of Technology, 1956.

Widom, C. S. :"The cycle of violence." *Science* 1989; 244: 162-166.

Wilford, J. N.: "Skulls found in Africa and in Europe challenge theories of human origins." *The New York Times,* August 6, 2002.

Wispé, L.: "History of the concept of empathy." In: N. Eisenberg & J. Strayer (Eds): *Empathy and its development.* Cambridge, New York, New Rochelle, Melbourne, Sydney: Cambridge University Press, 1987: 17-37.

Wong, D. F., E. P. Broussolle, G. Wand, V. Villemagne, R. F. Dannals, J. M. Links, H. A. Zacur, J. Harris, S. Naidu, C. Breastrup et al.: "In vivo measurement of dopamine receptors in human brain by positron emission tomography. Age and sex difference." *Ann NY Acad Sc.* 1988; 515: 203-14. Review.

Worman, C. B. and R. C. Silver````: "The myths of coping with loss." *J Consult Clin Psychol* 57 (1989), 57: 349-357.

Yamamoto, M.: "What time is not" in *The Study of Time II*, eds. J. T. Fraser, J. T. and N. Lawrence, 231-238, New York: Springer-Verlag, 1975

AUTHOR INDEX

A

Addison, P., 199
Adler, A., 201
Adler, L.L., 18, 119
Allport, G.W., 98
Altman, D.G., 265
Ames, L.B., 59
Anaximander, 240
Anaximenes, 240
Anderson, B., 266
Andreason, N.C., 18
Andrews, D.F., 18
Angus, J., 198
Anthony, E.J., 6
Argyle, M., 79
Aris, D.J.B., 80, 118, 119
Aristotle, 240, 241
Arnstein, R.L., 178
Aronson, E., 198
Asbury, K., 216
Attlee, C., 198, 199
Azari, N.P., 18

B

Bachofen, J.J., 245
Baddeley, A., 58
Bahn, P.G., 247
Balint, M., 214
Ban, M.R., 215
Barmé, G.R., 119
Barnett, L., 160
Bar-Yosef, O., 246
Bass, E.G., 266
Baumgartner, P., 98
Beahrs, J.O., 98

Beard, R.M., 59, 178
Becker, E., 80
Bengtsson, S., 18
Berger, A.M., 266
Berger, M., 215
Bergman, A., 98
Berk, L.E., 58, 246
Berne, E., 59
Bettelheim, B., 178
Billy, J.O., 149, 266
Binford, S.R., 246
Birch, H.G., 79, 118
Bland, R.C., 266, 267
Blizard, D.A., 244
Block, J.A., 79
Blotkey, M., 178
Blume, S., 266
Boernstein, W.S., 160
Bolt, R.O., 198
Bouchard, T.J., 79
Bowman, M.L., 79
Brady, J.V., 59
Bragg, M., 198
Brandon, S.G.F., 245, 246
Bray, W., 246
Brechner, G.A., 58
Breuil, H., 246
Brown, G.R., 266
Browne, A., 266
Brunel Deschamps, E., 246, 247
Bryer, J.B., 266
Busby, H., 199
Buss, A.H., 98
Butzer, K.W., 246

ISBN 141208843-7